W9-BPI-035

HEALTH CARE SERVICES, RACIAL AND ETHNIC MINORITIES AND UNDERSERVED POPULATIONS: PATIENT AND PROVIDER PERSPECTIVES

RESEARCH IN THE SOCIOLOGY OF HEALTH CARE

Series Editor: Jennie Jacobs Kronenfeld

Recently Published Volumes:

RESEARCH IN THE SOCIOLOGY OF HEALTH CARE   VOLUME 23

HEALTH CARE SERVICES, RACIAL AND ETHNIC MINORITIES AND UNDERSERVED POPULATIONS: PATIENT AND PROVIDER PERSPECTIVES

EDITED BY

JENNIE JACOBS KRONENFELD

Department of Sociology, Arizona State University, USA

ELSEVIER
JAI

Amsterdam – Boston – Heidelberg – London – New York – Oxford
Paris – San Diego – San Francisco – Singapore – Sydney – Tokyo

ELSEVIER B.V.
Radarweg 29
P.O. Box 211
1000 AE Amsterdam,
The Netherlands

ELSEVIER Inc.
525 B Street, Suite 1900
San Diego
CA 92101-4495
USA

ELSEVIER Ltd
The Boulevard, Langford
Lane, Kidlington
Oxford OX5 1GB
UK

ELSEVIER Ltd
84 Theobalds Road
London
WC1X 8RR
UK

First edition 2005

British Library Cataloguing in Publication Data
A catalogue record is available from the British Library.

ISBN-10:   0-7623-1249-1
ISBN-13:   978-0-7623-1249-8
ISSN: 0275-4959 (Series)

∞ The paper used in this publication meets the requirements of ANSI/NISO Z39.48-1992 (Permanence of Paper).
Printed in The Netherlands.

CONTENTS

SECTION 5: POLICY CONCERNS

LIST OF CONTRIBUTORS

David W. Baker	Feinberg School of Medicine, Northwestern University, Chicago, IL, USA
Cecilia Benoit	University of Victoria, Victoria, B.C., Canada
Zachary W. Brewster	Department of Sociology and Anthropology, North Carolina State University, Raleigh, NC, USA
Sarah Jane Brubaker	Department of Sociology, Virginia Commonwealth University, Richmond, VA, USA
Michèle Companion	Department of Sociology, University of Colorado-Colorado Springs, Colorado Springs, CO, USA
Rita K. Cydulka	Case Western Reserve University School of Medicine, Cleveland, OH, USA
Neal V. Dawson	Center for Health Care Policy Research, Case Western Reserve University School of Medicine, Cleveland, OH, USA
Kim Ebert	Department of Sociology, University of California, Davis, CA, USA
Karen Farrell	School of Health and Human Performance, Dalhousie University, Halifax, NS, Canada
Valda Ford	President of Center for Human Diversity© and Director of Community and Multicultural Affairs, University of Nebraska Medical Center, Omaha, NE, USA

Beth Furlong   School of Nursing and Center for Health
                                Policy and Ethics, Creighton University,
                                Omaha, NE, USA

James W. Grimm   Department of Sociology, Western
                                Kentucky University, Bowling Green, KY,
                                USA

Drew Halfmann   Department of Sociology, University of
                                California, Davis, CA, USA

Susan W. Hinze   Case Western Reserve, Cleveland, OH, USA

Anthony Kouzis   Johns Hopkins University, Baltimore, ND,
                                USA

Jennie Jacobs   Department of Sociology, Arizona State
Kronenfeld   University, Tempe, AZ, USA

Richard S. Lockwood   Department of Sociology, Portland State
                                University, Portland, OR, USA

Eric Mykhalovskiy   Department of Sociology, York University,
                                Toronto, Ontario, Canada

Elyse R. Park   Department of Psychiatry, MGH, Institute
                                for Health Policy/General Medicine,
                                Boston, MA, USA

Rachel Phillips   University of Victoria, Victoria, B.C.,
                                Canada

Eileen J. Porter   MU Sinclair School of Nursing, University
                                of Missouri-Columbia, Columbia, MO,
                                USA

Stephen Reder   Department of Applied Linguistics,
                                Portland State University, Portland, OR,
                                USA

Ellen J. Reifler   Foundation for Informed Medical Decision
                                Making, Boston, MA, USA

Jesse Rude   Department of Sociology, University of
                                California, Davis, CA, USA

Karen Seccombe   School of Community Health, Portland
                         State University, Portland, OR, USA

Karen Sepucha   Foundation for Informed Medical Decision
                         Making, Bethesda, MD, USA

D. Clayton Smith   Department of Sociology, Western
                         Kentucky University, Bowling Green, KY,
                         USA

*Joshua H.   Department of Emergency Medicine,
Tamayo-Sarver*   Harbor-UCLA Medical Center, Torrance,
                         CA, USA

Pamela H. Wescott   Foundation for Informed Medical Decision
                         Making, Boston, MA, USA

Robert S. Wigton   College of Medicine, University of
                         Nebraska, NE, USA

SECTION 1:
HEALTH CARE DISPARITIES:
RACIAL AND ETHNIC MINORITIES,
UNDERSERVED POPULATIONS
AND HEALTH CARE SERVICES

HEALTH CARE DISPARITIES AND UNDERSERVED POPULATIONS: ISSUES OF SOCIAL FACTORS

Jennie Jacobs Kronenfeld

ABSTRACT

This chapter provides an introduction to the volume and reviews some issues related to provision of health care services to racial and ethnic minorities and other underserved population. In addition to this review of some of the material on underserved populations and what has often been called in the US "health care disparities" concerns, this chapter also serves as an introduction to the volume. As such, the chapter explains the organization of the volume and briefly comments on each of the chapters included in the volume.

The theme of this volume is Health Care Services, Racial and Ethnic Minorities and Underserved Populations: Patient and Provider Perspectives. The volume is divided into five sections. This first section discusses the overall issue of health care disparities and underserved populations and also provides introductory material about the rest of the volume. The second section focuses on issues that relate to gender. The third section provides

Health Care Services, Racial and Ethnic Minorities and Underserved Populations: Patient and Provider Perspectives
Research in the Sociology of Health Care, Volume 23, 3–13
ISSN: 0275-4959/doi:10.1016/S0275-4959(05)23001-6

chapters on some other specific examples of underserved populations: those with mental health concerns, those with concerns related to emotional well being, the elderly population and sex workers. The fourth section includes chapters that discuss treatment disparities and providers of care. The last section includes chapters that relate to policy concerns.

The topic of health care services and underserved populations is one of growing importance within the US health care system, and one of importance in health care systems across the world. Concern about equity in health care is not new, and in fact, many of the early origins of medical sociology in the US related to concerns about equity in health care, such as the early work of Davis on immigrant deficiencies in access to health care (Bloom, 2000). This type of work was followed by the work within social ecology as part of the Chicago school of sociology that formulated some early major hypotheses about the relation between social conditions and mental disorder (Leacock, 1957). Certainly, from the 1960s, one consistent interest of medical sociologists has been related to issues of access to health care services and social inequities in the receipt of health care services as well as research on social inequities in health (Robert & House, 2000; Pescosolido, McLeod, & Alegria, 2000). In the earlier decades of this time period, much of the attention was focused on issues of social inequities relating to the receipt of health care services, and some research from these perspectives became important in the passage of the government programs Medicare and Medicaid that then helped to improve access to health services among the elderly and some groups of the poor. After the passage of those programs and their implementation beginning in 1965, some sociological research focused on understanding the extent to which these programs did improve access to care. In more recent decades, while there has been much tinkering with federal programs to help improve access to care, and the passage of the SCHIP (state child health insurance program) that has helped provide coverage to almost all poor and near poor children in the US, research foci have expanded to examine issues of unmet need for care, underserved populations and health disparities.

MORTALITY AND HEALTH DISPARITIES, ESPECIALLY LINKED TO RACIAL AND ETHNIC DIFFERENCES

Mortality measures, while imperfect, are generally recognized as helping us to understand broad, major impacts in health of an overall population and differentials in health of subgroups within those overall populations. The recognition that racial disparities in health in the US today are still substantial is illustrated by differences in overall mortality rates. The overall death rate for blacks in the US today is comparable to the white rate from 30 years ago, with almost 100,000 more blacks dying each year than would be true if death rates were equivalent (Levine et al., 2001). One recent article has examined social sources of racial disparities in mortality from 1995 through 2000 for five causes of death (Williams & Jackson, 2005). For three of these, homicide, heart disease and cancer, there are wide disparities between black and white populations. For two of the causes of death, pneumonia and flu and suicide, there are virtually no disparities.

For homicide, the rate in 2000 was almost six times greater for African Americans as contrasted with whites. This might make us conclude that this is an area of critical and perhaps even growing differences. The comparisons across time show that homicide deaths were almost 30 percent lower for blacks in 2000 than in 1950, and that the racial gap in these death rates was smaller in 2000 than in 1950 (Williams & Jackson, 2005). Importantly, the authors also point out that homicide is a small contributor to racial differences in mortality as the 15th leading cause of death in the US, in contrast to the three leading causes of death of heart disease, cancer and stroke.

Looking at heart disease, the leading cause of overall death in the US, we find that death rates from coronary heart disease were comparable for blacks and whites in 1950, however instead of improving by 2000 (as in the case of homicide), blacks had a death rate that was 30 percent higher than whites. One should not interpret this to mean that heart disease issues are not improving among blacks. The growing disparity reflects that the decline for whites was more rapid than the decline for blacks, leaving both relative and absolute racial differences larger in 2000 than in 1950.

What is the picture for cancer, the second leading cause of death currently in the US? Blacks have shifted from having a cancer death rate in 1950 that was lower than whites to having a rate 30 percent higher in 2000 (Williams & Jackson, 2005). For cancer, we find a different picture than for homicide or heart disease. For whites, cancer mortality rates have been stable over time, while for blacks they have been increasing (almost 40 percent higher in 2000 than in 1950).

One important overall factor to better understand these trends is linkage with socioeconomic status (SES). SES is a very strong predictor of variations in health, including mortality, whether measured by income, education or occupational category, the three classic ways within sociology to measure

SES differences. These SES indicators are related to racial and ethnic patterns. In fact, differences in SES within each racial group may often be more important than overall racial differences in health. Thus, understanding health disparities in mortality requires an appreciation of complexity in social factors.

How does this relate to the two conditions, flu and pneumonia and suicide, for which Williams and Jackson (2005) report no racial differences in mortality? Flu and pneumonia is a success story for improving medical care and its role in decreasing racial mortality differentials. Flu and pneumonia remains an important cause of death in the US, currently ranking as the seventh leading cause of death. While in 1950 there were large racial differences, with black mortality being 70 percent higher than that of whites, by 2000 there were only minimal differences. Flu and pneumonia is an acute respiratory illness that can be prevented at times by vaccination and can be treated with antiviral medications. Behavioral components are not that important, and diffusion of technology, facilitated by Medicare and Medicaid, is the major explanation (Williams & Jackson, 2005).

In some ways, for racial disparities, suicide is also a success story. Suicide rates for both major racial groups (blacks and whites) have been fairly stable over time. Suicide illustrates a health problem for which socially disadvantaged groups do not have elevated rates. Thus, the overall relationships between SES and health outcomes are different for this health problem.

Another way to consider the health impact of racial disparities is to compare the number of deaths attributable to excess mortality among African Americans with the number of lives saved by medical advances. Given the great emphasis on technology in the US health care system, and the large amounts of dollars spent in the US to improve health outcomes linked to such technologies as better drugs, devices and procedures, Woolf and his colleagues examined this comparison (Woolf, Johnson, Fryer, Rust, & Satcher, 2004). Using age-adjusted mortality rates, they estimated that technology related declines averted 176,633 deaths from 1991 to 2000. As of the year 2000, given that the mortality rate for African American infants and adults aged 25–54 was more than double the white rate, they applied age-specific mortality rates of the two ages to understand what the outcomes would have been using an assumption that age-specific mortality rates of the two races were comparable between 1991 and 2000. They find that 886,202 deaths could have been averted. They conclude that five deaths could have been saved for every life saved by medical advances (Woolf et al., 2004).

LINKAGES WITH HEALTH PRACTICES AND HEALTH SERVICES UTILIZATION

Over the past 10–20 years, there have been many studies that have documented the race and SES influence the use of health care services. Important questions that have been raised in recent years is how is it that factors such as income, education and race/ethnicity lead to less use of health care and worse health outcomes. Are these factors due to issues of use of health care services, or are they linked to health practices and social determinants? Several different lines of research have come up with somewhat different sets of explanations.

One set of studies has looked at people with Medicare, since similar basic coverage is available to most elderly, whatever their race or SES. A conclusion of a number of these studies is that less advantaged people economically and socially and black Americans use fewer preventative and cancer screening services, fewer common surgical procedures, and more procedures associated with poor outcomes of chronic diseases (Ayanian, Udvarhelyi, Gatsonis, Pashos, & Epstein, 1993; Gornick, 2000; Gornick, Eggers, & Riley, 2004). Some experts have pointed out that barriers relating to coinsurance requirements might explain disparities in services use such as for mammograms, however, among the largest disparities are those for services such as flu shots for which there is no fee under Medicare (Gornick et al., 2004). In a detailed study of the relationship between use of preventive services as linked with the probability of late stage cancer diagnosis and the impact of race and education, the most important finding was that for six of eight studied cancers, Medicare beneficiaries who used more of the available preventive services were less likely to have cancer diagnosed at a later stage than their counterparts who used fewer services (Gornick et al., 2004). A concern that these authors raise, especially important for those under 65 and without Medicare coverage, is that for those without good health insurance, the costs of health care will probably present significant barriers to use of preventive services which could impact the health of those people not only at that specific time, but many years into the future, thus helping to understand one of the linkages between low SES, racial and ethnic disparities, and overall poorer health outcomes.

A different approach has emphasized that practices of eating, sleeping, and exercise link social factors to biological practices that maintain health (Young, 2005). In Berkman and Breslow (1983) argued for the causal relevance of health behaviors on poor health outcomes. These arguments include social integration/social support approaches (Berkman & Syme,

1979), and arguments that individuals have both the power and the moral responsibility to maintain their own health by observing appropriate rules of health behavior (Knowles, 1977). A more sociological approach has been the fundamental cause argument of Link and Phelan (1995) and its argument that SES is a fundamental cause and social variables determine the intervening health practices. In a recent review of social factors and their linkage to health, Young (2005) argues that the medical establishment and the media generally reject the fundamental cause argument and accept the notion that practices are causal. This remains an important area for further research and debate.

MORE COMPLEX EXPLANATIONS, LINKED TO RESOURCES

One recent article argues that the residential concentration of African Americans is high and distinctive as compared to other racial ethnic groups (Williams & Jackson, 2005). These inequities in neighborhood environments, socioeconomic circumstances and medical care, they believe, are important factors in why racial disparities in health exist and persist. They do not believe these will be easy factors to overcome. While racial discrimination in the sale and rental of housing, for example, was made illegal in the US in 1968, there is evidence that such discrimination continues to persist. These authors believe it may require a major infusion of economic capital to improve the social, physical, and economic infrastructure of disadvantaged communities.

Other authors agree that African Americans often experience the most serious health disparities (Mechanic, 2002, 2005). Mechanic argues that eliminating racial disparities in health will be a very complicated effort, although clearly a worthwhile goal. He believes that concerned effort will be required in many areas, including access to high quality medical care, support for healthy social and educational development, and enhancement of environmental and neighborhood infrastructures.

Perhaps the best way to conclude this review of chapters related to health disparities, health outcomes and health services utilization is to examine the question of the importance of race versus class in health disparities. In a recent review essay, three competing causal interpretations of racial disparities in health were reviewed (Kawachi, Daniels, & Robinson, 2005). One approach emphasizes race as a biologically meaningful category and thus views racial disparities in health as reflecting inherited susceptibility to disease. This approach is generally rejected by most social scientists, since within sociology and other social sciences, race is viewed as a socially constructed category. Even the rush of enthusiasm to look for genetic explanations of diseases linked to the success of the human genome project has concluded that it is a gross simplification to assume that differences in genetic susceptibility explain observed racial disparities. A second approach views race as a proxy for class. This approach thus views socioeconomic stratification as the true explanation for racial disparities in health. One problem with using race as a proxy for social class is that it is only a rough proxy. The majority of the poor in the US are still white (about two-thirds). A third approach treats race as neither a biological category nor as a simple proxy for class, but rather as a distinct concept, almost akin to caste in some other social systems. In more technical terms, this approach argues that the most defensible view of racial disparities needs to simultaneously account for the independent and interactive effects of both class and race. Kawachi et al. (2005) argue for this approach, and present three propositions that follow from this approach. Race must not be conceptualized as a proxy for class. Racial disparities cannot be analyzed without at the same time considering the contribution of class disparities. Lastly, researchers must consider potential interactions between race- and class-based disparities. According to the same authors, to be able to do this consistently in studies, the US data infrastructure must be improved, both by improving the accuracy of race/ethnicity data and by collecting more complete information on SES. These suggestions will help to improve future research.

REVIEW OF THE OTHER SECTIONS OF THE BOOK AND THOSE CHAPTERS

Following this introductory essay, there are four additional sections of the book, focusing on the impact of gender and women as recipients of health care, on a variety of special groups with concerns about being underserved by the health care system, on policy concerns and on treatment disparities and providers of care. Section 2 of the volume includes two papers that focus on gender-related concerns unique to women. Brubaker examines issues of African American teen mothers and reproductive health concerns. She argues that racial/ethnic minority, low-income teens represent an important underserved group, and especially in terms of reproductive health care including birth control and prenatal care. She prepares insights based on in-depth interviews with 51 teen mothers. She views gender ideologies as important, as well as behavioral expectations and mothers' decisions around these issues. In the second paper, Westcott and her colleagues explore a different aspect of women's health concerns, breast cancer treatment decision making. Focus group interview data were obtained from African American, Hispanic and rural breast cancer survivors. One of the major research questions in this paper is whether there were important differences across these groups, or more similarities, especially as related to the use of decision aids to help make treatment decisions about how to handle one's breast cancer. An important finding is the importance of similarities across the different groups.

Section 3 includes four papers each of which examines a different aspect of underserved populations. The first paper in the section by Kouzis deals with mental health services utilization and investigates the role of social factors, health status and psychiatric disorders with this specialized group in the population. He uses multivariate logistic regression analysis with a nationally representative household survey to explore this issue. People with greater socioeconomic resources or those with comorbid psychiatric disorders are more likely to visit the specialty mental health sector for services. The fourth paper deals with a related issue, the relationship between physical and emotional well-being. This paper, unlike the previous paper that used a nationally gathered database, uses data from a specific county in Kentucky. Smith, Grimm, and Brewster use data collected from a random sample of insured, primarily working-aged adults in Warren County, Kentucky, to test the effects of insurance on respondents' emotional and physical health. In addition, a variety of demographic and household variables were examined. Being married and being widowed were more important to improved physical health than were education and being religiously affiliated. Less emotional distress was reported by those with no religious identification. People in households that restructured themselves to acquire or maintain health coverage reported higher emotional distress.

In contrast to the first and fourth papers that related to mental and emotional health concerns, the second and third papers in this section focus on elderly widows as an underserved population and sex industry workers. Porter explores the access problems that older women living in medically underserved areas in the US experience through in depth reports with six frail older women, varying in age from 82 to 93 years. Residence location becomes an important factor for this group of women. Phillips and Benoit draw on both closed- and open-ended interview data with 79 sex industry workers in a medium sized metropolitan area in British Columbia, Canada. Several respondents reported feeling intimidated and shamed in health care settings, and some withheld information relevant to their health care linked to their occupation because of fear of discrimination by health care workers. Unlike in the US, Canada has a universal system of health care. What this paper demonstrates is the complex system of structural and individual social variables that relate to differential access to health care within the framework of a universal system of care as is found in Canada.

Section 5 examines a variety of policy concerns and includes four papers. Seccombe and her colleagues explore the role of literacy on access to and use of health care services. They point out that the presence of substantial number of persons with low levels of literacy in the US presents major problems with access to care. Adults with lower levels of literacy are less likely to have a usual provider of care, to have health insurance, have trouble understanding written directions, and more difficulty getting needed medical care. In addition, they report poorer health than other population groups. An important policy point is that literacy is conceptually distinct from education, and independently impacts the ways in which adults seek health care. Companion explores the policy issues related to Native Americans and tribal health care management. She explores the impact of participation in programs that increase Native American control over their health care management. While this would appear to be a positive thing, participation in this program has ended up being detrimental for tribal self-determination. The paper reviews why approaches that emphasize bottom-up development models may work better both within the US for Native Americans and outside the US as part of international development models.

The second and third papers in Section 5 deal with some other policy aspects of health care disparities and underserved populations. Both of these papers take a broader perspective than the first two papers. Halfmann uses content analysis to trace the relative prominence of biomedical and public health approaches in congressional bills aimed at improving the health of racial and ethnic minorities over a 28-year period. The paper details the ways in which policy legacies shape the interests, opportunities and ideas of interest groups and policy makers. Ford and Furlong argue that one cannot have a successful health system without the inclusion of culturally competent health promotions programs. Moreover, a system cannot have such programs without an understanding of the role that cultural and linguistic competence play in the provision of clinically competent and cost effective services. The paper reviews research studies that relate to this topic, and is divided into two major parts. The first part addresses the need for culturally and linguistically appropriate care and the applicable laws and standards. The second part of the paper provides an ethical analysis of these issues.

Section 4 of the volume includes two chapters that examine treatment disparity issues as related to providers of care. Tamayo-Sarver and colleagues establish a theoretical framework for clinical decision making that includes non-medical factors such as race/ethnicity and places this within the ways physicians make decisions in the practice of medicine. They propose a model that is entitled the "Rapid Clinical Decision in Context" (RCDC) model which they argue will provide a basis for future studies to move beyond documentation of areas where disparities exist to understanding the causes of the disparities and the design of interventions to address the causes. Mykhalovskiy and Farrell explore the informal learning process through which family physicians develop an understanding of social context shaping the health of marginalized patients. The geographical context for the paper is a qualitative study that includes individual interviews with 10 family physicians around Halifax, Nova Scotia, Canada. One of the concerns of the paper is that formal education cannot fully prepare or equip medial students to successfully work with marginalized patients. Issues of time concerns and pressures to "clinically process" patients in as timely a fashion as possible are concerns factors that inhibit learning more about aspects of marginalized people's lives that are important for the delivery of good clinical care.

REFERENCES

Ayanian, J. Z., Udvarhelyi, I. S., Gatsonis, C. A., Pashos, C. L., & Epstein, A. M. (1993). Racial differences in the use of revascularization procedures after coronary artery angioplasty. *Journal of the American Medical Association, 269*, 2642–2646.

Berkman, L. F., & Breslow, L. (1983). *Health and ways of living: The Alameda County study.* Oxford: New York.

Berkman, L. F., & Syme, S. L. (1979). Social networks, host resistance and mortality: A nine-year follow-up study of Alameda County residents. *American Journal of Epidemiology, 109*, 186–204.

Bloom, S. (2000). The institutionalization of medical sociology in the United States, 1920–1980. In: C. E. Bird, P. Conrad & A. M. Fremont (Eds), *Handbook of medical sociology*, (5th ed.). Upper Saddle River, NJ: Prentice-Hall, Inc.

Gornick, M. E. (2000). *Vulnerable populations and medical care services: Why do disparities exist.* New York: Century Foundation Press.

Gornick, M. E., Eggers, P. W., & Riley, G. F. (2004). Associations of race, education and patterns of preventive service use with state of cancer at time of diagnosis. *Health Services Research, 39*, 1403–1427.

Kawachi, I., Daniels, N., & Robinson, D. E. (2005). Health disparities by race, and class: Why both matter. *Health Affairs, 24*, 343–352.
Knowles, J. (1977). The responsibility of the individual. *Daedalus, 106*, 57–80.
Leacock, E. (1957). Three social variables and the occurrence of mental disorder. In: A. Leighton, J. A. Clausen & R. N. Wilson (Eds), *Explorations in social psychology*. New York: Basic Books.
Levine, R. S., Foster, J. E., Fullelove, R. E., Fullelove, M. T., Briggs, N. C., Hull, P. C., Husani, B. A., & Hennekins, C. H. (2001). Black-White inequalities in mortality and life expectancy 1993–1999: Implications for healthy people 2010. *Public Health Reports, 116*, 474–483.
Link, B. G., & Phelan, J. (1995). Social conditions as fundamental causes of disease. *Journal of Health and Social Behavior, 36*(extra issue), 80–94.
Mechanic, D. (2002). Disadvantage, inequality and social policy. *Health Affairs, 21*, 48–59.
Mechanic, D. (2005). Policy challenges in addressing racial disparities and improving population health. *Health Affairs, 24*, 335–338.
Pescosolido, B., McLeod, J., & Alegria, M. (2000). Confronting the social contract: The place of medical sociology in research and policy in the twenty-first century. In: C. E. Bird, P. Conrad & A. M. Fremont (Eds), *Handbook of medical sociology*, (5th ed.). Upper Saddle River, NJ: Prentice-Hall, Inc.
Robert, S. A., & House, J. S. (2000). Socioeconomic inequalities in health: An enduring sociological problem. In: C. E. Bird, P. Conrad & A. M. Fremont (Eds), *Handbook of medical sociology*, (5th ed.). Upper Saddle River, NJ: Prentice-Hall, Inc.
Williams, D. R., & Jackson, P. B. (2005). Social sources of racial disparities in health. *Health Affairs, 24*, 325–334.
Woolf, S. H., Johnson, R. E., Fryer, G. E., Jr., Rust, G., & Satcher, D. (2004). The health impact of resolving racial disparities: An analysis of US mortality data. *American Journal of Public Health, 94*, 2078–2080.
Young, F. W. (2005). How social factors improve health. *Social Theory and Health, 3*, 61–73.

SECTION 2:
GENDER AND RELATED ISSUES

AFRICAN AMERICAN TEEN MOTHERS AND REPRODUCTIVE HEALTH CARE SERVICES: GENDER AND THE CONTEXT OF INTENTION

Sarah Jane Brubaker

ABSTRACT

Racial/ethnic minority, low-income teens represent a significantly under-served group in terms of reproductive health care including birth control and prenatal care. This paper provides patients' perspectives through analysis of in-depth interviews with 51 African American teen mothers about their reproductive health care and focuses on the influence of gender ideologies and behavior expectations on teens', and their perceptions of their mothers', decisions around these issues. The findings suggest that attention to cultural influences of gender on teens' decisions around sexuality and reproduction is critical to our theoretical and practical approaches to expanding health care services to underserved populations.

Health Care Services, Racial and Ethnic Minorities and Underserved Populations: Patient and Provider Perspectives
Research in the Sociology of Health Care, Volume 23, 17–33
Copyright © 2005 by Elsevier Ltd.
ISSN: 0275-4959/doi:10.1016/S0275-4959(05)23002-8

INTRODUCTION

Although teen pregnancy rates have continued to decline over the past decade, adolescent sexual activity remains a social issue of great concern and
public debate. From a health perspective, the immediate problematic consequences of early sexual activity can include sexually-transmitted infections
(STIs), unintended or early pregnancy, and inadequate prenatal care, not to
mention long-term health and economic problems for babies born to teens
and for the teens themselves. Of those at greatest risk for experiencing these
negative health outcomes of sexual behavior are adolescents from racial
ethnic minority and lower income groups (Bird & Bogart, 2005; Frieden,
2000; Halpern et al., 2004; SIECUS, 2003).

Efforts to understand the causal influences on these groups' increased risk
for these health outcomes related to sexual behavior have focused on structural issues such as access to contraception and other health care services
(Frieden, 2000; Veit et al., 1996); individual factors such as levels of self-
efficacy or psychological motivations, attitudes or beliefs, perceived risk, or
relative amounts of social capital (Basen-Engquist et al., 1999; Crosby,
Holtgrave, DiClemente, Wingood, & Gayle, 2003; Kershaw, Ethier,
Miccolai, Lewis, & Ickovics, 2003); and cultural issues such as health beliefs, perceptions of racism, and sexual and family values (Basen-Engquist et
al., 1999; Bird & Bogart, 2005; Scholly, Katz, Gascoigne, & Holck, 2005).

An important factor related to adolescent sexuality and reproductive
health that addresses multiple levels of influence is pregnancy intention.
Recent studies have begun to challenge conventional definitions of pregnancy intention and wantedness that traditionally overlooked important
contextual distinctions among differently located groups of women. While
these studies have identified and described important structural and cultural
dimensions of pregnancy intention, they have focused primarily on differences among various groups of women. Understanding these differences is
critical to improving our understanding of how decision-making processes
work, and to creating better methods of measuring intention and providing
services to women at various social locations. What is still missing from this
scholarship, however, is attention to the commonality of gender as an influence on women's reproductive decision-making.

In this article, I focus on reproductive health care, specifically contraception and prenatal care, as described by African American teen mothers
through in-depth interviews, and the role that gender as a cultural context of
ideology and behavioral expectations plays in shaping their (as well as their
interpretations of their mothers') decisions and behaviors regarding these

health care services. Teens' narratives addressed issues of intention not only with respect to pregnancy, but perhaps even more important to both their decisions to seek prenatal care and decisions around birth control, was their intention (or lack thereof) to engage in sex. Specifically, girls and their mothers approached reproductive health care within the normative gender contexts of morality that negatively define unmarried young women's engagement in sex. In many ways, their decisions and behaviors had the potential to dramatically harm the health and well-being of teens and their babies, yet they were consistent with positive cultural ideals of femininity. Teens' narratives about becoming pregnant and seeking prenatal care challenge simplistic conceptualizations of intention as a causal factor in the reproductive health care of underserved populations such as teens, poor women, and women of color, and suggest that greater attention be given to the role of culture, specifically gender culture, in shaping their relationship to the formal reproductive health care system.

BACKGROUND

One of the factors that researchers routinely identify as critical to understanding adult and adolescent women's reproductive decisions and behaviors, and ultimately improving health outcomes of sexual activity, is the issue of pregnancy intention. Typically researchers address intention with respect to pregnancy. Recently, some have begun to question simplistic notions of pregnancy intention, planning and desire, and to argue that each of these issues is distinct and shaped by structural, cultural, individual, and interpersonal factors. In general, "Pregnancy unintendedness is a complex concept, and has been the subject of recent conceptual and methodological critiques" (Santelli et al., 2003). Although generally believed to be directly related to women's use of contraceptives, as well as decisions to engage in sexual activity, women's pregnancy intention and wantedness as evaluated by conventional measures is not consistent with these assumptions (Kives & Jamieson, 2001; Trussell et al., 1995; Barrett & Wellings, 2000).

In response to the ambiguity surrounding the meaning of pregnancy intention and the need to better understand how women make reproductive decisions, Kendall et al. (2005) conducted a qualitative study of women attending prenatal care and family planning clinics. Their findings identify a number of factors that are related to pregnancy intention including contraception, motherhood, relationship dynamics (identified in other studies as well), and views toward adolescent sex and abortion.

The findings of this study similarly challenge conventional notions of pregnancy intention, but rather than addressing multiple factors shaping this concept, this article focuses on gender ideologies and norms surrounding sexual behavior as providing powerful cultural influences on the meanings young women give to reproductive health care and their related decisions and behaviors. Attention to gender provides important insights into how poor African American teen mothers become members of "underserved" populations, specifically with respect to contraceptive and prenatal care services.

METHODOLOGY

Recruitment and Data Collection

The data supporting this paper are based on a convenience sample comprised of 51 African American teen mothers enrolled in a Teen Parenting Program at an inner-city public school in the mid-southern region of the United States. The teens volunteered to participate in face-to-face semi-structured interviews conducted by the author during school hours. The interviews lasted from 25 to 90 min, averaging 50 min.

The original focus of this research was on teens' interpretations of prenatal care in the context of widespread stigmatization of teen mothers. Because of this focus, I did not ask teens to provide details about their sexual activity specifically, but to describe their knowledge of and decision-making around seeking prenatal care. In order to address the issue of pregnancy intention as an important factor shaping these decisions, I asked teens whether or not they were surprised when they found out they were pregnant. Most of their responses included narratives about their own and others' general perceptions of their engagement in sexual activity and often they addressed decision-making around birth control as well. If they did not address birth control, I followed-up with a question about whether they had even thought about doing anything to keep from getting pregnant. It is through analysis of teens' responses to these questions and narratives of these issues that the impact of broader cultural ideologies of gender emerged.

Sample

The teens all self-identified as Black or African American, and this racial group constituted 99% of the school's population. Their ages ranged from

14 to 19 at the time of the interview, averaging 17. Forty-one of the teens had already given birth at the time of the interview (31 had one child; 10 had two), seven teens were pregnant for the first time, and three teens were both mothering a child and pregnant.

Overall, 28 (54%) teens' families' primary source of income was from wages. Of these teens, all but one were either enrolled in the state health care program (formerly Medicaid), received WIC (The Special Supplemental Nutrition Program for Women, Infants, and Children), or received a "free lunch," suggesting that their families were at a low-income level. Twelve (23%) teens' incomes were based on both wages and AFDC (Aid to Families with Dependent Children), and 11 (21%) teens' families relied solely on AFDC. Based on the various indicators of social class, I consider the majority of teens to be at low-income levels.

Thirty-three (63%) teens were from female-headed households, 15 (29%) from two-parent households (biological or blended), and one lived only with her father. The composition of the family of origin for three teens was unclear. At the time of the interview, 23 (44%) of the teens were living only with their mothers, 20 (38%) with two parents or guardians, five with a female relative, three with their babies' fathers, and one with her father.

I conducted all of the interviews myself, and I spent a great deal of time at the school during the 3 months of data collection. I observed many classes ate lunch in the cafeteria and participated in various school-related events. I was 30-years-old at the time, married, white, and had no children, however, and I recognize the challenges to interviewing across social location and the potential limitations on the data. Based on lengthy conversations with the school administrators and teachers on this topic, I am fairly confident that the teens were as forthcoming with me as they were with their teachers and the principal, the majority of whom were adult African American women. The teens often seemed amused by the fact that I was so "old" and did not yet have children, and many seemed to enjoy the opportunity to enlighten me on various issues related to pregnancy, childbirth, and parenting.

Because the majority of the teens participated in a Teen Parenting Program, they are not representative of the general population of pregnant teens. Their participation in the program suggests that they may receive additional support mechanisms in their lives that enable them to find such a program and to continue attending school. As Brindis suggests, "It is important to note...that young women who remain in school while they are pregnant (especially those who stay in school throughout the pregnancy and birth) are a self-selected and motivated group." (Brindis, 1993, p. 259).

FINDINGS

Teens' responses to my initial question about whether or not they were surprised when they found out they were pregnant addressed and contextualized a number of different reproductive processes and decisions related to formal health care. I discuss the two primary issues separately – birth control use and seeking prenatal care – and how teens talked about intention around each. Across both issues, teens' narratives about how they became pregnant and how they made the decision to seek prenatal care were filled with notions of appropriate gender norms, the most common theme of which was that good girls do not have sex. Despite the powerful cultural messages that girls should be sexually desirable, the contradictory message is that they should not be sexual (Tolman, Striepe, & Harmon, 2003). This theme was invoked and illustrated as a major influence on girls' construction of accounts of both birth control use and prenatal care.

Using Birth Control

In this section, I examine two aspects of the "good girl" identity that shaped teens' narratives about intention and were related to their decisions regarding birth control use. Although, the initial focus of this section of the interview was on pregnancy intention, teens' responses quickly shifted to the issue of intention to engage in sex. Other researchers have addressed contraceptive behavior and access in terms of both pregnancy intention and intention to engage in sex, but in general, they have not focused on how larger cultural norms and ideologies related to gender shape issues of intention.

Good Girls do not (Plan to) have Sex

Most of the teens told me that their pregnancies were unplanned, supporting these claims in various ways. For example, most said that they were surprised when they found out that they were pregnant. Others admitted that although they "had a feeling" they were pregnant, they tried to deny the pregnancy because of their own disappointment or out of fear of others' reactions so that although they were not surprised, neither had they planned to become pregnant. All of these teens provided detailed descriptions of their negative reactions to their pregnancies in support of their claims that they were unplanned. Aware of the strongly negative views of teen pregnancy and adolescent sexual activity common among members of the general population, many teens were clear in their denial that they had intentionally chosen to join the stigmatized community of sexually active or pregnant teenaged girls.

In response to questions about their surprise in learning that they were pregnant, many teens presented a good girl identity by emphasizing that they did not routinely engage in sex. For example, three teens indicated that they became pregnant the first time they had sex, none of whom was using birth control since they had not planned to engage in sex beforehand. Others insisted that they were not planning to have sex when they became pregnant. For example, Olivia,[1] 15-years-old and 8 months pregnant explained, "*I wasn't…you know…it was like it came up all of a sudden that I was pregnant and I, you know, I wasn't doing anything, so why should I think about [pregnancy] at that time?*"[2] Similarly, Joyce insisted that there was no "best thing" about being pregnant, because she "*wasn't sexually active.*" I thought that she was referring to the time during the pregnancy and asked her, "Did somebody tell you not to while you were pregnant?" Joyce responded, "*No, I just never was.*"

These teens deny their intention to engage in sex or to become pregnant by emphasizing that they usually do not have sex. Despite evidence to the contrary, their narratives present the culturally accepted image of the good girl who is not promiscuous and suggests that even had they planned to engage in sex, or had consciously wanted to prevent pregnancy, these gender norms would not allow them to reveal their behavior and intentions in a way that would allow them to promote their health and well-being through the use of contraception.

Good Girls do not know about Birth Control

Another way in which teens responded to gender ideologies that define young women's sexual activity negatively was their attempt to claim the good girl identity through emphasizing their ignorance and naivete about birth control. In describing this absence of information, most teens identified their mothers or "othermothers" (Hill Collins, 2003) as the most likely source of, and therefore responsible for denying them, this information. Teens' narratives about their mothers' roles in providing or denying contraceptive information provide additional examples of how cultural gender ideals and norms constraining young women's sexuality shaped mothers' and their daughters' perceptions and decisions.

Overall, very few teens recalled their mothers providing them with information about birth control or about sex, but many were aware of their mothers' strong opposition to their engaging in sex. For example, 16-year-old mother of twins, Rochelle, recalled her grandmother's advice to "*keep your pants up.*" Lenora, a 17-year-old mother of two, describes her efforts to obtain birth control and her mother's reaction:

> *I had asked my mama once before because her friend was on them and I asked my mama like, "Are you gonna' get me some pills?" "What are you talking about, 'some pills?' Now you're ready to have sex aren't you?" I was like, "Oh, Lord." It was like I couldn't even talk to my mama about anything. She was like, "No, you don't need any pills. You aren't doing anything, are you doing anything?" "Nope, I'm not doing anything."*

Olivia explains why her mother never talked to her about birth control. "*My mom, you know, she didn't talk to me about it, because I wasn't the type that'll just come up pregnant, you know. And then when I started having sex, I got pregnant.*" Narratively, distancing herself from girls who are "the type that'll just come up pregnant," Olivia justified her mother's decision not to talk to her about contraception. Similarly, LaToshia's account illustrates this point:

> And, ok, before you got pregnant the first time, had anybody talked to you about trying not to get pregnant? *Yeah, my mama talked to me, but she didn't talk about any birth control.* What kinds of things did she tell you? *She didn't tell me anything, she just asked was I having sex, that's it.* What'd you tell her? *Nope.*

Kaplan (1997), who also conducted qualitative research with African American teen mothers, suggests that mothers may be afraid that teens will interpret discussions of birth control as a license to have sex. Consistent with this observation, many teens in this study identified their mothers' negative views about sex as a reason for their mothers' reluctance to tell them about birth control.

In addition to attempting to prevent their daughters from engaging in sex, becoming pregnant, and damaging their reputations, teens' mothers also are likely aware that they will be held accountable by others if their daughters do become pregnant and hope that by expressing their opposition to their daughters' engagement in sex, they will avoid blame. For example, Niki attempted to explain her mother's attempts to convince her to have an abortion, "*I kind of felt like the reason why she wanted me to have an abortion was because she was worried about what people said.*"

When mothers express their opposition to their daughters' engagement in sex and their pregnancies, they uphold dominant gender ideologies, aligning their beliefs and behaviors with cultural expectations by placing the blame on their daughters for becoming pregnant. One example of this strategy was provided by Davina, who recalls that after she moved in with her mother, at her mother's request, when she learned of her pregnancy, her mother "dogged" her to all of their relatives, "putting her down" for becoming pregnant. By supporting popular gender ideologies, her mother could align her own beliefs and practices with those of other responsible mothers who did not encourage or condone teen sexual activity or pregnancy.

African American mothers' attempts to control their daughters' sexuality suggest that perhaps because of racism and widespread stigmatization of Black teen mothers, marginalized families' and communities' views and behaviors related to sexuality may be even more influenced by dominant gender ideologies than those from more privileged groups. Violations of such norms by marginalized groups likely receive even harsher negative reactions than do those of privileged groups. As Kaplan (1997) comments about her study, "These teen mothers attempt to cope as best they can be redefining their situation in terms that involve the least damage to their self-respect… Black teenage mothers…struggle against being considered morally deviant, underclass, and unworthy." (1997, pp. xxi, xxiii).

Even if teens did have knowledge about and structural access to birth control, the powerful gender ideologies preventing young women from taking control of their sexuality likely limited their abilities to obtain birth control. This is illustrated by 17-year-old Veronica' story, who knew about a clinic where she could get birth control that required her to bring a parent. Veronica explained that she was "too ashamed" to tell her mother that she was having sex.

Seeking Prenatal Care

In this section, I explore teens' accounts of seeking prenatal care that are also related to intention and illustrate how their decision-making around this reproductive health issue is shaped by gender ideology. As reported in other studies, pregnancy "wantedness" or intention did seem to play a role in the teens' decisions to seek prenatal care, but the attention to cultural influences of gender help to contextualize this issue and further explain that connection in the context of teen pregnancy. The majority of the teens' pregnancies were unintended, but an additional and perhaps even stronger influence on their reactions to the pregnancy and willingness to acknowledge and reveal their pregnancies was the cultural expectation that unmarried, young women not engage in sexual activity. This gender norm shaped two significant aspects of their decisions and behaviors around seeking prenatal care – recognizing pregnancy symptoms and disclosing their pregnancies.

Good Girls do not know about Pregnancy Symptoms

The majority of teens, including 30 (58%) at first, and half at second, pregnancy, explained that they did *not* realize that they were pregnant until someone else told them. Although not all of these teens initiated prenatal care late, many teens who did begin prenatal care after the first trimester offered this explanation. Teens' stories of ignorance about and inability to recognize their pregnancy symptoms further supported their claims that they had not planned to become pregnant.

Teens identified two primary groups who typically noticed that they were pregnant: mothers or female guardians (mentioned by 12 or 41%); and doctors (mentioned by 10 or 34%). The remaining 25% said that the baby's father, other relatives, or friends had informed them that they were pregnant.

Many teens' mothers took responsibility for monitoring their daughters' menstruation cycles and other physical signs of pregnancy, often recognizing the pregnancy before their daughters. Carla, who was 16 when she became pregnant, described how her mother noticed what Carla did not see.

> Really I didn't know. I didn't know. It was like, I didn't have any period, I wasn't on, I didn't come on my cycle. I used to have morning sickness all the time, but I didn't think I was just pregnant, I'd think I was just sick. And I used to throw up. And that was about all. What made you decide to see if you were pregnant? Really, I didn't want to. I wasn't thinking anything about it. But my mom, she came home, and she noticed that my clothes were getting too little. I used to go shopping and buy me these different outfits all the time, and she was like [Carla], you just stay at home. I'm fixing to go to the store and get a pregnancy test. So she went to the store and got a pregnancy test. And that's it.

An interesting comment included in Carla's narrative was her response, "*Really, I didn't want to. I wasn't thinking about it.*" This comment suggests that in addition to her claim that she had no idea that she might be pregnant, at some level she was avoiding consideration of that possibility and others' likely negative responses to it.

Marquita, 16 and 3 months pregnant, recalled how her mother discovered her pregnancy:

> How I first found out I was pregnant? My period hadn't come and my period comes on at a certain time of the month and my mama asked me, always asked me, "[Marquita], has your period come yet?" I said, "No ma'am." She said, "You're pregnant." So that's why she knew. And I knew too then. My period didn't come, it comes every month, it doesn't skip any.

Marquita's narrative is consistent with her claim that she did not recognize her pregnancy symptoms and suggests that she had learnt important information about her body through the experience of becoming pregnant unintentionally. Although many teens' mothers were not able to prevent their daughters' pregnancies through appeals to gender norms and denial of their daughters' sexuality, many did play an important role in discovering their daughters' pregnancies and enabling them to receive care early in the pregnancy.

Twelve teens at first pregnancy, and four at second, credited medical providers with discovering their pregnancies at a doctor's visit when they were sick or having a checkup. Those who were sick typically attributed the problem to something besides pregnancy, like hepatitis or the flu. Camisha, who was 15 when she became pregnant, describes how the doctor discovered her pregnancy.

> I started throwing up, because, okay I had cravings for something, some greens, then when I ate that, I got home and started throwing up. My mama asked me, "What's wrong?" I didn't know, and so we went to the emergency room, and they asked me was there a possibility that I could be pregnant, and I was like "yeah." And my mom was upset, because she just didn't figure I was the type of person to have sex.

Again, we see the stigmatized gender identity teens strive to avoid, "the type of person to have sex" and how this ideology shaped teens' and their mothers' reactions to their pregnancies. Striving to claim the good girl identity, teens and their mothers were sometimes blind to the signs of pregnancy.

These teens' stories reveal their routine use of health care services and challenge research assumptions and individual-level explanations for teens' failure to adequately use health care services that focus on their undervaluing of health care. Furthermore, their accounts supported their claims that their pregnancies were not intended by explaining that they were completely unaware that their physical symptoms were indicative of pregnancy. Some also may have been in denial about their pregnancies. Either explanation for their failure to recognize their pregnancy symptoms on their own reflects the gender norm that young unmarried women not be sexual. Teens either lacked information and knowledge about pregnancy symptoms, because social institutions and socialization agents failed to provide this information in accordance with that gender ideology, or teens ignored the symptoms in an effort to appear naïve and innocent with respect to sexuality and therefore, a good girl.

Good Girls do not get Pregnant – Delayed Disclosure

In addition to those who recognized pregnancy symptoms late in the pregnancy, some teens explained that they chose to wait to tell others that they were pregnant long after their initial realizations. At first pregnancy, 11 teens suggested that they did not attempt to confirm their pregnancies as soon as they recognized pregnancy symptoms, and of these, nine waited until after the first trimester. At the second pregnancy, only two delayed disclosure, but both still confirmed the pregnancy in the first trimester. One possible interpretation of this pattern among the latter group of teens is that because they had already been pregnant before and were no longer attempting to uphold the image of the good girl, this gender ideology had less of an impact on their decisions and behaviors than on first-time mothers.

Some teens explained that they delayed confirmation because they did not believe others who said they were pregnant. Others knew early in the pregnancy that they were pregnant, but they were postponing the disclosure, typically out of fear of negative reactions. Again, both explanations suggest an awareness of their violations of gender norms, the likely negative reactions they would receive to their pregnancies and engagement in sexual activity, and an effort to avoid or at least delay revealing their actions. Their accounts of delayed disclosure draw on some of the same gender norms and ideologies that emerged in their accounts of contraceptive decisions and behaviors. Faced with negative reactions to the evidence of their sexual activity, teens attempted to retain their positive images and avoid the negative consequences of their pregnancies for as long as possible. Their accounts suggest that like their interpretations of pregnancy prevention issues, teens' decisions about seeking prenatal care are shaped by their awareness of dominant gender ideologies that define young unmarried women who engage in sex as deviant.

Most teens who explained how they delayed pregnancy confirmation suggested a hesitancy to tell their mothers about the pregnancy, some specifically stating that they feared their mothers' reactions. Some indicated that their mothers did not know they were engaging in sex, either because they had blatantly denied it when their mothers asked, or because their mothers did not suspect that they were "the type" to have sex or become pregnant. Teens' descriptions of their mothers' reactions to their pregnancies supported their fears of negative repercussions from disclosing the pregnancy. For example, Olivia described her mother's reaction, "*She went off, she was acting crazy… She got mad, said 'you're having an abortion'… And then she finally learned to accept it.*" Gloria's mother sustained her negative feelings until the baby was born.

> *Well, my mom said she knew, but she was shocked. She didn't want to know her little girl was gonna' have a baby, stuff like that.* So, would you say that she was upset at first? *Yeah. She was definitely – the whole eight months. She didn't say anything to me. Not a word.*

Gloria's account suggests that similarly to teen mothers themselves, their mothers may be in denial about their daughters' violation of gender norms and hesitant to face the consequences of their behaviors.

In the end, teens' inability to recognize pregnancy symptoms, as well as their efforts to conceal their pregnancies, threatened their own and their babies' health as they delayed prenatal care. Again I would argue that these factors are both shaped by the larger cultural norms that define ideal femininity as sexually innocent and ignorant, and that they have a powerful impact on teens' decision-making around reproductive health care irrespective of teens' access to services.

DISCUSSION AND CONCLUSION

The ideal image of femininity in the good girl who does not engage in sex was invoked in teens' narratives as they accounted for their decisions regarding the use of birth control as well as seeking prenatal care. Teens' accounts suggest that dominant gender ideologies prohibit girls from being active agents of their sexuality by preventing and prohibiting them from expressing, admitting, and responding to their intentions to engage in sex or to actively plan, prevent, or disclose pregnancy.

The teens' accounts that deny their sexual agency and knowledge are consistent with those of other researchers (Polakow, 1993; Thompson, 1995; Zabin & Hayward, 1993), who have found that teens talk about sex that "just happened," indicating that they had not planned to engage in sex. Rhode and Lawson (1993) suggest that appearing unprepared for sex is a way for girls to accommodate our culture's

> double message and double standard concerning female morality. Women are expected to be sexually alluring but not too sexually available, illustrating the double bind of sexuality for teenage girls. By letting intercourse "just happen," female adolescents seek to avoid being stigmatized as either prudish or promiscuous (1993, p. 8).

Many researchers have argued that lack of information about contraception, pregnancy, and other reproductive issues is an important factor in teens' inadequate use of birth control (Fennelly, 1993; Freeman & Rickels, 1993; Hardy, 1988; Ladner & Gourdine, 1992; Sidel, 1996; Zabin & Hayward, 1993), that teens must receive information about birth control that is clear and accurate, they must be able to internalize and use this knowledge (Moore et al., 1986; Zabin & Hayward, 1993), and that this information must include where to obtain birth control methods and how to use them (Fennelly, 1993; Freeman & Rickels, 1993; Hardy, 1988; Moore & Rosenthal, 1993). Although all of these factors are undeniably important, the findings of this research suggest that they are necessary but insufficient to promote young women's power and agency over their reproductive lives in the absence of widespread changes to the dominant gender ideology of the nonsexual good girl.

Despite popular assumptions to the contrary, this gender ideology does not appear to be limited to white middle-class ideals of femininity. Rather, as suggested by the data from this study, Elise (1995) suggests that they are common across racial ethnic groups.

> Black girls in my own and other studies admit an awareness of sexual conservatism in their communities. Although their awareness of strictures against premarital sex does not preclude their sexual activity, it does dissuade them from actively taking responsibility for becoming sexual subjects (Elise, 1995, p. 68).

Another researcher suggests that the

> traditional position many low-income Blacks take toward the use of contraceptives [is] the moral opposition based upon the assumption that nothing should be done to prevent conception except abstinence from sexual involvement (Ladner, 1971, p. 254).

Addressing the influence of gender culture on young women's reproductive decision-making suggests that the issue overwhelmingly was less whether or not teens had access to birth control or prenatal care (a place to get it, money to pay for it, insurance coverage, medical providers, etc.), than how the cultural expectation that girls not be sexual, shaped their reproductive power and agency. If young women are to accept and follow dominant gender norms that prohibit engagement in sexual activity, while also embracing the gender ideology that they be sexy and desirable, they are left with a limited set of options, illustrated in these teen mothers' stories. Ultimately, while engaging in sexual activity in order to be feminine, i.e., sexy and desired by men, young women:

1. do not (and do not appear to) prepare for sex – they do not seek out or use birth control or information about sex, birth control or pregnancy;
2. are not seen by their mothers as in need of information about sex or birth control or pregnancy;
3. do not recognize pregnancy symptoms – they either truly lack information about pregnancy symptoms or they pretend not to know what they are; and/or
4. delay disclosing their pregnancies.

These decisions involve enormous health risks as they leave young women vulnerable to pregnancy, STI's and unwanted sexual encounters, and they leave themselves and their babies vulnerable to late initiation of prenatal care.

While dominant gender ideologies that prohibit young women from engaging in sex shape teens' and their mothers' decision-making in these personal and interpersonal ways, they also deny young women access to information and birth control by larger social institutions. For example, while not the specific focus of this analysis, educators and medical providers often fail to provide young women with important information about sexuality and reproduction and how to promote sexual health.

These findings suggest that issues of pregnancy intention and access to birth control and prenatal care are better understood in the context of gender ideologies that define young women's engagement in sexual activity negatively, than outside that context. At least as important as access to prenatal care and contraceptive services is young women's access to information about their bodies, positive outlets for sexuality, positive identities, and sexual agency. As suggested by Tolman et al. (2003), there is a

> need to keep gender central in conceptualizing adolescent sexual health. For instance, for girls this means being able to acknowledge their sexual desire, feeling sexually empowered, and having access to contraception and condoms, all of which are "punishable" offenses under compulsory heterosexuality (p. 11).

The findings of this study similarly suggest that the constraints of normative gender ideologies limit young women's ability to access critical health care services. Other efforts to provide health care services to underserved populations should similarly address the power of culture as a contextual constraint.

NOTES

1. All names are pseudonyms.
2. Italicized quotes indicate teens' responses to interviewer questions.

ACKNOWLEDGMENTS

I would like to thank my dissertation chair, Ruth Horowitz, for guiding the research project. I would also like to thank Diana Scully, Ilene Speizer, and the volume editor, Jennie Kronenfeld, for their helpful comments on earlier drafts. Most of all, thank you to the 51 teen mothers who shared their stories with me and helped me better understand their worlds.

REFERENCES

Barrett, G., & Wellings, K. (2000). Understanding pregnancy intentions: A problem in evidence everywhere, letter to the editor. *Family Planning Perspectives, 32*(4), 194.

Basen-Engquist, K., Masse, L., Coyl, K., Kirby, D., Parce, G., Banspach, S., & Nodora, J. (1999). Validity of scales measuring the psychosocial determinants of HIV/STD-related risk behavior in adolescents. *Health Education Research, 14*(1), 25–39.

Bird, S. T., & Bogart, L. M. (2005). Conspiracy beliefs about HIV/AIDS and birth control among African Americans: Implications for the prevention of HIV, other STIs, and unintended pregnancy. *Journal of Social Issues, 61*(1), 109–127.

Brindis, C. (1993). Antecedents and consequences: The need for diverse strategies in adolescent pregnancy prevention. In: A. Lawson & D. Rhode (Eds), *The politics of pregnancy : Adolescent sexuality and public policy* (pp. 257–283). Cambridge, MA: Yale University Press.

Crosby, R. A., Holtgrave, D. R., DiClemente, R. J., Wingood, G. M., & Gayle, J. A. (2003). Social capital as a predictor of adolescents' sexual risk behavior: A state-level exploratory study. *AIDS and Behavior, 7*(3), 245–252.

Elise, S. (1995). Teenaged mothers: A sense of self. In: B. J. Dickerson (Ed.), *African American single mothers: Understanding their lives and families* (pp. 53–79). Thousand Oaks, CA: Sage.

Fennelly, K. (1993). Barriers to birth control use among hispanic teenagers: Providers' perspectives. In: B. Bair & S. E. Cayleff (Eds), *Wings of gauze: Women of color and the experience of health and illness* (pp. 300–311). Detroit, MI: Wayne State University Press.

Freeman, E. W., & Rickels, K. (1993). *Early childbearing: Perspectives of black adolescents on pregnancy, abortion, and contraception.* Newbury Park, CA: Sage.

Frieden, J. (2000). Prenatal care and race. *OB GYN News, 35*(2), 16.

Halpern, T., Hallfors, D., Bauer, D. J., Iritani, B., Waller, M. W., & Cho, H. (2004). Implications of racial and gender differences in patterns of adolescent risk behavior for HIV and other sexual transmitted diseases. *Perspectives on Sexual and Reproductive Health, 36*(6), 239–247.

Hardy, J. B. (1988). Teenage pregnancy: An American dilemma. In: H. M. Wallace, G. Ryan Jr. & A. C. Ogleby (Eds), *Maternal and child health practices* (pp. 539–553). Oakland, CA: Third Party Publishing.

Hill Collins, P. (2003). Bloodmothers, othermothers and women-centered networks. In: E. Disch (Ed.), *Reconstructing gender: A multicultural anthology* (3rd ed., pp. 317–323). Boston: University of Massachusetts.

Kaplan, E. B. (1997). *Not our kind of girl: Unraveling the myths of black teenage motherhood.* Berkeley and Los Angeles, CA: University of California Press.

Kendall, C., Afable-Munsuz, A., Speizer, I., Avery, A., Schmidt, N., & Santelli, J. (2005). Understanding pregnancy in a population of inner-city women in New Orleans – results of qualitative research. *Social Science and Medicine, 60*, 297–311.

Kershaw, T. S., Ethier, K. A., Miccolai, L. M., Lewis, J. B., & Ickovics, J. R. (2003). Misperceived risk among female adolescents: Social and psychological factors associated with sexual risk accuracy. *Health Psychology, 22*(5), 523–532.

Kives, S., & Jamieson, M. (2001). Desire for pregnancy among adolescents in an antenatal clinic. *Journal of Pediatric and Adolescent Gynecology, 14*(3), 150–151.

Ladner, J. A. (1971). *Tomorrow's tomorrow: The black woman*. Garden City, NY: Doubleday & Company, Inc.

Ladner, J. A., & Gourdine, R. M. (1992). Adolescent pregnancy in the African-American community. In: R. L. Braithwaite & S. E. Taylor (Eds), *Health issues in the black community* (pp. 206–221). San Francisco, CA: Jossey-Bass Publishers.

Moore, K. A., Simms, M. C., & Betsey, C. L. (1986). *Choice and circumstance: Racial differences in adolescent sexuality and fertility*. New Brunswick, NJ: Transaction Books.

Moore, S., & Rosenthal, D. (1993). *Sexuality in adolescence*. London: Routledge.

Polakow, V. (1993). *Lives on the edge: Single mothers and their children in the other America*. Chicago, IL: University of Chicago Press.

Rhode, D. L., & Lawson, A. (1993). Introduction. In: A. Lawson & D. L. Rhode (Eds), *The politics of pregnancy: Adolescent pregnancy and public policy* (pp. 1–22). New Haven, CT: Yale University Press.

Santelli, J., Rochat, R., Hatfiled-Timajchy, K., Gilbert, B. C., Curtis, K., Cabral, R., Hirsch, J. S., & Schieve, L. (2003). The measurement and meaning of unintended pregnancy. *Perspectives on Sexual and Reproductive Health, 35*(2), 94–101.

Scholly, K., Katz, A. R., Gascoigne, J., & Holck, P. S. (2005). Using social norms theory to explain perceptions and sexual health behaviors of undergraduate college students: An exploratory study. *Journal of American College Health, 53*(4), 159–166.

Sexuality Information and Education Council of the United States. (2003). *The truth about adolescent sexuality*. Washington, DC: Fact Sheet.

Sidel, R. (1996). *Keeping women and children last: American's war on the poor*. New York, NY: Penguin Books.

Thompson, S. (1995). *Going all the way: Teenage girls' tales of sex, romance and pregnancy*. New York: Hill and Wang.

Tolman, D. L., Striepe, M. I., & Harmon, T. (2003). Gender matters: Constructing a model of adolescent sexual health. *The Journal of Sex Research, 40*(1), 4–12.

Trussell, J., Vaughn, B., & Stanford, J. (1995). Are ALL contraceptive failures unintended pregnancies? Evidence from the 1995 National Survey of Family Growth. *Family Planning Perspectives, 31*(5), 246–247, 260.

Veit, F., Sanci, L., Coffey, C., Young, D., & Bowes, G. (1996). Barriers to adolescent health care: Family physicians' perspectives. *Journal of Adolescent Health, 18*(2), 156–157.

Zabin, L. S., & Hayward, S. C. (1993). *Adolescent sexual behavior and childbearing*. Newbury Park, CA: Sage.

BREAST CANCER TREATMENT DECISION MAKING: DOES THE SISTERHOOD OF BREAST CANCER TRANSCEND CULTURE?

Pamela H. Wescott, Ellen J. Reifler, Karen Sepucha and Elyse R. Park

ABSTRACT

Disparities in health care for underserved populations have raised questions about the quality of decisions made by these patients. We explored the decision-making experiences and reactions to a decision aid in focus groups of African American, Hispanic, and Rural breast cancer survivors. All groups were taped, transcribed, and thematic analysis was performed. Individual differences were more common than differences among demographic groups. Decision aids appear to be acceptable without extensive targeting to specific groups. However, translating the decision aid would increase its usefulness for Hispanic populations.

Health Care Services, Racial and Ethnic Minorities and Underserved Populations: Patient and Provider Perspectives
Research in the Sociology of Health Care, Volume 23, 35–53
Copyright © 2005 by Elsevier Ltd.
ISSN: 0275-4959/doi:10.1016/S0275-4959(05)23003-X

INTRODUCTION

Disparities in health care for underserved populations have led to concerns about the quality of decisions made by these patients. Disparities in diagnosis, treatment, and outcomes in breast cancer are pronounced for African American and Hispanic women, and those with lower socio-economic status (Peragallo, Fox, & Alba, 1998; Joslyn & West, 2000; Mandelblatt et al., 2002). For example, minorities are more likely than whites to be diagnosed with late stage breast cancer (AHRQ, 2003). African American women who have a lumpectomy are less likely than white women to receive radiation therapy. African American and Hispanic women are much less likely to have breast reconstruction after mastectomy compared to white women (Alderman, McMahon, & Wilkins, 2003). Low-income women, those who are less educated and those without insurance, are less likely to have a lumpectomy (Dolan & Granchi, 1998; Roetzheim et al., 2000; Gilligan et al., 2002). Regarding follow-up care among ethnic minorities after a breast cancer diagnosis, and even when access is not an issue, minorities still do not receive adequate levels of breast cancer care (Bickell, 2002).

African Americans and Hispanics are more likely than Caucasians to have difficulty communicating with clinicians, and to feel that they are treated with disrespect in health care encounters (Collins et al., 2002). Hispanics are more likely to report unmet health needs (e.g. difficulty getting appointments or delays in care), and to report difficulty in understanding written materials from their doctor's office (AHRQ, 2003). Minorities are more likely to report being less involved in medical decision making than they would like to be (Doescher et al., 2000; AHRQ, 2003).

Rural American patients tend to be older, poorer, and less educated than their urban counterparts (Vellozzi, Romans, & Rothenberg, 1996; Schootman & Fuortes, 1999; Gaston, 2001). Other factors influencing rural health care include lack of transportation, lack of insurance or underinsurance, and fewer physicians. Rural women are likely to face geographic isolation, have limited informal- or formal-support systems, and be the primary healers of their families, often utilizing self-care strategies developed over generations. Rural women are less likely than urban women to receive breast cancer screening, although few studies have evaluated the impact of screening on health outcomes in rural women (Schootman & Fuortes, 1999).

These studies reflect what has been reported by the Institute of Medicine and the President's Cancer Panel that strongly suggest that the quality of care is not as good as it could be, especially for underserved populations

(The President's Cancer Panel, 1999; Committee on Quality Health Care in America, 2001). In particular, these studies suggest that quality of the decisions made by patients and their doctors is poor. The quality of a decision is the extent to which it reflects the preferences of an informed patient and is implemented.

A growing field of research has been dedicated to developing tools, called decision aids, to improve the quality of decisions. These tools are often geared toward patients to provide easily understandable information about the diagnosis, treatment choices, and possible benefits and side effects. They are created in different media and can be computer-based, video, audio and/or paper-based. The aids also help patients clarify values, either explicitly through exercises or implicitly through providing representative vicarious experience. In randomized trials, decision aids have been shown to reduce uncertainty, increase knowledge, reduce decisional conflict, and increase patients' desire to participate in decision making, without increasing anxiety (O'Connor et al., 1999; Molenaar et al., 2000). However, there is only a limited understanding of how decision aids may work for different populations.

We recently revised a decision aid, *Early Stage Breast Cancer: Choosing Your Surgery* (©Foundation for Informed Medical Decision Making and Health Dialog, Inc., 2004). It is a 55-min video program with a booklet that describes the decision between mastectomy and lumpectomy with radiation for women with early-stage breast cancer. The program features 10 patients and two doctors, and is narrated by an African American physician. While Foundation policy is to recruit diverse patients for the programs, there has been limited diversity among the patients who participated in the evaluation of this program.

Specifically, we wondered whether there might be differences in ways of coping, attitudes about having cancer, experiences with the health care system, or communication styles that would suggest that decision aids should be customized. While the program currently includes some, but not an overwhelming amount of diversity in patients and providers, we wondered whether patients would note any cultural perspectives that were missing. If we evaluated our video using distinct demographic groups, would we learn anything about decision making that is culturally specific?

RESEARCH PROJECT

In September 2003, we received a grant from the Commonwealth Fund to study these questions. We planned focus groups targeting three distinct demographic groups, African American women, Hispanic women, and women who lived in a rural area. In addition, we recruited a comparison group of white women with some college education.

Research for this project included a review of the literature on racial/ethnic disparities in health care and relationships among culture, patient preferences, and patient decision making. Experts were consulted including an advisory group of individuals who are involved in community outreach, and in evaluating cultural competency and health literacy. They provided their expertise in the development of focus group instruments and met to review and critique the findings after the data was collected. Under their guidance, we decided to eliminate any questions in which we asked patients to speak directly about cultural or ethnic assumptions. Instead, we planned to do active listening, not to ask leading questions, but to let the evaluation of the video discussion unfold, with the assumption that if the participants were comfortable, they would begin to talk about these topics on their own. We used a structured focus guide that asked the questions we would ordinarily ask about content, clarity, and balance of the video.

We encountered a significant challenge in negotiating the issues that came up with patient recruitment and Institutional Review Board (IRB) approval. We sent sample documents (e.g. consent forms, proposal summaries, and confirmation letters) to aid in application preparation. We had frequent telephone and email contact to monitor progress and help troubleshoot problems as they occurred.

Two of our three original sites were able to get IRB approval and schedule focus groups. In Scarborough, Maine, we held 2 focus groups with rural women of mixed educational level. San Diego also got IRB approval, but then was only able to recruit three women for one focus group. When our third site, Detroit, Michigan, withdrew, we came up with a plan to recruit African American women in Atlanta, as well as the comparison group.

Because of the small turnout in San Diego, we decided to recruit a second Hispanic group in Boston. We contacted the Latin American Health Institute (LHI) in Boston with a request for assistance in recruiting Spanish speakers who would feel comfortable watching a video in English. We submitted a protocol, which their IRB reviewed and accepted. After watching the video, these participants completed questionnaires, which had been translated into Spanish. Dr. Dora Gutierrez, the Community Health Initiative Director for the Latino Health Institute, conducted the group in Spanish, which included two women diagnosed with early-stage breast cancer.

In total, we conducted eight focus groups at four sites, Scarborough, Maine; San Diego, California; Atlanta, Georgia, and Boston, Massachusetts. Our participants included 44 women and the breakdown is as follows:

- 11 African American women (2 focus groups in Atlanta, Georgia)
- 5 Hispanic women (1 focus group, conducted in English in San Diego, California; and 1 focus group, conducted in Spanish in Boston, Massachusetts)
- 18 women with mixed educational backgrounds, living in a rural area (2 focus groups in Scarborough, Maine)
- 10 comparison women, white with some college education (2 focus groups in Atlanta, Georgia).

All participants watched the decision aid *Early Stage Breast Cancer: Choosing Your Surgery* and filled out questionnaires. We conducted the focus groups using a structured interview guide. Each group was taped and transcribed. When we reviewed the transcripts, we identified themes such as: coping with cancer, attitudes about cancer, decision making, and criteria for evaluating the decision aid. Codes were assigned to enable us to document the themes in a systematic way. Three coders were enlisted and a pilot was undertaken: all read the same transcript and then met to discuss their interpretations; redefining and assigning codes as needed. They proceeded to code the remaining transcripts independently; then met twice to reconcile differences, creating one master transcript for each of the four demographic groups. On that master transcript, the codes assigned represented the final verdict after the three coders had independently coded each transcript, and then met to insure that the codes were in agreement.

Our findings were drawn from three sources of data: (1) questionnaires with patients' ratings of the decision aid; (2) themes from focus group transcripts; and (3) quotes which were compiled from the transcripts and organized according to themes related to making decisions about treatment of breast cancer, and feedback about the decision aid.

Based on our analysis, we identified specific similarities and differences that transcend culture in terms of the themes that were mentioned in our focus group discussions.

Coping and Attitudes: Range of Denial and Time to Begin Coping

There seems to be a range, transcending culture, of those who get stuck in denial before they can move on, and those who can deal with the enormity of the diagnosis from the beginning. A woman in the rural group said:

> One of the worst things when I got cancer was the absolute hopelessness and futility of doing anything. I mean, how did I get cancer? I don't smoke, I don't drink, I nursed four babies. I had kids before I was 30. I started my period at a normal age, not when I was seven. Every single criteria to not get breast cancer I did. I was never overly obese. I exercised every day. I ate well. I was at the normal weight. I was really angry when I got cancer, absolutely infuriated.

This was a reaction we heard from individuals across the different groups.

An African American patient expressed a related sentiment that cuts across all demographic groups:

> Cancer…is like being inducted into a club you never wanted to be part of.

We observed that individual temperament more than ethnic or cultural background seems to dictate how people deal with their diagnosis. The literature supports our finding that most coping responses are more similar than different across groups (whites, African Americans, and Hispanics) (Culver et al., 2002). In all demographic groups we heard some were overwhelmed by emotions in the beginning, others said they were numb until they had completed all of their treatments and only then did they start to have feelings about what they had been through. We heard from women who said they had wanted to know everything, and women who just wanted to know the next thing they needed to understand and nothing more.

In the African American demographic group the range included one patient who saw no reason to hold anything back:

> It took me less than a week to come to a point where I could deal with the diagnosis, but elected to talk freely with my family about it. This is my reality. There is no reason to be trying to hold anything back.

And we heard another African American woman who said it took two to three years to accept that breast cancer has happened to her:

> There is a denial factor. I mean I think that I was just trying to deny that this happened. So if I wake up from surgery and see myself reasonably whole from surgery, then maybe this didn't happen to me. For me, though, the true dawning was…two years down the road, maybe three years (recognizing) that this happened. Life has changed, and you are going to have to do things differently.

Gender Concordance with Health Care Provider important

Ethnic and racial concordance did not come across as much as gender concordance in being an important factor in forging a partnership with a health care provider. No one complained or was concerned about not having doctors or patients who looked like them. However, for the Hispanic women, having the tape in Spanish would have increased its helpfulness. Across demographic groups, participants mentioned how important it was to have women doctors/health care workers to talk to. They did have positive things to say about particular male doctors, but there was agreement that women in general are more understanding and many preferred women doctors. This observation is supported in the literature (Bickell, 2002) finding that Hispanic women, in particular, expressed the desire not to talk openly about or expose their breast to others, and particularly having issues with male doctors such as the perception of being disloyal to husbands if talking about their bodies with another man, even if that man is a doctor.

Participants articulated their feelings that women could understand more about what they were going through when confronting a disease like breast cancer. Women in the Hispanic group commented on the qualities of one particular female physician. One person said:

> She always answers the question and has the time for you.

Another added:

> She has the time for you and includes, if you don't understand...a drawing...And plus you go on the Internet and check up.

We heard these qualities being valued across all demographic groups: being willing to take the time, to answer all questions, to explain the process of what will happen, to find ways to make the concepts clear, being kind and caring, being comfortable with patients using the Internet and other sources of information.

Across demographic groups, we heard preferences for different communication styles of physicians. Some women across groups preferred "blunt and direct," while others found that style of expression offensive. Similarly, there were those who reacted across groups to "sugarcoating" or "Pollyanna stuff" while others felt comforted by it.

One woman in the rural demographic group explained exactly what she likes and does not like about how cancer is discussed in some of the literature that is handed out:

> It's good to know that people have survived it. But I don't want people making light of it. It's like this is the most devastating thing I have ever dealt with in my entire life, so far. And they're making light of it. They're saying, "Oh it's not that bad." Well you know what? Let me think it's really bad. Give me the options and give me some hope. But let me be really upset. Don't try to sugarcoat it.

A woman in the Hispanic demographic group described how she and her daughter reacted differently to the style of a female physician:

> I told my daughter, 'Well, this is the way I want her to (be)' because you don't want her to go around the bushes or hand it to you in a very sweet way. You want to know the reality because you are living in a world where you have to face reality as it comes. You cannot...be in the clouds and think 'It's going to be okay.' It helps to have a positive attitude, but it helps also to know the reality of things, what is the risk of everything that is involved.

DIFFERENT LEVELS OF SUPPORT ARE VALUED BY PEOPLE ACROSS DEMOGRAPHIC GROUPS

There were differences in how much family and friends support people received and how easy or difficult it was to ask for help. Each demographic group had people who were concerned about handling their family and friends relationships. In the African American demographic group it was noted that something missing from the decision aid was the interaction of a spouse who was involved in the decision making, and how cancer affects one's family and friends. One woman in this group described it this way:

> I saw a play which dealt with the community of people, and it was so powerful. And that's what we don't see, how it affects everybody.

Another recalled her husband's response:

> You do whatever you need to do, because it's not going to make a difference with me. I didn't marry you for that breast.

While a third said about her son:

> Everybody that he knew – knew that I had gone through something. And he was just so caring about the way – every morning before I got up – he was down at my bedroom door, knocking to make sure that I was O.K.

From the comparison and Hispanic groups, we also heard about the importance of having a supportive spouse. One Hispanic woman noted:

> They go with their wives to do the mammogram, and I think it's a good thing that they participate in that.

We have heard comments similar to this across all demographic groups.

Support can be Helpful or Burdensome

Women talked about how in addition to managing their own care and their own feelings about having cancer, they had to manage their family's feelings and reactions to the diagnosis. Again we observed a range – those family members who were able to provide helpful support right at the beginning, those who took a while to provide it, and those who could not be support-ive. All demographic groups could benefit by more discussion about man-aging family and friends' concerns.

The African American, Hispanic, and comparison groups mentioned much more often than the rural groups that they received support from family and friends. The African American and comparison groups also brought up managing the consequences of getting family support. One woman in an African American group said:

> I actually stopped telling people because I didn't know who I was going to have to console and who could console me and who could help me.

Similarly, another said:

> I did talk more positively to other people, generally, than I felt, just to keep them up. I ended up in the position of consoling other people.

A third described telling her three girls:

> We called all the girls in and we told them that I had been diagnosed. And immedi-ately…two of them really cried…I had to be strong for them and I kept saying, 'Well, you know, it's going to be okay. It's going to be okay. It's going to be okay.'

One who managed on her own said:

> I shared it with the family, Thanksgiving, the first time. And I'm kind of an independent person so I don't burden them. I'll tell them some of it.

In the Hispanic group, one woman was so comfortable with having her daughter provide support that she actually brought her to the group. In contrast, another Hispanic participant said she did not want to burden her children:

> Because I have three daughters and a boy, but they are in Florida. I am not going to be telling things to them. What are they going to do, suffer? What is the point, to cry and feel bad? They can't come.

The comparison demographic group exhibited a similar range in those who tried to involve others. This sometimes led to putting on a happy face, convincing everybody else that they were going to be okay, while others chose to manage family and friends by not telling all.

One comparison group participant tried to put her father's mind at ease by showing him her mastectomy scar. She said she had felt a thrill, like being 10 years old after her mastectomy:

> And I don't mind looking ten years old, she added. My father was so worried about what I was going to look like, I said, 'Dad, do you want to see it?' And he said, 'Yeah.' And I said, 'Okay,' so I undid my shirt and…he said, 'Oh that's okay.' And it just put him at ease. It…put me at ease.

Another member of that group who chose to present herself as self-sufficient in the eyes of her family and her neighborhood explained:

> I have two daughters…And I had to completely reassure them all the time, and I just make it my mission that I'm not going to have victim associated with my name…that's why I kept cutting the grass…not only helps other people see that, but helps you.

Coping Strategies Include Managing on One's Own, Religion, Support Groups

We heard the range in all groups from managing on one's own to leaning on others. One woman in the comparison group said:

> I wouldn't even let anybody go through chemo with me. I just didn't want to put my family through that because they looked so sad.

In the African American group we heard:

> I went through this during the Christmas holiday and I went by myself. I didn't want to bring anyone during the holiday. So it was just me and my doctor.

The African American demographic group mentioned managing on their own more than they mentioned prayer or going to church. However, they mentioned prayer and going to church more times than the comparison group, while the rural and Hispanic demographic groups did not mention this as a strategy at all. (Note: the literature reports that African Americans and Hispanics are more likely to use religious coping than Caucasians (Culver et al., 2002).

So, too, in our groups we heard least often from the comparison group on this topic, though one woman said:

> The Lord really sent me – He put me in the path of all these people who knew all the best doctors. I went to church.

We heard somewhat more about the power of faith from the African American women. As one put it:

I wanted to be healthy and I believe with all my heart that if God provided me with the opportunity to choose something that was going to allow me to live, then I would choose that.

And in the Hispanic group, the importance of faith was described in this way:

You have to...when they tell you that you have cancer...to trust God and to hold to God. When you are in the hands of the doctors, it's God that is with you doing surgery on you. You have to have faith and not think about the worst.

As expected, support groups were of enormous importance to the people who chose to belong to one. One African American woman referred to *the camaraderie* (of her support group)...*as one the best parts of the experience.* One possible cultural difference we noted was the ease with which the African American women talked about their feelings. We wondered if this was, in fact, cultural or because so many belonged to the same support group. There were also some women in the African American groups who were positive about their choices, and did not use a support group, because they felt they had enough support from family and friends. However, the African American and rural demographic groups mentioned going it alone as a useful strategy less often than the comparison demographic group.

Grieving/Loss Mentioned more Often by African Americans

Of all the demographic groups, the African American women had the highest number of mentions of grieving as a necessary part of moving on. One woman explained:

As strong as I thought I was, every now and then I would have a 'Woe is me day' where I would just let the water flow. And then I'd be all right. And then somebody told me it is all right to have those days. It is getting over these things that is important.

Another woman noted:

I had one breast. It was depressing to look in the mirror and not see anything.

While someone else realized:

I just had to get used to the idea that I actually had to go through those treatments.

INTERACTIONS WITH PROVIDERS VARIED
ACROSS GROUPS

African American, Hispanic and rural demographic groups had more comments about positive interactions with their health care providers than did the comparison group. Satisfaction was often expressed as praise of a physician who took the time to explain what was happening. One Hispanic patient noted:

> My doctor explained everything to me. He explained everything perfectly...and point by point he gave me all the explanations that I received. He presented me with everything because he is not a doctor who hides anything.

A woman from the rural group put it this way:

> I had wonderful doctors. I spent a lot of time with my oncologist, maybe an hour. He explained everything to me. I had a separate meeting with my radiologist. He told me exactly what would be done. And they are still there for me.

Hispanic, rural, and comparison groups had more comments than the African American demographic group about negative interactions with providers. This may have had to do with the fact that more of the African American women were recruited from support groups and had already discussed and processed those interactions.

Women who were dissatisfied with their providers often complained of getting information that was incomplete or "sugar coated." For instance, one woman in the comparison group reflected back about what the mastectomy experience had been like:

> I would say about the mastectomy, when the doctor presents it to you, he doesn't really tell you in detail what the surgery is.

Another patient from the comparison group put it this way:

> ...doctors present everything as good news. The good news is you can have a mastectomy and that will save your life. The good news is that you can have a lumpectomy and that will save your breast. And they don't tell you the side effects and the consequences of the chemo, the mastectomy and the radiation. They really don't.

While a third patient wished, she had taken a more active role because:

> ...doctors have their own agenda. Whether they admit it or not, they do. I learned it after the fact. I wish I had learned it during the process, that you really have to take your own health into your own hand and you be the decision maker, take his advice and weigh it and all that.

A patient from the rural group perceived her doctor as cold and authoritarian, not giving her the time or attention she needed when she spoke for the first time on the phone to her that evening:

> ...the oncologist that called me said, 'You have to do this.' I had never even seen her.

Reactions to the Decision Aid

Patients like Lively Patients who Express Humor
Regarding the patients and physicians in the program, women in all groups tended to notice and comment on the patients who used humor the most, and were the most "lively" – patients like Viola (African American), Theresa (white, "working class" Boston accent), and Tina (white, whose significant other gives her a "thumbs up" when he sees her mastectomy scar).

Patients Identify with Decisions made more than the Race/Ethnicity of the Patient
We heard across groups that women identified more with patients who made a decision similar to theirs rather than with patients who happened to be of a similar race or cultural background. One woman in the African American demographic group made these two observations:

> The person that stood out the most for me was the one who could care less about having breasts, or not, because that is kind of how I felt...anybody who didn't like me without breasts, didn't like me with breasts.

She went on to say:

> The other person who stood out was the one that said that her significant other, when she looked at him, she was looking at his expression before she looked at herself, and that gave her reassurance that she had made the right decision.

Another African American observed her process of identifying, or not, with patients on the screen:

> When somebody goes through that...it may touch (one person) a lot. And another person, it may make them be closed up and have nothing to say... We saw a person that was happy. We saw a person that was concerned about their looks. We saw another person that could care nothing about her breasts. And just (seeing) the different attitudes...(makes me feel that) we all today are totally different.

Across Groups Patients Respond to Similar Outlooks Regarding Hope and Optimism:
Someone in every group mentioned the patient in the program who exclaims that "cancer is a gift." Across groups, we heard some agreement, some

disagreement with that statement. In the rural demographic group, one woman (who happens to be in the same racial/ethnic and age demographic as the patient in the video) commented:

> I think for some people it can be a transformative time. But that doesn't mean for everybody. I mean other people may just think, 'This is just a pain in the butt.' And I never felt like, 'Oh I'm so happy I have cancer!'

Another woman in the same demographic group felt that the "cancer is a gift" quote should come out. Her rationale:

> You do not need to be diagnosed with death threatening illness to make you stop and think about what life is all about. That is ridiculous.

Decision Regret was Observed across Demographic Groups

We heard from patients who were unhappy with their surgery decisions in the comparison groups, the rural groups, and the African American groups. The Hispanic groups were the only ones that did not include a patient who experienced decision regret. A possible explanation for the lack of decision regret is the size and nature of these groups. That is, these groups were small and included only five women in total. Also, the women who did attend were remarkably open and comfortable about their treatment decisions. We hypothesize that this was a self-selected group of extroverts, and they were so comfortable with their decisions that they were willing to review a video in a second language.

We also observed that there are two types of decision regret. The first type can be characterized as unhappy because they did not realize they had a choice. Some women do not understand until after they had treatment that they could have chosen between mastectomy and lumpectomy with radiation. If they were told to have a mastectomy for instance, they can become dissatisfied with what they see was taken away. They can seem stuck in anger and mourning because they now believe they would have chosen differently. Decision aids are designed to reduce precisely this type of decision regret by delineating all the choices, with the risks and benefits.

The other type of decision regret is more complex. This type is experienced by a woman who had a bad outcome, even though she was aware of the risks. For example, one of the African American women chose lumpectomy and then had a mastectomy when the cancer came back. Even though she knew this was a possibility, when it became a certainty, she became uncomfortable with her informed decision. Although she understood this to be a risk, she still felt that if only she could have known ahead of time that this outcome was going to happen to her, she would not have chosen lumpectomy. Decision aids are also designed to reduce this type of decision regret by encouraging patients to think about how they might feel if certain risks happen to them.

Nothing in the way in which these women experience decision, regret seemed endemic to their cultural setting. They all seemed to have an urgent need to tell their story. These women, quite understandably, tended to be the group "dominators," the ones who need attention and the group seems to respond by active listening and by offering comfort and advice. This was true across the board.

ADVISORY COMMITTEE FEEDBACK

From our Advisory Committee, we received support for our finding that translating the program into Spanish, and including more about family issues would be valuable. They appreciated the patient quotes that were included and asked if we could add a few more (which we did). Finally, they offered two further research questions: (1) they hypothesized that the sisterhood of being diagnosed with breast cancer transcends culture. They wondered if more culture-specific tapes would be needed if the topic were breast cancer screening. (2) They suggested using this tape as an aid for screening. However, since the tape is targeted for women diagnosed with early-stage breast cancer, we felt perhaps a new tape would be more appropriate on the topic of the mammography decision.

CONCLUSIONS AND IMPLICATIONS

Overall, we did not find evidence that decision aids should be targeted to diverse groups. In general, when differences appeared in how women coped with cancer, sought support, experienced treatment, or responded to the testimony of patients and physicians in our decision aid, we noted that individual characteristics were more prominent than group characteristics. Every group had concerns about getting information that they could trust and that was easy to understand. Across demographic groups, we were struck more by similarities than differences. One exception was the recognition that translating our tape into Spanish would be of enormous value for women whose first language is not English, regardless of their education level. Other than that, there were few major demographic group differences and none that would cause us to tailor decision aids to different underserved groups.

Other recent research supports this finding. A more extensive study evaluating one of the Foundation's decision aids (for men making decisions regarding Benign Prostatic Hyperplasia) found, in fact, that "the hypothesized influence of race and education was modest, suggesting that decision aids may be effective in communicating information to diverse groups using a general, non-tailored approach." (Rovner et al., 2004). The researchers' findings suggest that "elaborate efforts to tailor decision aids to differences in ethnicity and education may not be the most important foci of future decision aid development."

Throughout this project, we have wondered, can cultural differences emerge when groups are led by people of a different cultural background? Were participants more willing to discuss gender differences than cultural because facilitators were of the same gender, but from different backgrounds?

We heard across demographic groups that women identified more with patients who made a decision similar to theirs rather than with patients who happened to be of a similar race or cultural background.

Ethnic and racial concordance did not come across as much as gender concordance in being an important factor in forging a partnership with a health care provider.

The concept of culture is difficult to define and may not be consistent among diverse groups or in the ways in which it is discussed in the clinical literature. Defining culture can be difficult because of the heterogeneity within groups (e.g. differences in acculturation, socioeconomic status, and other multiple influences). In attempting to identify cultural influences, there is always the risk of stereotyping and oversimplification of culture (Carrillo, Green, & Betancourt, 1999; Betancourt, 2003). This work reflects the experiences of a small number of women from varied cultures. Through their participation, we were able to learn a bit about how different women approach the decision-making process and how decision aids may work for them. This represents only a first step in an ongoing process to develop and refine our decision aids with the goal of improving the quality of decisions and the quality of care.

ACKNOWLEDGMENTS

Commonwealth Fund

The authors are grateful for the support provided by the Commonwealth Fund.

Advisory Committee Members

This group provided feedback on the evaluation instruments that were used with focus group participants. In October 2004, five members of the group met to review and critique the project findings. The entire group included the following:

Joseph Betancourt, MD, MPH (Director for Multicultural Education, Multicultural Affairs Office, Massachusetts General Hospital (MGH), Eileen Manning, RN (Clinical Director of the Breast and Cervical Cancer Screening Initiative for MGH Community Health Associates), Gwen Mitchell, LPN, MEd (Nurse Manager, MGH Comprehensive Breast Health Center), Deborah Washington, RN (Director of Diversity for MGH Patient Care Services), Ming Sun (Coordinator of Patient Education for MGH Community Health Centers), Loretta Holliday (Director, MGH Association for Multicultural Programs), Karin Hobrecker (medical interpreter for MGH Spanish-speaking patients), and Barbara Cashavelly, MSN, RN, AOCN (Nurse Manager, MGH Cancer Center).

Spanish-Speaking Focus Group Co-facilitators

Early in the project, we consulted Margaret Holmes-Rovner, Ph.D., Professor and Chief, Division of Health Services Research, Department of Medicine, Michigan State University, who has expertise in setting up focus groups for underserved and minority populations. Based on Dr. Holmes-Rovner's advice, we decided to ask Dr. Ana Navarro in San Diego to be a consultant to the project and a focus group co-facilitator.

Dr. Navarro is a native Spanish speaker whose expertise over the past 15 years has included qualitative research involving breast cancer patients. We would like to thank Dr. Navarro for reviewing the focus group guide, and for co-facilitating the focus group. This group was conducted in English and the questionnaires were in English. Dr. Navarro served as a translator as needed.

We also wish to thank Dr. Dora Gutierrez, the Community Health Initiative Director for the Latino Health Institute. Dr. Gutierrez had contacts at a local hospital (Beth Israel Deaconess Medical Center) and several community health centers, and she offered to help with recruitment of Spanish-speaking women diagnosed with early-stage breast cancer. She facilitated the focus group while translation of the questionnaire was done by Francisco Sastre. We would like to thank the Latino Health Institute for their collaboration in this project.

REFERENCES

A.H.R.Q. (2003). *National healthcare disparities report.* Rockville, MD: U.S. Department of Health and Human Services: Agency for Healthcare Research and Quality.

Alderman, A. K., McMahon, L., Jr., & Wilkins, E. G. (2003). The national utilization of immediate and early delayed breast reconstruction and the effect of sociodemographic factors. *Plastic Reconstructive Surgery, 111*(2), 695–703.

Betancourt, J. R. (2003). Cross-cultural medical education: Conceptual approaches and frameworks for evaluation. *Academy Medicine, 78*(6), 560–569.

Bickell, N. A. (2002). Race, ethnicity, and disparities in breast cancer: Victories and challenges. *Women's Health Issues, 12*(5), 238–251.

Carrillo, J. E., Green, A. R., & Betancourt, J. R. (1999). Cross-cultural primary care: A patient-based approach. *Annals Internal Medicine, 130*(10), 829–834.

Collins, K. S., Hughes, D. L., Doty, M. M., Ives, B. L., Edwards, J. N., & Tenney, K. (2002). Diverse communities, common concerns: Assessing health care quality for minority Americans. *Findings from The Commonwealth Fund 2001 Health Care Quality Survey.* New York: The Commonwealth Fund.

Committee on Quality Health Care in America, & I. O. M. (2001). *Crossing the quality chasm: A new health system for the 21st century.* Washington, DC: National Academy Press.

Culver, J. L., Arena, P. L., Antoni, M. H., & Carver, C. S. (2002). Coping and distress among women under treatment for early stage breast cancer: Comparing African Americans, Hispanics and non-Hispanic Whites. *Psychooncology, 11*(6), 495–504.

Doescher, M. P., Saver, B. G., Franks, P., & Fiscella, K. (2000). Racial and ethnic disparities in perceptions of Physician style and trust. *Archives Family Medicine, 9*(10), 1156–1163.

Dolan, J. T., & Granchi, T. S. (1998). Low rate of breast conservation surgery in large urban hospital serving the medically indigent. *American Journal Surgery, 176*(6), 520–524.

Gaston, M. H. (2001). 100% access and 0 health disparities: Changing the health paradigm for rural women in the 21st century. *Women's Health Issues, 11*(1), 7–16.

Gilligan, M. A., Kneusel, R. T., Hoffmann, R. G., Greer, A. L., & Nattinger, A. B. (2002). Persistent differences in sociodemographic determinants of breast conserving treatment despite overall increased adoption. *Medicine Care, 40*(3), 181–190.

Health Dialog Inc. (2004). Early stage breast cancer: Choosing your surgery. *A Shared Decision Making Program.* Boston: Health Dialog Inc.

Joslyn, S. A., & West, M. M. (2000). Racial differences in breast carcinoma survival. *Cancer, 88*(1), 114–123.

Mandelblatt, J. S., Kerner, J. F., Hadley, J., Hwang, Y. T., Eggert, L., Johnson, L. E., & Gold, K. (2002). OPTIONS (Outcomes and Preferences for Treatment in Older Women Nationwide Study). Variations in breast carcinoma treatment in older Medicare beneficiaries: Is it black or white. *Cancer, 2002*(95), 7.

Molenaar, S., Sprangers, M. A., Postma-Schuit, F. C., Rutgers, E. J., Noorlander, J., Hendriks, J., & de Haes, H. C. (2000). Feasibility and effects of decision aids. *Medicine Decision Making, 20*(1), 112–127.

O'Connor, A. M., Rostom, A., Fiset, V., Tetroe, J., Entwistle, V., Llewellyn-Thomas, H., Holmes-Rovner, M., Barry, M., & Jones, J. (1999). Decision aids for patients facing health treatment or screening decisions: Systematic review. *British Medical Journal, 319*(7212), 731–734.

Peragallo, N. P., Fox, P. G., & Alba, M. L. (1998). Breast care among Latino immigrant women in the U.S. *Health Care Women International, 19*(2), 165–172.

Roetzheim, R. G., Gonzalez, E. C., Ferrante, J. M., Pal, N., Van Durme, D. J., & Krischer, J. P. (2000). Effects of health insurance and race on breast carcinoma treatments and outcomes. *Cancer, 89*(11), 2202–2213.

Rovner, D. R., Wills, C. E., Bonham, V., Williams, G., Lillie, J., Kelly-Blake, K., Williams, M. V., & Holmes-Rovner, M. (2004). Decision aids for benign prostatic hyperplasia: Applicability across race and education. *Medicine Decision Making, 24*(4), 359–366.

Schootman, M., & Fuortes, L. J. (1999). Breast and cervical carcinoma: The correlation of activity limitations and rurality with screening, disease incidence, and mortality. *Cancer, 86*(6), 1087–1094.

The President's Cancer Panel. (1999). *The national cancer program: Assessing the past, charting the future.* 1999 Annual Report. Washington, DC.

Vellozzi, C. J., Romans, M., & Rothenberg, R. B. (1996). Delivering breast and cervical cancer screening to underserved women: Part I. Literature review and telephone survey. *Women's Health Issues, 6*(2), 65–73.

SECTION 3:
SPECIAL TYPES OF UNDERSERVED POPULATIONS: MENTAL HEALTH, EMOTIONAL WELL BEING, AGING AND SEX WORKERS

SOCIAL FACTORS, NEED, AND MENTAL HEALTH SERVICES UTILIZATION: FINDINGS OF THE NATIONAL COMORBIDITY SURVEY

Anthony Kouzis

ABSTRACT

To investigate the role of social factors, health status, and psychiatric disorders (DSM-III-R) on mental health services use, we utilized the National Comorbidity Survey (NCS), a nationally representative household survey (1990–1992) of the US (n = 5877). Multivariate logistic regression allowed estimation of the adjusted odds ratios and 95% confidence intervals on the likelihood of visiting the health or the specialty mental/addictive service sectors. Significant determinants included: gender, race, household income, work status, and quality of community-level health care resources. Those with greater socioeconomic resources or comorbid psychiatric disorders were more likely to visit the specialty mental health sector.

Health Care Services, Racial and Ethnic Minorities and Underserved Populations: Patient and Provider Perspectives
Research in the Sociology of Health Care, Volume 23, 57–78
ISSN: 0275-4959/doi:10.1016/S0275-4959(05)23004-1

SOCIAL FACTORS, NEED, AND MENTAL HEALTH SERVICES UTILIZATION IN THE US

The focus of this paper is on the role that social factors play in the utilization of mental health services. This issue is related to a diverse, but still underdeveloped, literature concerning how such determinants are related to all aspects of health and health care. A range of questions in this field remain unanswered. Following Hollingshead and Redlich's (1958) study on the influence of social class structure and health status and Susser's (Susser, Watson, & Hopper, 1985) social causation model, researchers have debated the influence of social factors on health and illness (Krieger, 1993; Adler et al., 1994). Less attention from health researchers has been focused on questions of access, use patterns, and determinants of services utilization for health and illness (Myers and Schaffer, 1954).

Looking at the question of the utilization of health services, the most notable finding is that most persons suffering mental illness do not receive treatment (Kessler et al., 1999) while the use of services has grown rapidly (The Nation's Health, 2002). Similarly, while a variety of factors are thought to affect the decision to seek help (Wu, Kouzis, & Leaf, 1999) questions concerning the relative importance of these factors on the use of mental health services remain (Rosenheck & Stolar, 1998). In particular, the role of *social* influences on utilization of health services for mental health and illness has not been adequately examined (Krieger, 1993). This paper addresses that issue.

Research on this question has been limited by the use of limited, or inadequate, data sources that are not representative of the population. One difficulty in assessing social causes stems from an early reliance on hospital, administrative, or psychiatric registry data (Brennan, Kagay, Geppert, & Moos, 2001). Investigations have often examined subpopulations (Prigerson, Maciejewski, & Rosenheck, 1999) or *single* communities, disorders, or service sectors. In some studies, data on physical health status, which may steer patients to medical care, is often missing as is vital information on sociodemographic characteristics. Investigations have often relied on symptom scales, psychological distress or substance use (Horwitz, 1996), rather than standardized diagnostic criteria. Such limitations have led to complaints of the scarcity of population-based analyses which explore the social aspects of services use (Rosenheck & Stolar, 1998). One reason suggested is that the large surveys of the general population dealing with mental health have focused on rates and morbidity (Mechanic, 1979; Bijl & Ravelli, 2000) rather than on the utilization of services. A more complete examination of the social determinants of mental health services use in the general population has recently been conducted in the Netherlands. Utilizing the Netherlands Mental Health Survey and Incidence Study (NEMESIS), Bijl and Ravelli (2000) claimed the *first* examination of the social predictors of mental health use employing data from a national probability survey. In this report, we address related questions for the US. This analysis looks at the influence of social factors on different treatment sectors for single or multiple psychiatric disorders in an epidemiologic survey utilizing standardized diagnostic criteria in a representative sample of the *US population.*

To examine the social influences of mental health services use we employed the US National Comorbidity Survey (NCS). We examine a variety of social and economic factors that effect the distribution and use of health services and their influence on service sector choice. Included are standardized criteria for both psychiatric and physical health status. Andersen's (1968, 1995) model of health utilization is predicted to account for variation in use of mental health services and for differences between those using the general medical and those utilizing the specialty mental health sector.

Health Services Use Model

The utilization model developed by Andersen (1968) includes three overarching factors and their relationship with health utilization patterns. *Predisposing* variables exist prior to the onset of illness and include sociodemographic variables. *Enabling* variables provide the means to use health care services for members of the society. *Need* factors are typically considered the strongest predictor (Mechanic, 1979; Leaf, Bruce, & Tischler, 1988; Wolinsky, 1996) of health care use and include symptoms experienced, disability, or chronic diseases.

Predisposing

Sex, race, and *age* differences in the use of mental health services have been found (Rhodes, Goering, To, & Williams, 2002; Markides, Levin, & Ray, 1985; Pescosolido, 1998). *Minority* groups have underutilized services for mental health problems. *Living alone* has been associated with a greater likelihood of using the mental health sector (Badawi, Kramer, & Eaton, 1996). U*nmarried* persons are also more likely to seek help for emotional problems, while marital dissolution, particularly for women, has been associated with increased mental health service (Prigerson, Maciejewski, & Rosenheck, 1999).

Enabling

Structural factors such as income, health insurance (public or private), and
the availability of health care facilities are known to be important. *Employed*
persons have been less likely to use mental health services than those who
were unemployed (Catalano, Rook, & Dooley, 1986). Possessing higher
income (Holzer et al., 1986) or having health *insurance* (Landerman, Burns,
Schwart, Wagner, & George, 1994) was positively related to receiving mental
health services. Mechanic and colleagues (Mechanic, Angel, & Davies, 1992)
posit *education* to be the sole socioeconomic "correlate" in an examination of
social determinants predicting diagnosis, medications, or psychotherapy.
However, others have not found a significant relationship between education
and service utilization or sector choice (Wells, Manning, Duan, Newhouse, &
Ware, 1987).

While health and mental health status are important predictors of use,
they have little effect on type of provider chosen (Fortney, Rost, & Zhiang,
1998; Frank & Kamlet, 1989). Social variables have been asserted as predictors of sector visited. Women, unemployed and publicly insured persons
with minor psychiatric problems have been shown to visit their general or
primary care doctors (Cooper-Patrick, Crum, & Ford, 1994). Persons treated in the general medical sector have more likely been black, older, women,
and have low income and education; a greater likelihood of specialty care
existed for young, single, or non-African–Americans.

Community-level health care resources are also thought to influence use
of services. This may include: the availability of health personnel and services, the ratio of specialists to generalists, the volume and distribution of
resources, and geographic region. Andersen and Aday (1978) showed physician to population ratio to be an important factor, in addition to age and
need. Availability of services has significantly impacted sector choice and
the decision to seek care in rural communities (Fortney, Rost, & Zhiang,
1998). Geographic barriers (Gresenz, Stockdale, & Wells, 2000) may com-
plicate access to specialty care. However, Blazer, Landerman, Fillenbaum,
and Horner (1995) showed no significant variation in service use by urban
or rural residence.

Need

Physical health factors have been the most powerful predictors of health
care use and include such variables as symptoms, disability, or chronic

diseases. Emotional distress increases the probability of using the health care system (Kouzis & Eaton, 1998). People with the greatest need have been found to be more likely to enter the treatment sector (Leaf et al., 1985). Physical health problems are often the context under which patients may seek mental health treatment (Verhaak, 1988).

Service sector use has also been analyzed. Many receive mental health treatment from general practitioners. The Epidemiologic Catchment Area (ECA) surveys demonstrated that approximately one-half of all persons with a mental disorder received treatment exclusively from this sector (Shapiro, Skinner, Kramer, Steinwachs, & Regier, 1985). Patients with less complex, more common albeit, disorders are more likely to be treated in the general health service (HS) sector by physicians or be referred to nonpsychiatric mental health providers. Those suffering more severe disorders requiring more frequent and total visits (Shapiro, Skinner, Kramer, Steinwachs, & Regier, 1985) are referred to and treated by psychiatrists (Narrow, Regier, Rae, Manderscheid, & Locke, 1993).

In sum, while numerous investigators have examined the relationship between social factors and utilization of mental health services, findings appear mixed and often contradictory. The high levels of symptomatology for psychiatric disorders and distress evidenced by the large epidemiologic surveys in the 1980s and 1990s and concomitant increase in utilization of specialty services have not reduced the disparity between need and levels of health services use (The Nation's Health, 2002). This suggests that diagnosis is not a perfect indicator of need, or that need is not a sufficient determinant of the use of mental health services (Regier et al., 1998) despite the preponderance of research asserting this to be the case (Leaf, Bruce, & Tischler, 1988; Wolinsky, 1996). We argue that the overwhelming evidence of large numbers of the population needing but not receiving mental health services demonstrates the increasing importance of understanding the influence of social determinants of utlization in the society. With increasingly shrinking resources and an expanding population this has become increasingly important.

Hypotheses

The National Comorbidity Survey (NCS) was examined for factors influencing the use of general and specialty sectors for mental health care in the general population. These relationships are analyzed while controlling for the potential influence of significant social (age, sex, education, marital status, and race), economic (employment, income, insurance, and community resources), and health (physical and mental) factors on utilization behavior. We examined for the use of any mental health service, the health HS sector, and the specialty mental or addictive (SMA) health sector. We hypothesized that (1) social factors will influence the use of mental health services; (2) these relationships will exist independently of need or mental health status; (3) determinants will differ by use of treatment sector; and (4) the existence of dual diagnoses ("comorbidity") will influence use and sector selection. The NCS allowed an examination of measures of social determinants, health status, and standardized diagnostic criteria (DSM-III-R) for single and co-morbid psychiatric disorders in an epidemiologic survey of the US population. In this study, we test Andersen's theoretical model of health utilization behavior. The contribution of this research is the ability to use: a nationally representative survey, standardized diagnostic criteria for diagnosis of psychiatric disorders, a more complete array of social variables, and the full range of single and comorbid psychiatric disorders in the general population. This investigation attempts to examine the determinants of mental health services use in the US.

METHODS

The NCS is based on a stratified, multistage area probability sample of persons ages 15–54 in the non-institutionalized civilian population of the 48 coterminous United States between 1990 and 1992. Also included was a representative supplemental sample of students residing on campus. The response rate was 82.4% for 8,098 completed interviews; informed consent was obtained. Part I of the interview included the core diagnostic questions and was administered to all respondents. Part II, which contained a risk factor battery and questions about services utilization, was administered to a subsample of 5,877 respondents consisting of all who screened positive for any lifetime diagnosis in Part I, all those ages 15–24, and a random sample of other respondents.

Diagnostic Assessment

All diagnoses were operationalized using DSM-III-R criteria (American Psychiatric Association, 1987) and were generated from a modified version of the Composite International Diagnostic Interview (CIDI) diagnostic computer algorithm (World Health Organization, 1990). We identified the presence of one, two or more (comorbid), or no disorders. The CIDI is a structured interview designed for trained, lay interviewers. Modification included changes in question order to improve flow, and in the introduction of clarifications to complex probe questions (Robins et al., 1988). WHO field trials have documented acceptable reliability and validity of the CIDI (Wittchen, 1994).

Use of Outpatient Services

The outpatient services use questions presented respondents with a list of professionals and asked: "Not counting the times you were an overnight patient in the hospital [which was assessed separately], did you ever in your lifetime go to see any of the professionals on this list for problems with your emotions or nerves or your use of alcohol or drugs?" After eliciting reports about professionals of all types, including open-ended reports about those not on the list, probe questions were asked about recency of contact and number of visits during the past 12 months. A separate list was then presented of sites where professional help could be obtained and respondents were asked: "(W)hich of these places have you ever gone to for professional help with your emotions or nerves or your use of alcohol or drugs?" After eliciting reports about all places where treatment was obtained, probe questions were asked about recency of contact and number of visits to each setting.

Our analysis was in three stages. We examined services use for persons who utilized (1) *Any Service* sector; (2) the *Health Service* sector; and (3) the *Specialty Mental health or Addictive service* sector. *Any service* sector refers to the use in the HS sector for emotional reasons (either general medical or specialty mental, and addictive), the human service sector (social service, clergy, job counseling, school services, hotline, or other), or a self-help group. The *HS* sector refers to those persons who visited the *General Medical* (GM) sector for mental health treatment or the SMA sector. The *GM* sector was defined as either seeing (i) a physician anyplace or (ii) a nurse, occupational therapist, or other allied health professional in either a hospital emergency department or a doctor's private office. *SMA service* contact was defined as either (i) seeing a psychiatrist or psychologist regardless of place, (ii) a social worker or counselor in either an emergency room, a psychiatric outpatient clinic, a drug or alcohol outpatient clinic, a doctor's office, or a drop-in center or program for people with emotional or alcohol or other drug problems, or (iii) seeing a nurse in either a psychiatric outpatient clinic, a drug or alcohol outpatient clinic, or a drop-in center or program for people with emotional or alcohol or other drug problems.

Specific *physical health conditions* included: arthritis, asthma/bronchitis, AIDS, severe visual or hearing impairment, hernia, hypertension, diabetes, history of heart attack, kidney or liver disorders, lupus/thyroid/or any autoimmune disorders, MS/epilepsy/or other neurological disorders, stomach or gallbladder problems, stroke, or ulcer. Having cancer in the past 12 months or a history of heart disease was also included. Those answering, "yes" to any of these conditions were coded "1," all others a "0."

Social variables included age (in years), gender, race, household income, employment status, urbanicity, education (in years), and marital status. *Insurance* status was determined by asking whether a respondent had private health insurance or received publicly assisted health benefits. A county level health services availability rating was created using factor loadings based on indicators of poor vs. non-poor attributes of services available in each county in the US. The variables examined include individual (age, gender, race, employment status, urbanicity, years of education, marital status, and health status), household (income in dollars), and community (quality of health services availability rating) level data.

ANALYSIS

The data were weighted to adjust for variation in within-household and between-household probabilities of selection and differential nonresponse. A second weight adjusted for differential nonresponse based on the non-respondent survey and a comparison of the Part I data. Respondents in the Part II subsample were also weighted by the inverse of their probability of selection to make this sample representative of the total population (Little, Lewitzky, Heeringa, Lepkowski, & Kessler, 1997). Data were poststratified via an interactive procedure to approximate the national population distributions of the cross-classification of sociodemographic (age, sex, and race) characteristics as defined by the 1989 US National Health Interview Survey. The weighted Part II sample is used for our analyses with the sample distributions reported reflecting the weighted number of respondents rounded to the nearest whole number.

Results presented consist of prevalences and adjusted odds ratios (ORs) obtained by the exponentiation of the regression coefficients from multivariate logistic models. There are several predictor variables that are strongly associated with a particular type of service use. A multiple hierarchical logistic regression program was used to estimate the parameters in each replicate, and, owing to the complex sample design, while macros were used to calculate the jackknife repeated replications to estimate the variances of these parameter estimates in design-based subsample replicates (Kish & Frankel, 1970).

RESULTS

The observed rate of services use was 13.3% (SE = 0.73). Of these, 63.9% (SE = 2.69) utilized the HS sector and 68.5% (SE = 4.12) the SMA sector (Table 1). Persons meeting criteria for two or more psychiatric disorders had the highest (33.3%, 70.7%, and 77.8%) while those *without* a disorder had the lowest, rates of services use. One exception occurred for the specialty sector where 69.3% (SE = 9.34) of those with no lifetime psychiatric diagnosis, who sought treatment utilized this sector. Over 8% with no current or lifetime mental disorder utilized the mental health service sector.

Hierarchical logistic regression modeling was utilized to determine the *additivity* of each variable to the $-2 \log \chi^2$ value of the base regression model (Table 2). The likelihood of using each sector was the dependent variable. We subtracted the $-2 \log$ regression equation value of the base model from each increased model value sequentially using significant variables in separate equations. For each of the 10 sociodemographic predictors, two models were examined: First, a *main effects* model with each predictor variable with 15 variables representing mental disorder; second, a model with *interaction effects* for each predictor with one disorder and with two disorders.

Table 1. Percentage and Standard Errors for Number of CIDI–DSM-III-R Psychiatric Diagnoses by Type of Mental Health Service Sector in the Past 1 Year.

Sector	Prevalence Number of Disorders			
	0	1	2	Overall
Any	8.2	17.9	33.3	13.3
	(0.8)	(1.82)	(2.01)	(0.73)
Health	55.4	69.3	70.7	63.9
	(6.00)	(3.93)	(2.84)	(2.69)
Specialty	69.3	62.1	77.8	68.5
	(9.34)	(4.59)	(3.47)	(4.12)

Table 2. Hierarchical Logistic Regression Model Showing Additivity of Social Factors for Main Effects and Interaction with Need Models by Type of Mental Health Service Sector Use in the Past 1 Year.

	DF		1 Anyplace $-2\log\chi^2$		2 Health $-2\log\chi^2$		3 Specialty $-2\log\chi^2$	
	Main	Inter	Main	Inter	Main	Inter	Main	Inter
Age	1	2	3.8	7.3*	33.6**	0.2	1.7	4.8
Sex	1	2	22.7**	3.2	0.4	1.4	5.2*	10.5**
Race	1	2	16.9*	2.2	0.08	3.6	10.9**	5.0
Marital status	2	4	8.6*	8.8	18.7**	1.7	10.8**	6.0*
Education	1	2	8.7**	0.4	7.9**	1.8	48.2**	20.9**
Urban	5	10	33.5*	23.9**	11.8*	17.7	7.7	12.2
City health	1	2	33.1**	3.5	2.7	6.9*	0.9	2.3
Employment	3	6	19.2**	10.8	66.7**	4.6	12.7**	26.8**
Income	2	4	29.4**	4.1	9.2**	26.3**	6.1*	0.5
Insurance	1	2	20.4**	3.2	7.3**	4.0	4.4*	1.9

*$p \leqslant 0.05$.
**$p \leqslant 0.01$.

Thus, 20 separate regression models were examined for statistical significance of χ^2 values. Only variables reaching statistical significance in Table 2 appear in the logistic regression models (Tables 3A–C) which produce adjusted ORs and 95% confidence intervals.

Among those visiting *any sector* for mental health visits, all sociodemographic predictors were statistically significant, except age (column 3). The interactions for having a disorder and age ($p = 0.05$) and disorder with urbanicity ($p = 0.01$) (column 4) were significant. For those using the *HS* sector (column 5), age, marital status, educational level, urbanicity, employment status, household income, and insurance were significant (column 5). Income ($p = 0.01$) and poor county-level health services ($p = 0.05$) interacting with need were significant (column 6). Among those seen in the *SMA* sector (column 7), all socioeconomic variables except age, urbanicity, and poor county health services were significant irrespective of health status; this demonstrates the greater likelihood of use of specialty services by those with the greatest socioeconomic resources. Sex, marital status, education, and employment had statistically significant interaction effects (column 8) with psychiatric morbidity.

Table 3A. Adjusted Relative ORs and 95% Confidence Intervals of Visiting any Sector for Mental Health Purposes in the Past 1 year.

	Adj OR	95% CI
Sex		
Male	1.0	
Female	1.6	(1.16, 2.28)*
Race		
Non-white	1.0	
White	1.5	(1.02, 2.28)*
Employment		
Workers	1.0	
Student	2.0	(1.24, 3.08)*
Homemaker	1.3	(0.77, 2.20)
Other	1.7	(0.74, 3.78)
Insurance		
No	1.0	
Yes	1.3	(0.92, 1.76)
Marital status		
Married/Cohab	1.0	
Separated/Wid/Div	1.4	(1.05, 1.82)*
Never	1.5	(0.94, 2.28)
Income		
$0–15,000	0.5	(0.33, 0.80)*
$15–69,000	0.8	(0.53, 1.24)
$70,000+	1.0	
County-level health services		
Non-poor	1.0	
Poor	0.7	(0.52, 0.99)*
Education		
0–15	1.0	
16+	1.2	(0.79, 1.68)
Age		
0 Dx, 12 months	1.0	(0.99, 1.03)
1 Dx, 12 months	1.03	(1.01, 1.06)*
2 Dx, 12 months	1.03	(1.01, 1.06)*
Urbanicity		
Suburban, major metro	1.0	
City, major metro		
0 Dx	0.6	(0.31, 1.03)
1 Dx	2.3	(0.78, 6.74)

Table 3A. (*Continued*)

	Adj OR	95% CI
2 Dx	1.0	(0.45, 2.04)
Adj, major metro		
0 Dx	0.6	(0.26, 1.63)
1 Dx	1.0	(0.24, 4.31)
2 Dx	0.8	(0.30, 1.94)
City and suburban, other metro		
0 Dx	0.6	(0.39, 0.97)*
1 Dx	0.8	(0.40, 1.46)
2 Dx	1.2	(0.75, 1.93)
Adj, other metro		
0 Dx	1.0	(0.66, 1.63)
1 Dx	0.6	(0.25, 1.36)
2 Dx	1.2	(0.75, 1.76)
Rural (adj and outlying)		
0 Dx	0.6	(0.26, 1.13)
1 Dx	0.9	(0.50, 1.68)
2 Dx	0.9	(0.55, 1.38)
Chronic physical condition		
None	1.0	
1+	1.5	(1.03, 2.09)*
Psychiatric disorder		
None	1.0	
One	0.9	(0.40, 2.04)
Two or more	1.7	(0.59, 4.92)

*Statistically significant.

Multivariate logistic regression analyses to estimate the adjusted ORs, and 95% confidence limits of using *each* service sector were conducted (Tables 3A–C). For each dependent variable (visiting any mental health, the HS, or the SMA service sector) modeled, only the *significant* variables or interaction effects (with need) from the analysis in Table 2 were included as independent variables. The presence of single or comorbid psychiatric diagnoses was also included in the model.

Among those visiting *any health or mental health service* sector, women, whites, students, and unmarried persons had a greater likelihood of seeking help (Table 3A). Students were twice as likely (OR = 2.0, 95% CI = 1.24, 3.08) as full-time workers, to use mental health services. Having a chronic physical health condition was associated with a 50% greater likelihood of utilization. Persons from poverty income households, residing in a county with poor health services, or living in a city outside a metropolitan area were

Table 3B. Adjusted ORs and 95% Confidence Intervals of Visiting the Health Service Sector for Mental Health Reasons in the Past 1 Year.

	Adj OR	95% CI
Age	1.0	(0.97, 1.03)
Sex		
Male	1.0	
Female	1.2	(0.77, 1.86)
Race		
Non-white	1.0	
White	1.0	(0.56, 1.74)
Employment		
Workers	1.0	
Student	0.3	(0.14, 0.57)*
Homemaker	0.6	(0.22, 1.58)
Other	4.0	(1.33, 11.88)*
Insurance		
No	1.0	
Yes	1.9	(1.24, 3.27)*
Marital status		
Married/Cohab	1.0	
Sep/Wid/Div	0.7	(0.35, 1.32)
Never	0.7	(0.38, 1.30)
Income		
$0–14,999		
0 Dx	0.9	(0.32, 2.50)
1 Dx	0.9	(0.15, 5.71)
2 Dx	0.9	(0.20, 4.35)
$15,000–69,999		
0 Dx	0.3	(0.10, 0.68)*
1 Dx	0.8	(0.24, 2.67)
2 Dx	3.1	(0.78, 12.24)
$70,000	1.0	
Poor county-level health services		
Non-poor	1.0	
Poor		
0 Dx	1.1	(0.48, 2.42)
1 Dx	0.3	(0.12, 0.80)*
2 Dx	1.9	(0.59, 6.38)
Education		
0–15	1.0	
16+	1.5	(0.67, 3.26)

Table 3B. (*Continued*)

	Adj OR	95% CI
Urbanicity		
Suburban, major metro	1.0	
City, major metro	0.8	(0.37, 1.87)
Adj, major metro	0.5	(0.17, 1.48)
City and suburban, other metro	0.7	(0.41, 1.22)
Adj, other metro	1.2	(0.50, 3.04)
Rural (adj and outlying)	0.8	(0.29, 2.06)
Chronic physical condition		
None	1.0	
1+	1.0	(0.62, 1.73)
Psychiatric disorders		
None	1.0	
One	0.9	(0.20, 3.58)
Two or more	0.2	(0.03, 1.23)

*Statistically significant.

less likely to utilize services. The interaction of age with one or more mental disorders was also significant; the main effects for age were dropped, however, as age was not significant in Table 2. As predicted, most social variables were statistically related to mental health services use.

The strongest predictor of using the *HS sector* was for persons who were unemployed or who had a disability. These persons had a four times (95% CI = 1.33, 11.88) greater relative odds than full-time workers of visiting the HS sector (Table 3B). Persons having health (public or private) insurance were twice as likely (OR = 1.9, 95% CI = 1.14, 3.28) to visit this sector. Students, persons with need residing in a county with poor quality health services, and members of households earning $15,000–69,000 were less likely to use health services. Persons with a *comorbid* psychiatric diagnosis also had a reduced likelihood of utilizing the HS sector for mental health care. Both predisposing and enabling factors were found to influence use of services. This lends support for our hypothesis of social factors serving independently of need to influence use of health services.

Separate analyses were also conducted for visiting the *SMA sector* (Table 3C). This is critically important, as psychiatrists typically have more specialized training and are capable of offering more extensive and expensive treatment. Students without a psychiatric disorder were 72 times (95% CI = 8.00, 640.32), while unmarried persons without a diagnosis were 13 times (95% CI = 3.18, 53.00) as likely to see specialists as their reference

Table 3C. Adjusted ORs and 95% Confidence Intervals of Visiting the Specialty Mental Health Sector for Mental Health Reasons in the Past 1 Year.

	Adj OR	95% CI
Age	1.0	(0.95, 1.03)
Sex		
Male	1.0	
Female		
0 Dx	2.8	(0.53, 14.58)
1 Dx	1.0	(0.24, 3.73)
2 Dx	0.6	(0.22, 1.66)
Race		
Non-white	1.0	
White	1.9	(0.63, 5.69)
Employment		
Worker	1.0	
Homemaker		
0 Dx	0.9	(0.19, 4.56)
1 Dx	0.3	(0.04, 1.67)
2 Dx	1.0	(0.26, 3.42)
Student		
0 Dx	71.6	(8.00, 640.32)*
1 Dx	0.4	(0.07, 1.58)
2 Dx	2.4	(0.36, 15.77)
Other		
0 Dx	0.3	(0.01, 9.55)
1 Dx	2.7	(0.23, 31.57)
2 Dx	1.9	(0.52, 7.09)
Insurance		
No	1.0	
Yes	2.2	(0.83, 5.72)
Marital status		
Married	1.0	
Never		
Dx	0.8	(0.12, 4.95)
1 Dx	4.4	(0.89, 21.4)
2 Dx	0.6	(0.16, 2.69)
Sep/Wid/Div		
0 Dx	13.0	(3.18, 53.00)*
1 Dx	1.4	(0.23, 8.70)
2 Dx	2.8	(0.69, 11.08)

Table 3C. (*Continued*)

	Adj OR	95% CI
Income		
$0–14,999	0.7	(0.12, 0.80)*
$15,000–69,999	0.6	(0.25, 1.49)
$70,000	1.0	
County-level health services		
Non-poor	1.0	
Poor		
0 Dx	1.1	(0.48, 2.42)
1 Dx	0.3	(0.12, 0.80)*
2 Dx	1.9	(0.59, 6.38)
Education		
0–15	1.0	
16+		
0 Dx	48.3	(3.00, 778.34)*
1 Dx	0.8	(0.20, 3.63)
2 Dx	9.8	(2.06, 46.72)*
Urbanicity		
Suburban, major metro	1.0	
City, major metro	1.6	(0.40, 6.57)
Adj, major metro	1.0	(0.34, 3.23)
City and suburban, other metro	0.8	(0.30, 2.07)
Adj, other metro	0.9	(0.33, 2.67)
Rural (adj and outlying)	1.1	(0.37, 3.55)
Chronic physical condition		
None	1.0	
1+	0.4	(0.20, 0.68)*
Psychiatric disorder		
None	1.0	
One	4.9	(0.76, 31.77)
Two or more	12.2	(1.72, 87.06)*

*Statistically significant.

group of married persons. Yet, these may be unstable owing to the small numbers. Experiencing a physical health problem resulted in a 60% less likelihood of seeking treatment. Persons with a mental disorder who resided in counties with poor quality health care resources had a 70% *reduced* relative odds of visiting the SMA. As with the HS sector, persons with the lowest household income were *less* likely (OR = 0.7, 95% CI = 0.12, 0.80) than persons with the highest income to be seen by specialists. In contrast, the most highly educated or wealthy were more likely to utilize psychiatrists, even without a diagnosis. This finding for education, income, and community level resources is quite striking in its demonstration of social inequity in the allocation of health resources. Individuals with a comorbid disorder were 12 times as likely to visit the SMA sector, although this may be unstable due to small numbers. This lends support to our hypothesis of differences in utilization patterns for individuals with more than one psychiatric disorder.

DISCUSSION

Our hypothesis of the importance of social factors on health services use was supported in our analysis of an epidemiologic survey of the US population. As predicted, differences were found by type of treatment sector utilized for mental health care. Psychiatric morbidity was not the sole determinant of services use, nor was it consistently significant, despite the preponderance of research findings. For each HS sector, social factors, whether predisposing or enabling, predicted utilization patterns independent of levels of health or mental morbidity (Kulka, Veroff, & Douvan, 1979).

The persistence of *social class* as a major determinant in the distribution of mental health services points to the prescience of early studies (Hollingshead & Redlich, 1958; Kessler et al., 1999) on social inequality in health care. This dramatizes a disturbing pattern of those with the fewest resources having less access to treatment. Differential service sector use compounds this disparity. While many persons *without* a disorder were found to visit the specialty sector, unemployed, disabled, or residents of poor communities *with* a disorder, were *less likely* to utilize services. If morbidity were the sole criterion for receiving treatment than those with the greatest resources in the society, the lowest relative risk of a disorder would be *less* likely to utilize services (Holzer et al., 1986). The large numbers of people needing but not receiving health care and the presence of persons without a diagnosis in the specialty sector underscore the importance of social determinants in the use of mental health services.

Persons with a comorbid psychiatric diagnosis had an increased likelihood of receiving specialty care owing perhaps to the complexity of diagnosis and treatment of their problems. Recognition and treatment for mental illness in the health sector may not always be optimal (Wilkinson, 1986); specialty psychiatric care has been shown to be less costly over time (Fries, Koop, Sokolov, Beadle, & Wright, 1998). Efforts to reduce stigma may facilitate greater acceptability. Interventions may encourage availability and affordability of psychiatric services (Sturm & Wells, 2000). A drop in the rise of uninsured persons, who are at particular risk, is desirable. Our research suggests that incorporating social as well as clinical attributes of those seeking medical care could help inform efforts to improve access and quality of care.

An apparent shortcoming in our research is the cross-sectional nature of the data. Follow-up data from the same respondents would allow another panel with which to view respondents over time. The reliance on retrospective self-reports of illness and health sector contact, especially when asking respondents to recall visits during a specified time, is a limitation. Our diagnostic assessment is based on a single structured diagnostic interview by trained interviewers; clinical examinations (Eaton, Neufeld, Chen, & Cai, 2000) may contradict our findings. The lack of significance for age, independent of health status, may stem from the absence of older respondents in the NCS. Future research may help to overcome such shortcomings.

Another limitation was our inability to examine the determinants of mental health services use for different ethnic groups in the society. The small number of Hispanics subsample in our services prevented us from examining the type of service utilization. Data from epidemiologic studies have produced few differences in rates of mental illness between whites and Hispanic Americans (Robins & Regier, 1991). Reports from research on Mexican Americans by Vega, Kolody, Aguila-Gaxiola et al. (1999) and Canino et al. (1987) in Puerto Rico showed similar rates as those in the US. It has been demonstrated by Alegria et al. (2002) that Latinos living in *poor* income households were less likely to receive specialty services care. While this is consistent with prior research (cf. Hough et al., 1987), it was not established that this persists for all Latinos or for each mental health service sector utilized. Hopefully, further research will allow an examination for ethnic group differences by type of mental health service sector.

In a recent revision of his behavioral model of health care use, Andersen (1995) suggested that social and behavioral factors such as emotional distress, relationships with family and friends, and cultural beliefs and practices may influence the decision to seek help, frequency of contact, and sector choice. Inclusion, as predisposing or enabling factors, he argued, may reduce an overemphasis on need as the determinant of utilization. Research examining social causes of inequality and health disparities by groups within the society and the differential use of service sectors appears warranted.

ACKNOWLEDGMENTS

The National Comorbidity Survey (NCS) is a collaborative epidemiologic investigation of the prevalence, causes, and consequences of psychiatric morbidity and comorbidity in the United States. The NCS is supported by the National Institute of Mental Health (Grants MH46376 and MH49098) with supplemental support from the National Institute of Drug Abuse (through a supplement to MH46376) and the W.T. Grant Foundation (Grant 901351190). Ronald C. Kessler, Ph.D. is the Principal Investigator. The author is grateful to Ronald C. Kessler and William W. Eaton for their help with the analysis. Richard E. Ratcliff read an earlier version of the manuscript. Thanks is due the editor, Jennie Jacobs Kronenfeld, for critiquing the paper.

REFERENCES

Adler, N. E., Boyce, T., Chesney, M. A., Cohen, S., Folkman, S., Kahn, R. L., & Syme, S. L. (1994). Socioeconomic status and health: The challenge of the gradient. *American Psychologist, 49*, 15–24.

Alegria, M., Canino, G., Rios, R., Vera, M., Calderon, J., Rusch, D., & Ortega, A. N. (2002). Inequalities in use of specialty mental health services among Latinos, African Americans, and Non-Latino Whites. *Psychiatric Services, 53*, 1547–1555.

American Psychiatric Association. (1987). *Diagnostic and statistical manual of psychiatric disorders* (rev. 3rd ed.). Washington, DC: American Psychiatric Association.

Andersen, R. M. (1968). *Behavioral model of families' use of health services*. Research Series No. 25. Chicago: University of Chicago.

Andersen, R. M. (1995). Revisiting the behavioral model and access to medical care: Does it matter? *Journal of Health Social Behavior, 36*, 1–10.

Andersen, R., & Aday, L. A. (1978). Access to medical care in the US: Realized and potential. *Medical Care, 16*, 533–546.

Badawi, M., Kramer, M., & Eaton, W. W. (1996). Use of mental health services by households in the United States. *Psychiatric Services, 47*, 376–380.

Bijl, R. V., & Ravelli, A. (2000). Psychiatric morbidity, service use, and need for care in the general population: Results of the Netherlands mental health survey and incidence study. *American Journal of Public Health, 90*, 602–607.

Blazer, D. G., Landerman, L. R., Fillenbaum, G., & Horner, R. (1995). Health services access and use among older adults in North Carolina: Urban vs. rural residents. *American Journal of Public Health, 85*, 1384–1390.

Brennan, P. L., Kagay, C. R., Geppert, J. J., & Moos, R. H. (2001). Predictors and outcomes of outpatient mental health care: A 4-year prospective study of elderly medicare patients with Substance Use Disorders. *Medical Care, 39*, 39–49.

Canino, G., Bird, H. R., Shrout, P. E., Rubio-Stipec, M., Martinez, M., Sessman, M., & Guevara, L. M. (1987). The prevalence of specific psychiatric disorders in Puerto Rico. *Archives of General Psychiatry, 44*, 727–735.

Catalano, R., Rook, K., & Dooley, C. D. (1986). Labor markets and help-seeking: A test of the employment security hypothesis. *Journal of Health and Social Behavior*, *27*, 277–287.

Cooper-Patrick, L., Crum, R. M., & Ford, D. E. (1994). Characteristics of patients with major depression who receive care in general medical and specialty mental health settings. *Medical Care*, *32*, 15–24.

Eaton, W. W., Neufeld, K., Chen, L. S., & Cai, G. (2000). A comparison of self-report and clinical diagnostic interviews for depression. *Archives of General Psychiatry*, *57*, 217–222.

Fortney, J. C., Rost, K., & Zhiang, M. (1998). A joint choice model of the decision to seek depression treatment and choice of provider sector. *Medical Care*, *36*, 307–320.

Frank, R. G., & Kamlet, M. S. (1989). Determining provider choice for the treatment of mental disorders: The role of health and mental health status. *Health Services Research*, *24*, 83–103.

Fries, J. F., Koop, C. E., Sokolov, J., Beadle, C. E., & Wright, D. (1998). Beyond health promotion: Reducing need and demand for medical care. *Health Affairs*, *17*, 70–84.

Gresenz, C. R., Stockdale, S. E., & Wells, K. B. (2000). Common effects of access to behavioral health care. *Health Services Research*, *35*(Part II), 293–306.

Hollingshead, A. B., & Redlich, F. C. (1958). *Social class and mental illness*. New York: Wiley.

Holzer, C. E., Shea, B., Swanson, J. W., Leaf, P. J., Myers, J. K., George, L. K., Weissman, M. M., & Bednarski, P. (1986). The increased risk for psychiatric disorders among persons of low socio-economic status. *American Journal of Social Psychiatry*, *6*, 259–271.

Horwitz, A. V. (1996). Seeking and receiving mental health care. *Current Opinion Psychiatry*, *9*, 158–161.

Hough, R. L., Landsverk, J. A., Karno, M., Burnam, M. A., Imbers, D. M., Escobar, J. I., & Regier, D. A. (1987). Utilization of health and mental health services by Los Angeles Mexican Americans and non-hispanic Whites. *Archives of General Psychiatry*, *44*, 702–709.

Kessler, R. C., Zhao, S., Katz, S. J., Kouzis, A. C., Frank, R. G., Edlund, M., & Leaf, P. J. (1999). Past-year use of outpatient services for psychiatric problems in the National Comorbidity Survey. *American Journal of Psychiatry*, *156*, 115–123.

Kish, L., & Frankel, M. R. (1970). Balanced repeated replications for standard errors. *Journal American Statistical Association*, *65*, 1071–1094.

Kouzis, A. C., & Eaton, W. W. (1998). Absence of social networks, social support and health services utilization. *Psychological Medicine*, *28*, 1301–1310.

Krieger, N. (1993). Analyzing socioeconomic and racial/ethnic patterns in health and health care. *American Journal of Public Health*, *83*, 1086–1087.

Kulka, R., Veroff, J., & Douvan, E. (1979). Social class and the use of professional help: 1957 and 1976. *Journal of Health Social Behavior*, *20*, 2–17.

Landerman, L. R., Burns, B. J., Schwart, M. S., Wagner, H. R., & George, L. K. (1994). The relationship between insurance coverage and psychological disorders in predicting use of mental health services. *American Journal of Psychiatry*, *151*, 1785–1790.

Leaf, P. J., Bruce, M. L., & Tischler, G. L. (1988). Factors affecting the utilization of the specialty and general medical mental health services. *Medical Care*, *26*, 9–26.

Leaf, P. J., Livingston, M. M., Tischler, G., Weissman, M. M., Holzer, C. E., & Myers, J. K. (1985). Contact with health professionals for the treatment of psychiatric and emotional problems. *Medical Care*, *23*, 1322–1337.

Little, R. J. A., Lewitzky, S., Heeringa, S., Lepkowski, J., & Kessler, R. C. (1997). Assessment of weighting methodology for the National Comorbidity Survey. *American Journal of Epidemiology*, *146*, 439–449.

Markides, K., Levin, J. S., & Ray, C. A. (1985). Determinants of physician utilization among Mexican-Americans: A three-generation study. *Medical Care, 23,* 236–246.

Mechanic, D. (1979). Correlates of physical utilization: Why do multivariate studies of physician utilization find trivial psychosocial and organizational effects? *Journal of Health and Social Behavior, 20,* 387–396.

Mechanic, D., Angel, R., & Davies, L. (1992). Correlates of using mental health services: Implications of using alternating definitions. *American Journal of Public Health, 82,* 74–78.

Myers, J. K., & Schaffer, L. (1954). Social stratification and psychiatric practice: A study in an out-patient clinic. *American Sociological Review, 19,* 307–359.

Narrow, W. E., Regier, D. A., Rae, D. S., Manderscheid, R. W., & Locke, B. Z. (1993). Use of services by persons with mental and addictive disorders: Findings from the National Institute of Mental Health Epidemiologic Catchment Area Program. *Archives of General Psychiatry, 50,* 95–107.

Pescosolido, B. (1998). Social networks and patterns of use among the poor with mental health problems in Puerto Rico. *Medical Care, 36,* 1057–1072.

Prigerson, H. G., Maciejewski, P. K., & Rosenheck, R. A. (1999). The effects of marital dissolution and marital quality on health and health services use among women. *Medical Care, 37,* 858–873.

Regier, D. A., Kaelber, C. T., Rae, D. C., Farmer, M. E., Knauper, B., Kessler, R. C., & Norquist, G. S. (1998). Limitations of diagnostic criteria and assessment instruments for mental disorders: Implications for research and policy. *Archives of General Psychiatry, 55,* 109–115.

Rhodes, A. E., Goering, P. N., To, T., & Williams, J. V. (2002). Gender and outpatient mental health service use. *Social Science and Medicine, 54,* 1–10.

Robins, L. N., & Regier, D. A. (1991). *Psychiatric disorders in America: The epidemiologic catchment area study.* New York: The Free Press.

Robins, L. N., Wing Wittchen, J. H. U., Helzer, J. E., Babor, T. F., Burke, J. D., Farmer, A., Jablenski, A., Pickens, R., Regier, D. A., Sartorius, N., & Towle, L. H. (1988). The composite international diagnostic interview: An epidemiologic instrument suitable for use in conjunction with different diagnostic systems and in different cultures. *Archives of General Psychiatry, 45,* 1069–1077.

Rosenheck, R., & Stolar, M. (1998). Access to public mental health services: Determinants of population coverage. *Medical Care, 36,* 503–512.

Shapiro, S., Skinner, E. A., Kramer, M., Steinwachs, D. M., & Regier, D. A. (1985). Measuring need for mental health services in a general population. *Medical Care, 23,* 1033–1043.

Sturm, R., & Wells, K. (2000). Health insurance may be improving – but not for individuals with mental illness. *Health Services Research, 35*(Part II), 253–262.

Susser, M., Watson, W., & Hopper, K. (1985). *Sociology in medicine* (3rd ed.). New York: Oxford.

The Nation's Health. (2002). Mental disorders affect quarter of population: Illness among leading causes of poor health disability, 2001–2002. *The Nation's Health, 11.*

Vega, W., Kolody, B., Aguilar-Gaxiola, S., & Catalano, R. (1999). Gaps in service utilization by Mexican–Americans with mental health problems. *American Journal of Psychiatry, 156,* 928–934.

Verhaak, P. F. M. (1988). Detection of psychologic complaints by general practitioners. *Medical Care, 26,* 10009–10020.

Wells, K. B., Manning, W. G., Duan, N., Newhouse, J. P., & Ware, J. E. (1987). Cost-sharing and the use of general medical physicians for outpatient mental health care. *Health Services Research, 22,* 1–17.

Wilkinson, G. (1986). *Overview of mental health practices in primary care settings, with recommendations for further research.* National Institute of Mental Health. Series DN, No. 7 (ADM 186-1487), Washington, DC: Supt of Doc, US Govt Printing Office.

Wittchen, H. U. (1994). Reliability and validity studies of the WHO-Composite International Diagnostic Interview (CIDI): A critical review. *Journal of Psychiatric Research, 28,* 57–84.

Wolinsky, F. D. (1996). Advances in the measurement of health status. *Gerontologist, 36,* 570–601.

World Health Organization (WHO). (1990). *Composite International Diagnostic Interview (CIDI, v1.0).* Geneva: WHO.

Wu, L. T., Kouzis, A. C., & Leaf, P. J. (1999). Influences of comorbid alcohol and psychiatric disorders on utilization of mental health services in the National Comorbidity Survey. *American Journal of Psychiatry, 156,* 1230–1236.

SOCIAL DETERMINANTS OF HEALTH CARE ACCESS AMONG SEX INDUSTRY WORKERS IN CANADA

Rachel Phillips and Cecilia Benoit

ABSTRACT

Drawing on closed and open-ended interview data (n = 79), this paper explores the health care experiences of a purposive sample of sex industry workers in a medium-sized metropolitan area of British Columbia, Canada. The respondents reported high average health care utilization and many reported satisfactory access to health care, including a positive relationship with a regular health provider. However, several respondents reported feeling intimidated and shamed in health care settings (felt stigma) and many choose to withhold information relevant to their health care due to fear of discrimination (enacted stigma) by health professionals.

INTRODUCTION

Canada's publicly funded health care system is designed to ensure that all services deemed to be "medically necessary" (including physician- and

Health Care Services, Racial and Ethnic Minorities and Underserved Populations: Patient and Provider Perspectives
Research in the Sociology of Health Care, Volume 23, 79–104
ISSN: 0275-4959/doi:10.1016/S0275-4959(05)23005-3

hospital-based services) are universally available to Canadian citizens, regardless of their ability to pay. One indication of the relative success of this system is research showing that health *need*, rather than personal income, largely drives the utilization of health care services (Broyles, Manga, Binder, Angus, & Charette, 1983). However, utilization is but one indicator of health care access, and other research has shown that socially marginalized populations, including the poor and those with lower education, are less likely to access timely, appropriate and non-judgemental health service than other Canadians (Stewart et al., 2001; Roos & Mustard, 1997; Roos, Forget, & Wald, 2003). In other words, disadvantaged populations with greater health need consume more health care services, but they are less likely to derive the same satisfaction or positive outcome from service received as more advantaged Canadians. From a sociological perspective, this is an important paradox because it speaks to the complex system of structural and individual social variables that give rise to differential access to health care, even within an ostensibly universal system. Given that access to health care is a key social determinant of health and the provision of a universal health care system is specifically intended to achieve a pattern of care based on health need (CIHI, 2004), research on the social intricacies of accessing health services becomes crucial to ongoing efforts by policy makers and service providers to re-orient service delivery to meet the needs of target populations identified to be at risk or underserved by the existing health care system.

Sex industry workers[1] present a unique opportunity to examine the operation of social and cultural barriers to health care access because they are a clandestine population who are considered to be at high risk for health problems. In Canada, it is not illegal to sell sex services; however many of the practical activities associated with selling sex are illegal.[2] Moreover, there is a strong social stigma attached to this economic activity. Whereas the public tend to view sex industry workers as victims, or as contaminants to neighbourhoods and communities (Lowman, 1995), those schooled in public health and social work tend to view these workers primarily through the lens of *risk*. Such limited views impact workers' personal relationships, public activities, and access to public services such as health care because they overlook some of the more serious (hidden) problems they face (Lowman, 1991; Shaver, 1993; Benoit & Millar, 2001). In addition, stereotypical depictions of the industry most often portray those who work in it as always female and involved in the visible street trade. Consequently, relatively little is known about the population of male sex industry workers and the more predominant indoor-based sex industry of both genders.

Despite common consensus that health care access is crucial to sex industry workers because of the well-documented risks associated with their way of making a living, there has been little research on sex industry workers' perceptions of their health or on their experiences accessing care. This paper adopts a social determinants of health perspective to address this gap in the literature. This perspective draws attention to the distribution of social resources among populations and situates disparities in health and health care access within the broader socio-structural context (Evans, Barer, & Marmor, 1994; Canadian Population Health Initiative, 2002; Raphael, 2004). In this case, first-hand data from 79 adult female and male workers located in various parts of the sex industry in one of Canada's medium-sized metropolitan areas are analysed with a focus on understanding perceptions of health need, social factors shaping help seeking, and conditions that facilitate and impede access to satisfactory health care.

BACKGROUND LITERATURE

One of the driving forces behind the provision of health care in Canada and many other high-income countries is the *medicalization* of human behaviour and physical functioning. Sociologists have devoted considerable energy to understanding the social conditions under which behaviours and functions are *medicalized*, a concept which "consists of defining a problem in medical terms, using medical language to describe a problem, adopting a medical framework to understand a problem, or using a medical definition to 'treat' it" (Conrad, 1992, p. 211). Recently, it has been argued that medical dominance, most often exercised by physicians, is on the decline and consumers of health care are exercising greater control over their health and health services. The supposed decline in medical control over definitions of health and illness, help-seeking behaviour, and patient–provider interactions is said to be the result of widespread scepticism about the ability of medicine to solve health problems, the increasing knowledge of the general public about health matters (Blishen, 1991; Haug, 1988), and government efforts in countries such as Canada to reign in escalating physician-related costs by seeking less expensive methods of delivering health care (Coburn & Eakin, 1993). However, the likelihood that disadvantaged populations such as sex industry workers are able to participate in this consumer movement to the same extent as more privileged Canadians is doubtful.

What is for sure is that health professionals, particularly physicians, but also nurses, enter the service context armed with expert bio-medical knowledge and more socio-economic resources than many of their more vulnerable patients. The combination of both professional expertise in medical understandings of health and higher socio-economic status may present barriers to effective patient–provider communication, especially if the health provider and patient perceive one another as socially distant from their own experience. This social distance is not neutral, but rather hierarchical, placing the physician (or other provider) in a position of authority in relation to the socially marginalized patient. Therefore, when physicians convey ideological notions about desirable health behaviour, especially as these notions help shape patients' roles in the public and private spheres, medical encounters contribute to the broader hegemonic impact of dominant ideologies (Waitzken, 1998, p. 280). Given the stigma attached to sex industry work, it seems likely that one of the barriers faced by sex industry workers accessing health care is this social distance between the patient and provider, as well as the possibility that the provider will convey biases in the service context that mirror dominant social values that are disaffirming to the patient's experience.

The social stigma surrounding sex industry work results in other barriers to care that extend beyond patient–provider communication. Indeed, perhaps to avoid uncomfortable encounters with health professionals and discussions regarding stigmatized health conditions, people who sell sex services may choose to delay seeking health services (acting on *felt stigma*) until the point of health crisis (Watson & Corrigan, 2002). Alternatively, sex industry workers may access health services, but choose to withhold critical information, including their involvement in sex industry work, in order to avoid the possibility of discrimination (*enacted stigma*) (Scambler, Perswanie, Renton, & Scambler, 1990; Snell, 1991; Carr, 1995; Davies & Feldman, 1997).[3] When sex industry workers do not disclose their line of work, they increase their chances of non-judgemental care, yet some of their health service needs may go unmet and prevention opportunities may be missed (Maticka-Tyndale, Lewis, Clark, Zubick, & Young, 1999).

On the other hand, recent literature on the topic of stigma and health care suggests that there is a tendency among members of dominant culture – so-called "normals" – to assume that the effects of stigma are more pervasive in the lives of the stigmatized than actually is the case (Camp, Finlay, & Lyons, 2002; Shultz & Angermeyer, 2003; Kusow, 2004). Some structurally marginalized individuals have been found to develop effective means of managing stigma in public contexts. Others appear not to internalize stigma (i.e., they do not feel its impact) because they either question the truthfulness of dominant knowledge or because they develop alternative communities where stigma labels are interpreted differently. Therefore, despite the common perception that sex industry workers face formidable barriers to health care either because of shame or fear of discrimination from biased health professionals, it may be the case that some of these workers manage to bypass or overcome such hindrances and in doing so, provide crucial knowledge about the conditions that facilitate positive health care in the context of social marginalization.

Even if sex industry workers are able to avoid feeling stigmatized by health professionals, it does not mean that their health concerns will be addressed when they seek help. As noted earlier, the predominant focus by professionals and researchers alike on the health risks associated with sex industry work has resulted in a limited body of literature addressing other dimensions of sex industry workers' health. Recent social science studies have shown that this population has health concerns that extend beyond the public health focus on sexually transmitted infections (STIs), including as Alexander (1998) points out, the more mundane workplace health risks faced by sex industry workers such as exposure to other types of viruses, unclean work sites, urinary tract infections, and musculoskeletal strain. Other scholars have suggested that a greater investigation of the psychological risks faced by those who work in the sex industry is needed, not only because of the stigmatized social context in which they work but also because of the emotional toll on their mental health in providing personal services in what is often an unequal exchange with clients (Vanwesenbeek, 1994; Bruckert, 2002). Further research is also needed on how the structural and interactive contexts of both the workplace and the private sphere influence health practices, such as safer sex practices (Jackson, Highcrest, & Coates, 1992), and the development of subcultures of knowledge that inform help-seeking (Evans & Lambert, 1997). Finally, not unlike other Canadian citizens, workers in the sex industry describe concerns with the convenience and efficacy of treatment and with the personal characteristics of health providers (Maticka-Tyndale et al., 1999), such as whether an attitude of caring and attentiveness to their individual needs and concerns is shown.

Drawing on the extant literature described above, this paper attempts to further the research on social determinants of health care access among sex industry workers, with primary data from male- and female-sex industry workers located in both indoor and outdoor venues. In order to establish a context of health care need among the participants, background data is presented on social determinants of health status including, gender, education, ethnicity, early family life, and occupational risks. These data suggest that, on average, sex workers represent some of the most marginalized sub-populations of Canadian society and have reduced access to health resources, often beginning early in their lives. The findings also help us to understand why participants become involved in the sex industry in the first place and situate the health status of participants within a larger pattern of socio-economic stratification in population health (Evans, Barer, & Marmor, 1994; Marmot & Wilkinson, 1999; Marmot, 2003). Given the high health need among the respondents, it is reassuring that health care utilization is also high, attesting to the primary benefit of a publicly funded health care system. However, as will be discussed in greater detail, there is significant room for improvement with regards to providing sensitive and efficacious health care to sex industry workers. The data show that evidence of timely access to health care services and open relationships with health care professionals is mixed, with some describing positive experiences and others describing largely unsatisfactory experiences. Rather than economic barriers, respondents described primarily socio-psychological barriers to care. These include fear of discrimination, actual experiences of enacted discrimination by health professionals, and difficulty of finding health professionals who are perceived as possessing expertise in the needs of sex industry workers.

METHODOLOGY AND DATA

The data presented in this paper were collected by graduate student research assistants and experiential research assistants (persons with a history of sex industry involvement) in face-to-face interviews. The authors have reported on this unique methodological design elsewhere (Benoit, Jansson, Millar, & Phillips, 2005). The experiential research assistants were hired and trained as part of community–academic collaboration, led by the second author (Benoit), and initiated by the Prostitutes Empowerment Education and Resource Society (PEERS), a local social welfare service organization staffed in large part by former sex industry workers. Several methods were used to gather contact information on potential respondents – key informants, snowballing, and advertising. These recruiting methods are common to research on vulnerable populations and help overcome the limitations associated with having no sampling frame (Becker, 1963; Biernacki, 1986; Heckathorn, 1997). Although the research sample is relatively large (given the hidden nature of the population) and purposely includes both male and female workers from a wide array of venues (hence our use of the term sex *industry* workers), it is difficult to estimate the biases inherent in the respondent population. Thus, the findings from this purposive sample cannot be considered generalizable, even within the local setting of the research.

The research instrument consisted of 135 closed-ended questions covering background information and early childhood experiences, factors precipitating entrance into the sex industry, working conditions across the various venues, health and safety on and off the job, and for former workers, several questions on the process, challenges and benefits of leaving the sex industry. The closed-ended research instrument was completed by 201 respondents, 54 of whom had left the industry. In addition, 27 open-ended interview questions were administered to a sub-sample ($n = 79$) of the respondents, all of whom had experience working in indoor venues. These unstructured questions focussed on respondents' personal experiences in the sex industry, the social context of their work, the health risks they associate with their work, their health and use of local health services, and future training and career prospects. The reason for administering the open-ended interviews to persons with experience in indoor venues was to broaden knowledge on the more elusive body of indoor workers who are less frequently represented in academic literature than street-based workers. However, in the course of conducting the research it became apparent that it is difficult to neatly categorize workers based on venue, primarily because mobility within the industry is quite common and the distinctions between different types of work may be permeable, with some workers performing more than one service out of a single venue (Maticka-Tyndale et al., 1999), and others working in more than one venue at a time and/or in more than one venue over time (Benoit et al., 2005). Therefore, although the open-ended data presented here is informed by at least some experience in indoor venues such as escort agencies and home-based escort services, both the large sample and the sub-sample contain respondents representing a multitude of sex industry work experiences.

The research data are presented in six sections below. We begin with some key statistical data on the background and occupational characteristics of the sub-sample of respondents who completed the open-ended portion of the research instrument. These data are derived from the closed-ended survey portion of the interview and were analysed using the Statistical Package for the Social Sciences (SPSS). Following this, data on respondents' self-reported health are presented to help contextualize the data on health care utilization and health care access. Because the data set is relatively rich in descriptive information, only those data that are relevant to the specific topic of our paper are presented. Following some brief indicators of health care utilization, a more detailed analysis of the qualitative data on health care is presented. Methodologically speaking, the qualitative findings are based on a thematic analysis of the interview dialogue (Boyatzis, 1998; Denzin & Lincoln, 1994). In practice, the data were initially coded according to subjects inherent in the research questions. Following this, emergent codes were highlighted based on ideas, opinions, and topics raised by the respondents. Theoretically speaking, one of the aims of combining survey and interview data is to gain a better vantage point on the dialectic between socio-structural factors and personal contexts and individual health care behaviour. This perspective on the agency-structure dialectic is fitting within a broader social determinants of health framework because it highlights the recursive nature of individual practices and collective lifestyles by linking macro level determinants of health such as education and occupation to the knowledge, personal networks, and decision-making processes of individuals within a particular social location (Snow, 2001; Williams, 2003).

DEMOGRAPHICS AND BACKGROUND INFORMATION

The vast majority of those interviewed ($n = 160$) for the larger study identified themselves as female (80%), reflecting the gendered nature of the sex industry in Canada (Brock, 1998; Carter & Walton, 2000). Those identifying as male ($n = 36$) comprised just fewer than 18%. The remaining 2% ($n = 5$) identified as male to female transgendered. Respondents ranged in age from 18 to 63, and the mean age was 32 years. The gender breakdown was slightly different for the 79 people who completed the open-ended portion of the research instrument: 23% of respondents identified as male, 74% as female, and two ($<1\%$) as female-to-male transgendered. The mean age of this sub-group was 34 years, which was slightly higher than that of the overall sample.

The vast majority of respondents (89%) in the larger sample and sub-sample (91%) were born in Canada and none of those interviewed can be easily classified as victims of global trafficking (see Jiwani & Brown, 1999; Wonders & Michalowski, 2001). For the just over 10% of the larger sample who were born abroad, all but one person came from other high-income countries (United States, United Kingdom, and continental Europe). Furthermore, the 22 respondents in the larger sample who were born outside of Canada are best classified as long-term residents, having lived here between 13 and 50 years, with an average of 30 years. The respondents did not stand out in regards to visible minority status, and may even under represent this sub-population. In total, 6.5% of respondents fit the Canadian Employment Equity Act definition of visible minority persons – i.e., other than Aboriginal people, who are non-Caucasian in race or non-white in colour. At the time of 2001 census, Statistics Canada reported 11.3% of residents in the research site were visible minorities (Statistics Canada, Community Profiles, 2001a). Respondents with Aboriginal status (measured as status and non-status Indians, Metis, and Inuit people) were, however, notably overrepresented in the research sample. Nearly 15% of respondents placed themselves in this category. This figure is substantially higher than the percentage of Aboriginal people in the census metropolitan area as a whole – 2.8% in 2001 (Statistics Canada, Community Profiles, 2001b).

The level of educational attainment among respondents was mixed, but generally low in comparison to the general population. The median level of education was grade 10; less than 40% of the respondents had graduated from high school, whereas 77.4% of persons living in the census metropolitan area as a whole have graduated from high school (Statistics Canada, Community Profiles, 2001c). The sub-sample of respondents who completed the open-ended portion of the research had the same median level of education, but 41% said they had completed high school, indicating the possibility of a slightly higher level of education among the sub-sample who had experience working in indoor venues. Nevertheless, educational attainment among the respondent population appears to be notably lower in comparison to the general Canadian population.

For a large number of respondents, childhood was characterized by instability, with frequent changes in their family situation. Almost 40% of the overall sample had experienced four or more changes in their caregiving/living situation by the time they had reached 18 years of age. By contrast, just fewer than 25% of those who completed the open-ended questions had experienced four or more changes in their caregiving/living situation by the time they reached 18 years of age. This suggests that the primarily indoor-based sex industry workers who completed the open-ended portion of the research instrument may have had, on average, a slightly more stable childhood experience than their counterparts representing a more street-oriented sex industry experience. The average age at which the total sample of respondents said they first began living without a legal guardian was 16 years, with 11% reporting that they began living on their own before they were 14 years of age. Among those who completed the open-ended questions, the average age they began living without a legal guardian was 17 years, again suggesting a slightly more stable childhood among this sub-population of respondents.

Almost 90% of respondents reported having experienced one or more instances of physical, emotional or sexual abuse in their childhood. This figure was the same for the sub-sample of respondents who completed the open-ended questions. In regard to gender, females were more likely to report being sexually abused while males were more likely to report being physically abused. Although it is difficult to establish a point of comparison for these results because the incidence of child abuse in the general population is not known, it was evident in the narratives of the respondents that many of them had experienced difficult childhoods to a degree that is beyond the norm in the general population. As a case in point, the majority of respondents – 57% for the whole sample and 59% for the sub-sample – had at some point in their childhood resided in foster care, group homes, or other state-funded institutions. Approximately 1% of children in the research district are in government care at present, which suggests that the alarmingly high incidence of government care among the research respondents is far from the norm.(Ministry of Children and Family Development, Province of British Columbia, 2005).

The current living situations of the respondents varied considerably from the general population as well. In the study area, 63% of all householders own their own dwellings (Reitsma Street, Hopper, & Seright, 2000). However, only 3.5% of respondents owned their home/dwelling at the time of interview, and just under 3% of the sub-sample said they owned their own dwelling. While three-quarters of respondents reported having stable living situations – i.e., owned or rented an apartment or house or living with family/guardians, nearly one-quarter of both the overall sample and sub-sample of respondents reported that they resided in relatively unstable or very unstable circumstances. These included shelters/transition houses, the homes of others, hotels and the street. Although a survey question was not asked about government income assistance, it became apparent in the open-ended comments that many of the respondents were recipients of income assistance, including disability income assistance, which is further evidence of the on average lower socio-economic status of the respondents.

Within the overall sample, 70% of females and 58% of males had given birth to or fathered a child. Close to one-quarter of those children were born before the respondents reached the age of majority (19 years), indicating that young parenthood was not uncommon among the respondents. At the time of the interview, 28% of the females and 14% of the males were currently caring for dependent children. Among those who reported having had children, but not having children in their care, the "other parent" (either the father or mother), other relatives, or living independently were the most common alternative care situations. Many of the female respondents were single caregivers. Although it was not common, a small group of respondents noted that their children were living in government care or had passed away. The findings on births and dependents were not notably different among the sub-sample of respondents, and overall, provide tenuous evidence that for many of the respondents, difficulty in family-life extended beyond childhood and into adulthood.

The findings presented above suggest that the majority of respondents are structurally marginalized along a wide number of social determinants of health. These factors contextualize their involvement in the sex industry in the first place and foreshadow compromised health status, irrespective of the health risks encountered on the job.

WORKING IN THE SEX INDUSTRY: WHY AND HOW

The median age of entry into the sex industry was 18 years among the sample as a whole, and 17 among the sub-sample. Female respondents were slightly younger at age of entry in the sex industry (18 years) than male respondents (19 years). The median age of entry into the sex industry was younger (17 years) for Aboriginal respondents, mirroring broader patterns of inequality in Canadian society at large. Among the sub-sample the median age of entry for females was 17 years of age, for males it was 19 years of age, and for aboriginal respondents it was 15 years of age.

Respondents mentioned a variety of circumstances that precipitated their entry into this line of work. Just over one-third said that they entered because they were enticed by a presenting opportunity such as having peers who were involved, seeing an employment ad, or having someone approach them with an offer of money for sex. For over one-quarter of respondents, however, economic duress – "unable to find a job", "on welfare with small children", "living on streets with no income", "had bills to pay" – was the main motivating factor, and in many cases economic need overlapped with acting on a presenting opportunity. In addition to opportunity-based and economic reasons, a minority of respondents cited their dependency on illicit drugs and alcohol as a motivating factor. A few respondents described what might be characterized as forced or abuse-related involvement. This includes the few who reported that they had been "turned out" by an individual representing a power position such as a "pimp" or relative, and those who said that they become involved in the sex industry due to an earlier experience of childhood sexual abuse. Reasons for entering sex industry work varied by gender; whereas females were more likely to enter for economic reasons, males were more likely to enter because of enticement or curiosity, followed by drug and alcohol use.

The majority of respondents had been involved in the sex industry for more than 5 years at the time of interview. Among the sample as a whole, the average length of involvement in the sex industry was 8 years. Among those who completed the open-ended portion, the average number of years involved in the industry was slightly longer.

While some respondents in this study reported relatively high annual incomes from selling sex services (maximum reported was $84,000 CAD, including tips) and others reported virtually no income at all, the median income was a modest $18,000 CAD ($20,000 CAD per year for females and $10,000 CAD for males, many of whom worked less hours than their female counterparts). Among those who completed the open-ended portion of the interview, the median reported income was slightly lower than that of the respondent group as a whole.

There was substantial variation depending upon whether respondents worked full-time or part-time, but there was little reported variation in income across venues. In fact, one of the benefits of working independently indoors or outdoors was that all earnings were kept, which was not the case among the escort workers who took home only a portion of the money they earned after managers had taken their fees. Just over 16% of the respondents who were actively working in the sex industry at the time of the interview were concurrently working outside the sex industry in a mainstream job, suggesting that for the majority of the respondents, sex industry work was the main source of income (notwithstanding those who were also collecting income assistance benefits from the provincial government).

THE HEALTH CONTEXT OF SEX INDUSTRY WORK

As might be expected given the background presented above, respondents' self-reported health was mixed. While some of their health concerns could be linked with the social context of their work, others were more likely attributable to their societal marginalization. The majority of respondents (57%) who answered the open-ended questions said that working in the sex industry had affected their health, whereas the remaining attributed the health concerns to other factors. These figures were virtually the same for the study population as a whole. Among those in the sub-sample who said that their health had been affected, a few of them said that the impact had been positive (had resulted, for example, in weight loss, better self-care, safer sex practices, and increased exercise). However, the vast majority of respondents felt that the overall effects were negative. Respondents who felt their health was impacted by their work mentioned an array of occupational health concerns: fatigue, sleep disturbances due to the hours of work, bladder infections, increased substance use, STIs, lower self-esteem, anxiety, and difficulty in romantic relationships, among other concerns. The most pervasive theme of those in the sub-sample who reported that involvement in the sex industry had affected their health was the mental and emotional toil of the work, a finding that was also supported by the survey data: just over half of the respondents in the overall sample (51%) reported chronic depression and 45% reported feelings of anxiety. This finding was virtually the same among the sub-sample who completed the open-ended portion of the interview.

Although the minority of respondents reported dependent use of illicit drugs and alcohol, those who were frequent drug and alcohol consumers, particularly intravenous drug users (27.7% of males and 36.8% of females),[4] reported additional health concerns that could not be easily disentangled from their involvement in the sex industry.

Many of those reporting a history of intravenous substance use had acquired Hepatitis C Virus (HCV) and a few had acquired Human Immuno-Deficiency Virus (HIV). Overall, 36% of females and 28% of males reported having HCV, and the vast majority of these cases were attributed to substance use. Similarly, among the seven (3.5%) of respondents who reported HIV, the majority had a history of intravenous drug use, and none attributed their acquisition of HIV to sex industry work.

As elaborated on in the open-ended portion of the interview, respondents regarded the ever-present threat of violence and the possibility of acquiring STIs to be their greatest health concerns at work. Females reported an overall higher incidence of workplace injuries, including injuries requiring hospitalization (38%), than males (28%).

Although a high rate of condom use was reported for all commercial sexual encounters, just over half (54%) of the respondents reported having had an STI while working in the sex industry. The three most common STIs reported where Chlamydia, Gonorrhoea, and Syphilis, respectively. Some of the instances of STIs were likely the result of sexual encounters in the private sphere where condom use was reported to be far less frequent (Jackson, 1992).

UPS AND DOWNS OF ACCESSING HEALTH CARE SERVICES

The Good News: Few Barriers to Utilization

The vast majority of respondents (95%) indicated that they had a personal health care card that freed them from paying for physician and hospital services. The few respondents who reported not having a current BC personal health card (typically because they had moved to BC from another province and not yet applied for their BC card) indicated that they were still able to freely access services provided in local health clinics. This finding lends strong support to the contention that the Canadian publicly funded health care system goes some way in meeting the needs of marginalized citizens, which is less the case in countries such as the United States with pluralistic health care systems (Benoit, 2003; Kunitz & Pesis-Katz, 2005).

The median number of visits by respondents to a health professional in the last year was 10 times. Although at first glance this rate of utilization may appear high, given the broad nature of the measure and the absence of directly comparable statistics, it is difficult to assess whether or not this figure differs substantially from the population at large. However, as a general point of reference, Statistics Canada found that 68% of females and 51% of males aged 12 years and over have visited a health professional on two or more occasions in the previous year (Statistics Canada, 2000), whereas 96% of the respondents in this study had visited a health professional on two or more occasions in the previous year.

Utilization of health care services showed patterns based on gender as well as severity of illness, with females reporting, on average, more encounters with health professionals (median = 10) than males (median = 6) in the preceding year. Similarly, street-based workers, who by several accounts are at the most risk of injury, reported using more health care services (median = 12) than workers in indoor venues (median = 8). Persons who reported intravenous drug use also had a higher average rate of service utilization (median = 12), as did persons reporting one or more mental health conditions such as depression, or a chronic disease such as HIV (median = 24) and HCV (median = 12). The median number of visits reported by Aboriginal respondents was considerably lower than non-Aboriginal respondents (median = 5), possibly reflecting either cultural differences regarding conceptions of health, the desire among Aboriginal respondents for culturally sensitive health services, or both. Such concerns expressed by Aboriginal people seeking health services in other urban areas of Canada have been reported elsewhere (Waldam, Herring, & Young, 1995; Benoit et al., 2003).

The latter exception notwithstanding, these data on health care utilization among our study population provide evidence that being female, working on the street, consuming addictive substances, and having poor self-reported health were correlated with increased utilization of health care among sex industry workers. These results confirm other findings that disadvantaged populations are more likely to report higher overall average use of health care services in Canada and that utilization rates are also positively correlated with health need (Broyles et al., 1983; Roos & Mustard, 1997).

The Not so Good News: Participants' Health Service Experiences

Although it appears that the vast majority of respondents have regular contact with the health care system, the experiences they described conveyed the constraints associated with concealing or managing health and identity stigma(s) in public contexts. Among those reporting negative experiences, both *felt stigma* (located in the perceptions of stigmatized) and *enacted stigma* (observable instances of discrimination) regarding their occupation were dominant themes. As June,[5] a 36-year-old street-based worker, commented: "I would just like to see a doctor out there who will not judge and look more at the whole picture of what is going on with the woman or the man that they are looking at. There's a lot more than just what they're doing for a living." Referring to the nurse who worked in her physician's office, Sarah, a 45 year old escort worker, likewise commented: "I find that even with my own doctor, his nurse tends to look down on me [because of] what I do [sex industry work]."

Other respondents noted that physicians frequently overlooked the labour involved in sex industry work and the expertise of those involved in performing it, viewing it instead as a health risk activity. Another female agency-based escort, age 25, argued that doctors are "pretty closed minded; they don't respect what I do as hard work. It's a lot of lectures on safety. Chances are I'm safer than you. I'm well aware of the risks out there." Echoing a similar concern about the tendency for medical personnel to treat sex industry workers as the embodiment of contagion, Margo, a 42-year-old street-based worker poignantly remarked that she would like to see a physician who "you could actually go in, sit down and say, this is what I am, and not have to worry about them putting on the gloves just to talk to you".

These qualitative data suggest that the medicalization of sex industry workers as "vectors of disease" combined with the paucity of knowledge health personnel have of the working environment of the people who sell sex services, can negatively affect the provider–patient relationship (Alexander, 1998; Downe, 1997; Davies & Feldman, 1997). Whether or not these physicians actually held biased views is less important than the fact workers perceived discrimination and felt both demeaned and misunderstood in the service encounter. Several studies have demonstrated that felt stigma is more disruptive in the lives of the stigmatized and may exist independent of any instances of enacted discrimination (Cree, Kay, Tisdall, & Wallace, 2004; Crocker & Quinn, 2000; Norvilitis, Scime, & Lee, 2002). By way of illustration, a number of respondents reported feeling that they received inferior service once their physician became aware of their involvement in the sex industry. Sybille, a 29-year-old street-based worker put it this way: "there's a few doctors that I had to change because [when] they were familiar with my background, I felt like I was being treated secondary, like I really didn't count that much." John, a 34-year-old home-based escort worker, echoed Sybille's point: "A lawyer shouldn't be looked after better than a prostitute, or a judge shouldn't be treated better than a prostitute, or a cop [better than] a criminal. We are all human, we are all the same and we should all be treated the same."

Although most respondents articulated their experience of perceived and enacted stigma in general terms, a few respondents provided concrete examples of seemingly discriminatory encounters. Amy, a 26-year-old street-based worker, reported: "I had four doctors tell me basically that they don't want to be my doctors any more. They've never given me a reason. [I think it] has a lot to do with the stereotypical attitude." Respondents who exposed their illicit drug use also described their perception of discrimination when seeking medical care. Myra, a 28-year-old former street-based worker, was a case in point: "a lot of them [doctors] didn't want to deal with me because I'd been working and I had been using, and I had abscesses and stuff. [T]hey treated me like I was a piece of shit". Relatedly, Lisa, a 19-year-old massage parlour worker, described her emergency department experience this way: "at the hospital they didn't respect me at all. It was 'oh, you're a prostitute [and] what did you expect' and other negative things were said to me."

Several of our respondents also perceived other problems accessing health care services, including that sometimes providers appeared intimidating to people like themselves who had little disposable income and limited formal education. Joan, a 31-year-old agency-based escort worker, noted the following about her relationship with her current doctor and doctors in general: "he doesn't know what I do. The relationship has been okay. They're not jerks or anything and they know what they're doing, most of the time, but they're very patronizing." Expressing similar views to Joan, other respondents made comments such as "they [doctors] treat me like I am stupid" or they are often "intimidating". Sybille added that doctors can also be dismissive and uncaring about who their patients actually are: "they don't really talk to you. They just sit you down, they write a prescription, do their thing and just ignore you. I would like to be able to talk, even if it's about the sex trade." Admitting that she might not be an easy person to provide care for, Tina, a 33-year-old street-based worker, nevertheless argued that health providers should be able to look beyond her outward behaviour and try to realize that her personal circumstances are very difficult and she most overcome barriers to access service:

> [They] say come on in, we'll help you, we're here for you. [And], you go in and you say why your there. [They] don't treat you well and a lot of the times they get angry because you say no, no, and you get the personal boundary thing happening. Then they say you're an aggressive person and we don't want that here, or we can't have that here. Well what [ ] do you think I'm going to be like after living the life I've lived? I'm coming to you for help and you have no perception of where I've been, and you treat me like crap. [They] have to realize that there is a lot of pain coming in when you walk in that door or you wouldn't be walking in there.

The strong emphasis that respondents placed on having a health provider who demonstrated care and compassion and took the time to listen, as opposed to being strictly professional, could, in part, be explained by their level of health need in combination with their diminished access to social and economic resources – in short, their vulnerability.

In addition to feeling rushed in health care settings by providers who did not take the time to genuinely interact with them, several respondents noted that physicians and nurses often appeared to lack knowledge, not only about the work sex industry workers do for a living, but also about their specific occupational and other health concerns. Margo described her main problem with the health care system this way: "the reason that I'm not (satisfied) is that I don't feel that my doctor is educated in substance abuse issues. I would never talk to her about my prostitution ever. I've never been satisfied with any doctor that I've ever had because none of them seem to be educated in my issues, which are substance abuse and prostitution." Echoing a similar theme, Nicole, a 24 year old woman working in the street-based trade, commented that nurses in an alternative clinic located in the downtown core provided more sensitive service because they were specifically trained in health issues associated with street life: "[I went] to the street nurse when I didn't feel comfortable going to the doctor because I didn't feel comfortable building a relationship with my doctor and I felt the street nurses had the most compassion for people in our kind of [work]. They're completely non-judgmental."

Finally, given the pervasive societal stigma associated with the sex industry and the prevalence of stigmatizing health conditions among the respondent population – mental illness, substance dependency, STIs, blood borne infections – it is not surprising that several respondents voiced concerns about both confidentiality and discretion in accessing health care services. As noted earlier, the prevalence of felt stigma results in widespread use of information management strategies – secrecy, covering, instrumental disclosure – with the objective of avoiding enacted stigma (Gray, 2002; Scambler & Hopkins, 1986; McRae, 2000). In order to avoid complications, many respondents indicated that they did not disclose their involvement in the sex industry to their health providers, even those they had known for many years. A case in point was Mary-Anne, a 42-year-old agency-based escort who reported: "I had a doctor for thirty-six years, so I looked at him like my father too. He never knew that I was in the sex trade and I never told him. I was too ashamed." Another respondent commented in more succinct terms that "my doctor doesn't know what I do, so I get treated the same as anybody else". Choosing not to disclose involvement in the sex industry was not confined to health professionals; respondents mentioned that in many cases they chose not to disclose to parents, friends, their children, and, in some cases, their romantic partners. Susan, 21-year-old agency-based escort stated that "none of my friends know. I have a boyfriend and I promised him that I would never tell our friends". Information management, including not disclosing is perhaps the most common and practical technique for avoiding enacted stigma (Gray, 2002; Scambler & Hopkins, 1986; McRae, 2000). Unfortunately, non-disclosure limits access to both informal social support, including from extended family and friends, and limits the efficacy of the health care services sought.

Even though privacy and discretion in health care settings was crucial to respondents, the organization of local services did not always ensure this, resulting in discomfort on the part of the patient. Sybille commented that "it makes me feel very small to go in and get the test [HIV and HCV] done. It's such a professional place and you feel out of touch. You don't feel like you belong there at all. Maybe they should have some way to give blood tests privately. They could do checkups privately in a place where no one has to know this is going on." In addition to feeling out of place in the health service environment, Sybille was also likely nervous about being tested for communicable diseases. The combination of test anxiety and an unfriendly, indiscrete environment would be sufficient to keep many from accessing the service.

Up to this point we have focussed on the myriad of difficulties respondents encountered in seeking formal care for their health needs, difficulties that involve felt stigma (feeling intimidated or ashamed), enacted stigma (instances of overt discrimination such as being refused service or having ones health needs repetitively typecast by providers), and corollary behaviour such as information management in health service settings. It has likewise been noted that lack of education on the part of the service provider, a cold bedside manner, a rushed service environment, and indiscrete services for stigmatizing health conditions are also barriers that compel some to avoid service and leave others feeling harmed by or dissatisfied with the health service encounter. However, it is also important to note that many respondents described positive experiences with individual health providers who were seen as caring, non-judgemental, and knowledgeable about the situation of sex industry workers. However, finding such a provider was easier said than done: John, a 26-year-old agency-based escort, told us that "there's two doctors that I've seen that I don't want to be with because I didn't really think that they respected my lifestyle and my wishes. Through trial and error, I've found a great doctor. She's really cool and she really understands and she's on a street level. She knows what is going on and she is not naïve."

Respondents who reported positive relationships with physicians described them not only as caring and respectful but also as encouraging and willing to advocate on their behalf. Allison, age 22 and involved in the street trade, said that "My doctor was very helpful to me when I told him that I was a hooker on the street... He was very respectful and gave me pamphlets about what diseases you could get and how you can get them. That's why I like him."

It is interesting to note that while this doctor appeared to also adopt a risk behaviour perspective on sex industry work, unlike those who were quoted earlier, Allison did not feel affronted by her physician's negative take on what she does for a living, possibly because the physician was also very caring and encouraging.

Thoughts on Improving Health Care

As already noted in some of the quotes above, the respondents in our study had numerous suggestions on how to improve the health care system and were interested in having their voices heard. These included easy access to non-judgemental health providers, who present as caring and attentive to 'individual patient needs and concerns. Helga, an agency-based escort worker, age 37, said that her ideal health worker "would be someone who was non-judgmental and helps as best they could to their ability, regardless of my profession." John a 37-year-old freelance escort (bars, clubs, park) suggested that there should be more health professionals "like street nurses; they have an attitude that they care about the people they work with. I think they're really valuable to the community. I think that if most health care providers had their attitude that we'd be in a lot better shape than we are in now."

More than one individual suggested that it would be helpful if 'doctors advertised that they take sex workers', as this would cut down on the process of having to see multiple providers before finding one that was experienced in health and the sex industry. Better yet, would be a list of 'sex worker friendly' physicians. Respondents also spoke about the need to ensure that services were easily accessible in terms of both hours of operation and timely service. Jim, a 24-year-old street-based worker said that for him "the ideal health care worker would be one that is there when you needed them to be there, rather than having to phone up for an appointment for two or three weeks from now."

Once again raising the issue of professional expertise, a few respondents mentioned the need for health providers to acquire additional training about the issues and concerns of sex industry workers. As Chad, a 24-year-old escort noted, such training would allow providers to "to teach [health prevention techniques] in a manner that is not belittling or accusatory". A few respondents noted that service providers who had a history of working in the sex industry themselves would be ideal, though not necessarily for everyone. John put it like this: "I don't know if it would work for everyone but for people in the sex trade, I would like someone that came from that background. Someone that could relate to me not only from a book or training, but also through life experiences." Articulating a similar view on the value of experiential knowledge for addressing the social distance between provider and patient, and at the same time noting the value of a provider who was skilled in assessing both physical and mental well-being, Charles, a 28-year-old home-based escort, wanted "someone that could relate to me. Someone that's been through the same things that I've been through [and] can sit down with you and look at your physical well being and your mental health. Someone that won't just diagnose you off the cuff. Someone with a little more compassion."

The ability to easily access additional medical and health prevention services were also suggested by the respondents, including providing sex workers with disability, sickness, and extended medical and dental benefits not covered by the public health care system. A few respondents, including James, a 28-year-old home-based escort, thought that a clinic specifically for sex industry workers would be a great asset, one that provided counselling services in addition to regular primary care services: "Probably some sort of clinic that's exclusive to sex trade workers, with set up therapy groups and [where you could] sit down and talk with someone for an hour a week. Someone that you can just clean your head with. Someone that's been through it and been around."

Acknowledging existing alternative services, another respondent comment-ed that a service specifically for those who work off the street, including in escort agencies or out of their own home, would be ideal. The local alternative clinics, as highly valued as they were by some respondents, were seen by many off-street workers as most appropriate for persons with health problems related to illicit drug use and life on the street. Natasha, a 31-year-old agency-based escort put it this way:

> You have to go down to the needle exchange right now, and to me that's a very threat-ening place because of my life style. When I see people dropping off needles, like right in front of me and getting new ones it just makes me feel really uncomfortable. I think they should give us our own [service environment]. I'm not saying have leather couches and stuff but leave that as the needle exchange and have a separate place for escort workers who aren't there to exchange needles and stuff. That bothers me."

Other respondents noted that 24-h mobile services were required, particu-larly for indoor agency workers who had less access to free condoms than persons who used the local street-level health clinics. Summing up the views of some of the other off-street workers, Lisa, introduced above, expressed a need for "more places for girls and guys out there to get condoms for free [and that] condoms should be at the escort agencies... Condoms are ex-pensive, and not everybody wants to spend six bucks on a pack of them, especially when it's somebody you don't enjoy sleeping with."

DISCUSSION AND CONCLUSION

This paper has adopted a social determinants of health perspective to con-ceptualize primary data on the self-reported health and access to health care concerns of sex industry workers in one region of Canada. The respondents in this study reported histories of marginalization that dated back to their childhood years, long before they entered the sex industry. Many had low educational attainment and other barriers to gainful employment in the mainstream labour force. Given the compromised social conditions of their lives, it is not entirely surprising that a sizable minority of respondents felt that their health concerns originated outside of the sex industry. For those who felt their health had been negatively impacted by their work, many described associated emotional and mental health strains, but a wide array of other health effects was also noted. Although fear of violent customers and contracting a contagious infection were considered the primary risks of sex industry work by almost all of the respondents, their daily health needs extended far beyond these issues. Among other things, they hoped to find professionals who they could speak openly with, without receiving lectures on risks they were already well aware of.

Respondents' self-reported health was in many cases poor (often because of the presence of chronic conditions) and their health care utilization rates were high compared to the general Canadian population, attesting to the success of the pubic health care system in reaching the neediest. However, despite active use of the health care system, satisfaction with services was in many cases less than adequate. Felt and enacted stigma emerge as important barriers to satisfactory health care. Respondents associated such stigma with, among other things, the negative view of their work by the majority of members of society, the social distance between themselves and their health providers and possession of one or more discrediting health conditions such STIs and substance addiction.

These findings on sex industry workers' relatively poor health status according to select indicators confirms that access to health services, including mental health services, is a crucial social determinant of health for this vulnerable population (Andrulis, 1998; Heaman, 2001). Although the publicly funded, universal health care system in Canada takes us a long way in the equitable provision of health care (Kunitz & Pesis-Katz, 2005), other strategies are required to sensitize health services to the needs of marginalized and stigmatized populations.

NOTES

1. For the purposes of this research, a wide rather than narrow definition of *sex industry work* has been adopted. The term 'sex industry worker' has been employed because it is broad in nature, but also because it is less stigmatizing than the more common term 'prostitute', which in our society evokes images of defilement and debasement (Shrage, 1994; Falk, 2001). Those who participated in the research included street-based and other freelance (bars, strip clubs, parks) workers, agency-based escorts, independent home-based escorts, exotic entertainers, exotic masseuses. Some of these individuals had also worked in pornography and telephone sex.

2. See the Canadian Criminal Code Sections 210 through 213, 163, 174, and 167 through 173. Broadly speaking, the following are legislated as illegal activities: public solicitation or communication for the purpose of selling sexual services, operating a bawdy house, and living off the avails of prostitution. Researchers have noted that enforcement of these laws varies from city to city across Canada (Lowman, 1995; Shaver, 1993).

3. The term *felt stigma* refers to the perceptions of the stigmatized and the term *enacted stigma* refers to observable instances of discrimination of discomfort on the part of non-stigmatized individuals (Scambler & Hopkins, 1986).

4. These percentages indicate the number of persons who reported that they had consumed illicit substances intravenously in the "last 6 months" prior to the interview and may exclude persons who have a history of intravenous drug use prior to the 6-month period referred to in the question.

5. We use pseudonyms throughout to refer to individual respondents to help protect their identities.

REFERENCES

Alexander, P. (1998). Sex work and health: A question of safety in the workplace. *Journal of the American Medical Women's Association, 53*(2), 77–82.

Andrulis, D. (1998). Access to care is the centerpiece in the elimination of socioeconomic disparities in health. *Annals of Internal Medicine, 129*(5), 412–416.

Becker, H. (1963). *Outsiders: Studies in the sociology of deviance*. New York: Free Press.

Benoit, C. (2003). The politics of health care policy: The United States in comparative perspective. *Perspectives in Biology and Medicine, 46*(4), 592–599.

Benoit, C., Dena, C., & Munaza, C. (2003). In search of a healing place: Aboriginal women in vancouver's downtown eastside. *Social Science and Medicine, 56*, 821–833.

Benoit, C., Jansson, M., Millar, A., & Phillips, R. (2005). Community-academic research on hard-to-reach populations: Benefits and challenges. *Qualitative Health Research, 15*(2), 263–282.

Benoit, C., & Millar, A. (2001). *Dispelling myths and understanding realities: Working conditions, health status and exiting experiences of sex workers*. Report prepared for the Michael Smith Foundation for Health Research (formerly the BC Health Research Foundation): Victoria.

Blishen, B. (1991). *Doctors in Canada: The changing world of medical practice*. Toronto: University of Toronto Press.

Boyatzis, R. E. (1998). *Transforming qualitative information: Thematic analysis and code development*. Thousand Oaks, CA: Sage.

Broyles, R. W., Manga, P., Binder, D. A., Angus, D. E., & Charette, A. (1983). The use of physician services under a national insurance scheme. *Medical Care, 21*(11), 1037–1054.

Bruckert, C. (2002). *Taking if off, putting it on: Women in the strip trade*. Toronto: Women's Press.

Camp, D. L., Finlay, W. M., & Lyons, E. (2002). Is low self esteem an inevitable consequence of stigma: An example from women with chronic mental health problems. *Social Science & Medicine, 55*(5), 823–834.

Canadian Institute for Health Information (CIHI). (2004). *Improving the health of Canadians*. Ottawa: Canadian Institute for Health Information.

Canadian Population Health Initiative (CPHI). About Population Health. Canadian Institute for Health Information (CPHI). Webpage:http://secure.cihi.ca/cihiweb/disp Page.jsp?cw_page = cphi_aboutph_e[Last Accessed October 10, 2002.]

Carr, S. (1995). The health of women working in the sex industry – A moral and ethical perspective. *Sexual and Marital Therapy, 10*(2), 201–213.

Coburn, D., & Eakin, J. (1993). The sociology of health in Canada: First impressions. *Health and Canadian Society, 1*(1), 83–110.

Conrad, P. (1992). Medicalization and social control. *Annual Review of Sociology, 18*, 209–232.

Cree, V. E., Kay, H., Tisdall, K., & Wallace, J. (2004). Stigma and parental HIV. *Qualitative Social Work*, 3(1), 7–25.

Crocker, J., & Quinn, D. M. (2000). Social stigma and the self: Meanings, situations, and self-esteem. In: T. F. Heatherton, R. E. Kleck, M. R. Hebl & J. G. Hull (Eds), *The social psychology of stigma* (pp. 153–183). New York: Guilford Press.

Davies, P., & Feldman, R. (1997). Prostitute men now. In: G. Scambler & A. Scambler (Eds), *Rethinking prostitution: Purchasing sex in the 1990s* (pp. 29–55). Routledge: London.

Denzin, N. K., & Lincoln, Y. S. (Eds) (1994). *Handbook of qualitative research*. Thousand Oaks, CA: Sage.

Downe, P. J. (1997). Constructing a complex of contagion: The perceptions of aids among working prostitutes in Costa Rica. *Social Science & Medicine, 44*(10), 1575–1583.

Evans, C., & Lambert, H. (1997). Health-seeking strategies and sexual health among female sex workers in urban India: Implications for research and service provision. *Social Science & Medicine, 44*(12), 1791–1803.

Evans, R. G., Barer, M. L., & Marmor, T. R. (Eds) (1994). *Why are some people healthy and others not?* New York: Aldine de Gruyter.

Falk, G. (2001). *Stigma: How we treat outsiders*. Amherst, NY: Prometheus Books.

Gray, D. E. (2002). Everybody just freezes. Everybody is just embarrassed: Felt and enacted stigma among parents of children with high functioning autism. *Sociology of Health and Illness*, 24(6), 734–739.

Haug, M. (1988). A re-examination of the hypothesis of physician deprofessionalization. *Milbank Memorial Fund Quarterly*, 54, 83–106.

Heaman, M. (2001). Conducting health research with vulnerable women: Issues and strategies. *Canadian Journal of Nursing Research*, 33(3), 81–86.

Heckathorn, D. (1997). Respondent driven sampling: A new approach to the study of hidden populations. *Social Science & Medicine*, 35(3), 281–286.

Kunitz, S., & Pesis-Katz, I. (2005). Mortality of white Americans, African Americans, and Canadians: The causes and consequences for health of welfare states institutions and policies. *The Milbank Quarterly*, 83(1), 5–39.

Kusow, A. M. (2004). Contesting stigma: On Goffman's assumptions of normative order. *Symbolic Interaction*, 27(2), 179–197.

Lowman, J. (1991). Prostitution in Canada. In: M. A. Jackson & C. T. Griffiths (Eds), *Canadian criminology: Perspectives on crime and criminality* (pp. 137–164). Toronto: Harcourt Brace Jovanovich.

Marmot, M. (2003). Understanding social inequalities in health. *Perspectives in Biology and Medicine*, 46(3 Suppl.), S9–S23.

Marmot, M. G., & Wilkinson, R. G. (Eds) (1999). *Social determinants of health*. Oxford: Oxford University Press.

Maticka-Tyndale, E., Lewis, J., Clark, J., Zubick, J., & Young, S. (1999). Social and cultural vulnerability of sexually-transmitted infection: The work of exotic dancers. *Canadian Journal of Public Health*, 90(1), 19–22.

McRae, H. (2000). Managing courtesy stigma: The case of Alzheimer's. *Sociology of Health and Illness*, 21(1), 54–70.

Ministry of Children and Family Development, Province of British Columbia. (2005). Email correspondence with Anne Batchelor, Acting Regional Research Analyst.

Norvilitis, J. M., Scime, M., & Lee, J. S. (2002). Courtesy stigma in mothers of children with attention-deficit/hyperactivity disorder: A preliminary investigation. *Journal of Attention Deficit Disorder*, 6(2), 61–68.

Raphael, D. (Ed.) (2004). *Social determinants of health: Canadian perspectives.* Toronto: Canadian Scholars Press Inc.

Reitsma Street, M., Hopper, A., & Seright, J. (2000). *Poverty and inequality in the capital region of British Columbia.* Victoria: Capital Urban Poverty Project.

Roos, N., Forget, E., & Wald, R. (2003). *Socioeconomic status, health status, and healthcare costs: Can medical savings accounts meet the healthcare needs of Canadians.* Ottawa: Canadian Health Services Research Foundation.

Roos, N., & Mustard, C. (1997). Variation in health and health care use by socioeconomic status in Winnipeg, Canada: Does the system work well? Yes and no. *The Millbank Quarterly*, 75(1), 89–111.

Scambler, G., & Hopkins, A. (1986). Being epileptic: Coming to terms with stigma. *Sociology of Health & Illness*, 8(1), 26–43.

Scambler, G., Perswanie, R., Renton, A., & Scambler, A. (1990). Women prostitutes in the AIDS era. *Sociology of Health & Illness*, 12(3), 260–273.

Shaver, F. (1993). Prostitution: A female crime? In: E. Adelberg & C. Currie (Eds), *Conflict with the law: Women and the Canadian justice system* (pp. 153–173). Vancouver: Press Gang Publishers.

Shrage, L. (1994). *Moral dilemmas of feminism: Prostitution, adultery, and abortion.* London, NY: Routledge.

Shultz, B., & Angermeyer, C. (2003). Subjective experiences of stigma: A focus group study of schizophrenic patients, their relatives, and health professionals. *Social Science & Medicine*, 56, 299–312.

Snell, C. L. (1991). Help seeking behaviour among young street males. *Smith College Studies in Social Work*, 61, 293–304.

Statistics Canada. (2000). *Women in Canada 2000: A gender-based statistics analysis.* Ottawa: Ministry of Industry.

Statistics Canada. (2001a). Community Profiles. Website: http://www12.statcan.ca/english/ profil01/Details/details1pop2.cfm?SEARCH = BEGINS&PSGC = 59&SGC = 59935&A = &LANG = E&Province = 59&PlaceName = Victoria&CSDNAME = Victoria&CMA = &SEARCH = BEGINS&DataType = 1&TypeNameE = Census%20Metropolitan% 20Area&ID = 1298 [Last Accessed December 19, 2004.]

Statistics Canada. (2001b). Community Profiles. Website: http://www12.statcan.ca/english/ profil01/Details/details1pop2.cfm?SEARCH = BEGINS&PSGC = 59&SGC = 59935&A = &LANG = E&Province = 59&PlaceName = Victoria&CSDNAME = Victoria&CMA = &SEARCH = BEGINS&DataType = 1&TypeNameE = Census%20Metropolitian% 20Area&ID = 1298 [Last Accessed December 19, 2004.]

Statistics Canada. (2001c). Community Profiles. Website: http://www12.statcan.ca/english/ profil01/Details/details1edu.cfm?SEARCH = BEGINS&PSGC = 59&SGC = 59935&A = &LANG = E&Province = 59&PlaceName = Victoria&CSDNAME = Victoria&CMA = &SEARCH = BEGINS&DataType = 1&TypeNameE = Census%20Metropolitian% 20Area&ID = 1298 [Last Accessed December 19, 2004.]

Stewart, M., Fast, J., Letourneau, N., Love, R., Raine, K., Raphael, D., Ruetter, L., Rootman, I., Shorten, D., Thurston, S., & Williamson, D. (2001). *Low income consumers' perspectives on determinants of health services use.* Ottawa: Canadian Health Services Research Foundation.

Vanwesenbeek, I. (1994). *Prostitutes' well-being and risk*. Amsterdam: VU University Press.
Waitzken, H. (1998). A critical theory of medical discourse. In: W. C. Cockerham, M. Glaser & L. S. Heuse (Eds), *Readings in medical sociology*. Eaglewood Cliffs, NJ: Prentice, Hall.
Waldam, J., Herring, D., & Young, T. K. (1995). *Aboriginal health in Canada: Historical, cultural and epidemiological perspectives*. Toronto: University of Toronto Press.
Watson, A., & Corrigan, P. (2002). *The impact of stigma on service access and participation*. Behavioural Health Recovery Management Project. Website: http://www.scholar. google.com/scholar?hl = en&lr = &q = cache:Iw690DP0N9UJ:www.heart-intl.net/ Hepatitis,%2520AIDS,%2520Research%2520Trust/Stigma/Complete/Impact%2520of %2520 Stigma.pdf + watson + and + corrigan + guideline + developed + for + the + Behavioral + Health + Recovery + Management + project last viewed August 2, 2005.
Williams, G. H. (2003). The determinants of health: Structure, context and agency. *Sociology of Health & Illness, 25*, 131–154.

PRESENTING AND ANTICIPATORY NEEDS FOR ACCESSIBILITY TO PROVIDERS AND SERVICES: THE EXPERIENCES OF SIX FRAIL OLDER WIDOWS LIVING IN MEDICALLY UNDERSERVED AREAS

Eileen J. Porter

ABSTRACT

Older women living in medically underserved areas (MUA) might have particular problems with access to health care. This is an in-depth report of the accessibility issues raised by six frail older women (age 82–93 years) during a longitudinal descriptive phenomenological study of the experience of home care. Three White women lived in the same rural MUA, and three Black women lived in the same urban MUA. The need for health service was understood subjectively and prospectively as the personal perception of a situation requiring relief or supply. Some women reported presenting needs for accessibility to providers, whereas others

Health Care Services, Racial and Ethnic Minorities and Underserved Populations: Patient and Provider Perspectives
Research in the Sociology of Health Care, Volume 23, 105–132
ISSN: 0275-4959/doi:10.1016/S0275-4959(05)23006-5

reported needs for their future accessibility to providers or services. Some intentions were likely linked to residence location, and residence in a rural MUA was relevant to the phenomenon of securing the help that I might need down the road. Feasibility was proposed as a new parameter of access. Research and practice implications were proposed.

The prediction of home-care use based upon need has been a staple thrust in research on health services use of older adults (Grabbe et al., 1995; Porter, 2000; Wolinsky, 1994). However, only a small proportion of frail elders utilize in-home and community-based services, probably due to limited availability and difficulties with access (Mui, Choi, & Monk, 1998). Older women are at risk for being underserved; compared to older men, they have greater requirements for care at home (Hobbs & Damon, 1996). Older rural women (Coward, McLaughlin, Duncan, & Bull, 1994), women of color (Mui et al., 1998), and poor women (Ettner, 1994) are at a particular disadvantage. Indeed, the population parameters of low income and advanced age are factors in the designation of a medically underserved area (MUA) (Bureau of Health Professions, n.d.).

The designation of a vicinity as an MUA cannot be considered as a direct inference that older poor women living in such areas have difficulty accessing health services. However, there have been few descriptive studies of the health service needs perceived by older women who live in MUAs. That gap is addressed in this paper. Certain perceptions of three frail women living in a rural MUA are considered alongside comparable data shared by three frail women living in an urban MUA. To elaborate the personal–social context of their perceptions, their views about their communities are shared. Interview data are cited to detail the principal health problems reported by the women, their presenting concerns about service needs, and their worries about obtaining the services that they thought they would need in the future to continue living alone at home.

REVIEW OF THE LITERATURE

Predicting the Use of Home Care Based on Need

A central focus of home-care research has been predicting service use (Benjamin, 1992; Chappell, 1994) using the Anderson–Newman model

(ANM) (Andersen & Newman, 1973). The model posits that service use is contingent on need, enabling factors, and predisposing factors. Andersen (1968) defined need as the "most immediate cause of health service use" (p.17) and suggested that need be "measured by the amount of illness perceived by the family" (p. 17). Need, which often has been understood as functional disability (Porter, 1995b), has been measured with tools designed to tap (a) activities of daily living (ADL), (b) ADL and instrumental activities of daily living (IADL) (Wolinsky, 1994), or (c) ADL and health status (Kart, 1991). Defined and measured in those ways, need has been the best predictor of home-care use (Benjamin, 1992; Chappell, 1994; Kane & Kane, 1987).

Enabling and Predisposing Factors: Influences on Access to Service

In the ANM, home-care need is influenced by enabling factors (such as family income and service cost) that "condition both the opportunity and the choice to use given services" (Benjamin, 1992, p. 26). Poverty has been cited as a major influence on the opportunity to access home-care services (Skinner, 1995; Wallace, Levy-Storm, Kington, & Andersen, 1998), particularly for women (Ettner, 1994), because their risk of poverty increases with age (Barusch, 1994). White-Means and Rubin (2004) found a U-shaped association between income and formal home-care use among both Blacks and Whites. Among persons with lower incomes, incremental income increases of $1,000 were linked to decreased use of care, but an income above $49,500 was associated with a higher probability of home-care use.

According to the ANM, "predisposing" factors, such as demographics and health-related beliefs (Wolinsky, 1994), are influences upon enabling factors. Home-care use has been associated with living alone (Choi, 1994; Jenkins & Laditka, 2003; Katz, Kabeto, & Langa, 2000; Mitchell & Krout, 1998), geographical stability (Wolinsky & Johnson, 1992), older age (Branch et al., 1988; Calsyn & Winter, 2000; Lun, 2004), female gender (Katz et al., 2000; Miner, 1995; Jenkins & Laditka, 2003), and ethnicity (Mui et al., 1998). White-Means and Rubin (2004) found that older Black and White persons had comparable access to home care, but that Blacks were more likely to use formal home care when income levels were equal. Racial differences in home-care use have been explained by structural factors such as accessibility, availability, and acceptability (Wallace et al., 1998). Lun (2004) concluded that older persons who perceived structural barriers to community-based and in-home services used fewer services.

Residence Location: Influence on Access to Service

Andersen and Newman (1973, p. 109) viewed a community's "rural-urban nature" as an enabling variable because of variations in community values or norms of medical practice. However, some researchers have treated residence location as a predisposing variable. For instance, Lun (2004) found that in-home and community-based service use of older persons varied with the type of service as well as residence location. Compared to rural older persons, older urban people were more likely to use congregate meal services and transportation and less likely to use housework services and personal care/nursing. Higher levels of home-care use have been associated with residing in an urban area (Grabbe et al., 1995; Soldo, 1985). Compared to urban elders, rural elders have been viewed as lacking access to formal care, which is provided by a privately hired helper or an agency (Coward & Dwyer, 1991) paid by the older person, the family, the public, or some combination thereof (Penrod, Harris, & Kane, 1994).

Indeed, using data from the 1994 National Health Interview Survey, Auchincloss, Van Nostrand, and Ronsaville (2001) found that older Americans living in rural areas and impoverished areas had more difficulty accessing care. Access to primary health care is a critical variable in designating an MUA. Geographic areas eligible for consideration as an MUA are: (a) an entire county in a non-metropolitan area, (b) a group of contiguous counties or similar units in non-metropolitan areas with population centers no more than 30 min apart in travel time, and (c) a group of census tracts in a metropolitan area that constitute a neighborhood due to the common demographic and socioeconomic characteristics of residents. For eligible areas, the Index of Medical Underservice (IMU) is calculated based upon these parameters: (a) ratio of primary care physicians per 1,000 people, (b) infant mortality rate, (c) percentage of the population with an income below the poverty level, and (d) percentage of the population age 65 or older (Bureau of Health Professions, n.d.). Thus, criteria for designation of an MUA have been associated with home-care use – low income (Mui et al., 1998), advanced age (Branch et al., 1988), and residence location (Grabbe et al., 1995; Krout, 1988; Soldo, 1985).

The Research Problem

Scholars have emphasized the complexity of home care (Gubrium & Sankar, 1990), but relatively little progress has been made in understanding that complexity. As a group, the enabling and predisposing factors of the ANM have explained little of the variance in home-care use (Benjamin, 1992; Chappell, 1994; Grabbe et al., 1995; Porter, 2000; Wolinsky, 1994). These difficulties can be traced, in part, to unchallenged assumptions grounded in the ANM and its research methods. Two such assumptions, bearing directly on this study, are reviewed next.

First, most researchers have assumed that home-care need should be defined as Andersen (1968) defined it some 35 years ago, as a cause of health-care use. That definition has had a marked influence on methods in home-care research. It has established the premise for a retrospective approach in which the effect (use) is identified before the cause (need). Although this strategy has been paramount in quantitative studies (Wolinsky, 1994), some qualitative researchers also have adopted it. For instance, Forbes and Hoffart (1998) explored beliefs, attitudes, and values considered by elders and caregivers as influences upon the decision-making process about using community-based services. They referred to "health need [as] events such as diabetic coma . . .[that] prompted the need for services and nursing home placement" (p. 743). Because their view of need was retrospective, they could not consider the influence of ongoing events or concerns for the future.

However, Andersen and Newman (1973, p. 110) also opened a different window upon the idea of need when they referred to the "need for service" Twenty years later, in a review of literature about the ANM, Yeatts, Crow, and Folts (1992, p. 25) revived that interpretation; they defined need simply as "the individual's perceived need for a service". That definition seems straightforward enough, but beyond its tautological format, it is problematic in several ways. Some older persons are not aware of available services, and in such cases, they are not likely to perceive a need for a specific service. Furthermore, a focus upon service is consistent with the perspective of providers rather than the viewpoint of older persons (Porter, in press).

To guide descriptive studies, scholars must select more general interpretations of key constructs, such as need, that are not directly tied to long-standing scholarly views. For this descriptive phenomenological study, this definition of need was adopted: personal perceptions about a situation "requiring relief or supply" (Neufeldt, 1997, p. 906). That definition is oriented to the present as well as the future. It establishes the premise for prospective studies designed to explore underlying influences on current use of services as well as presenting concerns and worries about future accessibility to health services.

As explained elsewhere (Porter, 1998b), a second problematic assumption grounded in the ANM (Porter, 1998b) is that access to care, as a component of the health care system (Andersen & Newman, 1973), can be measured in terms of distance to a service site (Love & Lindquist, 1995), actual use of a service (Comer & Mueller, 1995), or barriers to service delivery such as transportation (Gillanders & Buss, 1993). In contrast, however, Yeatts et al. (1992) proposed that certain structural barriers (in knowledge, access, and intent) could influence service use of poor minority elders. In contrast to other views of access, this is a more person-centered interpretation akin to "accessibility" (Andersen & Newman, 1973, p. 109). However, a person-centered perspective of accessibility has not been fully articulated in many studies about structural barriers. For instance, although Lun (2004) asked older persons about perceived structural barriers, responses were categorized as indicative of "no barriers, not aware of service, and other barriers" (p.128), in effect, masking respondents' personal views about accessibility.

Older persons who live in urban and rural areas that have been designated as MUAs might face barriers and challenges in accessing health services; as noted earlier, older women might be at a particular disadvantage. Unfortunately, few researchers have sought to reveal complexities in the health-related experiences of older women who live in MUAs by describing their presenting concerns and worries about future accessibility to services.

A concern about the underlying complexity of experience was paramount to Husserl, the founder of the philosophy of descriptive phenomenology. Husserl (1913/1962) concluded that psychologists had a limited understanding of experience because constructs had not been grounded in lived experience. He encouraged scholars to explore phenomena (structures of experience) as sources of scientific knowledge (Spiegelberg, 1994). The aim of descriptive phenomenological research is to discern the empirical structure of the experience (Husserl, 1913/1962; Porter, 1998a) and its context (Porter, 1995a; Schutz & Luckmann, 1973) by identifying similarities and differences in the details of a person's experiences.

Descriptive phenomenological studies are to emerge from a critical analysis of extant constructs so that the empirical, experiential perspective of findings can be compared to constructs relevant to the experience of interest (Porter, 1995a, 2000). For instance, the formal–informal dichotomy of home care has been criticized for various reasons (Rubinstein, Lubben, & Mintzer, 1994), including its principal orientations to compensation and the identity of the care-provider (Porter, Ganong, Drew, & Lanes, 2004). A descriptive study of the home-care experiences of 25 older widows was undertaken in part to explore the empirical basis of the dichotomy. Associated with the finding that a feature of the personal–social context of the experience was counting on my standby helpers to stand by me, a typology of four standby helpers was discerned. Each woman's helpers were differentiated according to the frequency of help and the nature and duration of interactions with the woman. Because data revealed that formal and informal helpers were represented among all four types of standby helpers, the typology was posed as a counterview to the formal–informal dichotomy (Porter et al., 2004).

Using data drawn from the larger home-care study, this paper is a description of the accessibility issues raised by six frail older widows who were living in rural and urban MUAs. They reported presenting needs for relief associated with accessibility to specific health care providers. They also reported anticipatory needs for relief or supply associated with accessibility to health services in the future. The intentions of some women concerning these presenting and anticipated situations were influenced, in part, by aspects of personal–social context, including residence location and residence in an MUA.

METHOD

A longitudinal, prospective design was used for the descriptive phenomenological study of the home-care experience. Over 3 years, 25 older women were to participate in a series of tape-recorded interviews. A three-stage sampling strategy was used (Porter, 1999). First, older women living in a six-county region of central Missouri were invited to participate through contacts with local service agencies. A second sampling stage was purposive; the inclusion criteria were: (a) being 80 years or older, (b) living alone at home, (c) being widowed, (d) having children, and (e) continuing to live in the community where one had lived while married. Finally, quota sampling (Luborsky & Rubinstein, 1995) was done, as is indicated when an experience might vary due to a demographic characteristic (Sandelowski, 1995). Volunteers who met the inclusion criteria were further screened based on ethnicity and place of residence. In 1990, 5% of Missouri's population of older women was African-American and 25% of the population was rural, living in or outside a community of less than 2,500 persons. Urban persons were living in an urbanized area or in a place of 2,500 or more persons outside of an urbanized area (US Department of Commerce, 1992). In a sample of 25 women, African-American women were over-sampled at 25% and rural women were over-sampled at 50%. For case-by-case comparisons (Cutler & Coward, 1989) on widowhood, parenthood, and relocation, three rural women met criteria (a) and (b), but just two of the criteria (c), (d), and (e).

Sample

For this particular study, data were selected from interviews with six women who were residing in MUAs. Three Black women lived in an urban area composed of 16 census tracts that were first designated as an MUA in 1994, and three women lived in a rural town in a county first designated as an MUA in 1978 (Bureau of Primary Health Care, n.d.). The IMU scale ranges from 0 (completely underserved) to 100 (best served or least underserved), with an IMU of 62.0 or less required for a service area to be designated as an MUA (Bureau of Health Professions, n.d.). At the most recent renewal of the MUA designation, the IMU for the urban MUA was 44.1, whereas the IMU for the rural MUA was 44.6 (Bureau of Primary Health Care, n.d.).

All three urban women and two rural women met all inclusion criteria. One rural widow had relocated after her spouse's death, and unlike the other women, who were living in their own homes; she was living in a rented home. The six women ranged in age from 82 to 93 years (M = 88.9). All six women were considered frail; they needed help to climb stairs and an assistive device for walking (Arfken, Lach, Birge, & Miller, 1994). Specific data about income was not sought, but the women volunteered it. One urban woman owned property in addition to her own home, and the rural woman who had relocated had savings from the sale of her home. Two of the three urban women and two of the three rural women reported that they were enrolled in Medicaid.

The study was deemed exempt from review by the Health Sciences Institutional Review Board of the University of Missouri because data were to be maintained without identifiers. Informed written consent was secured prior to the initial interview. Four of the six women were retained for 3 years. One urban woman stopped participating due to declining health, and the rural woman who had relocated moved again out of the six-county area.

Data Collection and Data Analysis

Seven open-ended interviews were to be conducted with each woman in her home, with additional interviews after major events such as a hospitalization or a brief nursing home stay. For these six women, the number of interviews ranged from three to nine. The main interview topics were seeking help and having help while living alone at home. As reported elsewhere, the women were asked to name their helpers, to describe the help received, and to talk about their interactions with helpers (Porter et al., 2004). To tap perceptions about the personal–social context of the home-care experience, I asked the women to share any concerns about their ongoing home care and about the help they might need to continue living alone at home.

The average length of the tape-recorded interviews was 90 min. Although a few interviews were conducted by trained research assistants, I conducted all interviews reported here. After each interview was transcribed to disk, I checked the data file for accuracy. To facilitate data management, interviews were entered into NUDIST v. 4. Before the third and last interviews with each woman, I discussed her experience with a co-investigator; due to staggered enrollment into the study, these discussions occurred over a 4-year period.

Data analysis was guided by a descriptive phenomenological method (Porter, 1994, 1995a, 1998a) that I developed from Husserl's (1913/1962) book, Ideas. When persons describe what they are trying to do relative to an experience (an intention), they often refer to contextual factors, such as why a particular event, object, or activity is important (Schutz & Luckmann, 1973). Data pertaining to context (Porter, 1995a) were differentiated from data pertaining to intentions and analyzed separately. The experiences of the three women at each residence location were compared; finally, the experiences of all the six women were compared. Commonalities and differences emerged; related intentions of the various women were understood as parts of larger phenomena that structured the experience (Porter, 1998a).

RESULTS

Supplemented by demographic data, the women's words are used as the principal resource for describing their residence locations. As the women talked about their major health problems and their helpers, they also described their presenting and anticipatory needs for relief and supply associated with accessibility to providers and services. Relevant data reported by each woman are cited or summarized, and relevant structures of experience and context are noted. As shall be explained, some intentions were considered relevant to residence location.

The Women and Their Residence Locations

Coward et al. (1994) noted that "a proper definition of residence, from a health care perspective, involves a combination of the number of people residing in a place, some aspect of geographical space and distance, and some recognition of the distance of the place from other nearby health and human services" (p. 4). These parameters, as well as others more personal to the women in this study, are considered in the descriptions below.

The Urban Location

The neighborhood has long been the residential center for Blacks in the city of Clarkton, a community of 80,000 people with one public hospital and two private hospitals. Several family clinics and convenience clinics are located in the neighborhood.

The three women, Mrs. A, Mrs. B, and Mrs. C, were long-time residents living within three blocks of each other. As professional persons living in an impoverished neighborhood, Mrs. A and her husband had been very active in the community. Mrs. A rarely left her home, but she actively supported efforts to maintain historical properties in the district. Mrs. B had cared for the children of prominent White families at their homes. She was born just a few blocks from her present home; she related childhood memories of the neighborhood as a rural place. Mrs. B went outside her home daily in part to "pick the trash up, 'cause sometime people throw trash and the wrappers for cocaine. And they'll pitch it right in the yard, too." Mrs. C proudly related that she had lived on her street all of her life, having moved to her present home 35 years earlier when "they cut through (her street) to build the (urban housing) projects." Like Mrs. B, she commented upon changes in the neighborhood. "We have them drug-houses now. The neighbors is all watching. We have that thing, what do you call it, neighborhood watch? We're all looking out to see what's going on, and we tell each other then."

The Rural Location

Bixford, a town of 2,400 people, is the county seat of Popard County. A small county hospital is located in a town about 15 miles away. Clarkton, with its three hospitals, is about 25 miles away. There are two family medical clinics in Bixford, one of which is affiliated with the public university in Clarkton. Four physicians are in practice in Bixford.

The three women, Mrs. D, Mrs. E, and Mrs. F, lived within a mile of each other on the same side of the highway that bisects the town. Mrs. F, who had clerked at a local store for years, lived on a well-traveled street near the main street. She thought that the neighborhood had changed. She expressed concern about a nearby robbery and spoke to the mayor about the legality of activities of her new neighbors. When she talked about having an auction, she said this. "We have an auctioneer over at Bixford, over in Bixford. (She paused.) This is Bixford. I sometimes feel like this is so different that it's hardly my home." Mrs. D, a homemaker, who had grown up in Bixford, left there after high school. She moved back after the death of her second husband, the father of her stepchildren, to live closer to her three sisters. She lived on the outskirts of the town across from a cultivated field. Her house, like the other nearby homes, appeared to be less than 50 years old. Mrs. E was a homemaker. Her impoverished neighborhood was equidistant to those of Mrs. D and Mrs. F. The streets were very narrow, poorly paved, and irregularly configured. Some homes, including farmettes with outbuildings, were very dilapidated.

Mrs. E and Mrs. F bemoaned the closing of the 50-bed hospital in Bixford a few years earlier. Mrs. F said, "Everybody that knows anything about the old hospital, just thinks it's sad, because now we have to go out of town after we go to the doctor." This issue was also salient to Mrs. D, who had been raised in Bixford. She said, "It's a cryin' shame. They could have used a hospital if they'd just left it here, but it didn't make the money they thought it should." The old hospital, which had been renovated for other uses, was within six blocks of each woman's home.

Helper Networks

Like the other women in the larger sample (Porter et al., 2004), these six frail women had some standby helpers at home, including their children, grandchildren, siblings, cousins, nieces, in-laws, neighbors, friends, privately hired helpers, government-subsidized helpers (for housekeeping and home-health care), volunteers, and business persons. Like helpers of all women in the larger sample, the helpers of this sub-sample were classified into four types (Porter et al., 2004). Regular helpers (RHs) came at specific times to do only specific jobs. The women contacted on-call helpers (OCHs) about specific tasks such as transportation or shopping. The can-will-doer (CWD) was willing to do more than one task and typically did a range of tasks within a certain facet of responsibility, such as financial management. The trusted mainstay, who did a variety of tasks and took on extra duties willingly, was someone without whom the women said they could not have lived alone at home (Porter et al., 2004). For each woman, the cadres of standbys varied by helper type and kinship. Every woman did not have every type of standby, but residence location was not an obvious influence upon network composition. Even in this small sample, kin and non-kin were represented among the RHs, OCHs, CWDs, and mainstays for both the rural and the urban women.

Presenting and Anticipatory Needs

Each woman had a major health-related problem with which her standby home-helpers and health-care providers were involved. Each woman reported needs for relief or supply relative to current accessibility to current providers, future accessibility to providers or services, or both. The presenting needs for supply or relief were basic to these intentions: (a) getting help with what I think I can do, (b) keeping a regular home-care nurse, (c) reaching the home-care nurse, and (d) reaching the doctor quickly. Those intentions were parts of one of the two phenomena of mobilizing my helper or keeping my helper. A contextual feature – expecting the helper to do what the helper is supposed to do – was basic to both phenomena.

In contrast to the presenting needs, anticipatory needs for relief and supply were associated with data about the overriding intention to continue living alone at home for as long as possible – an intention that these six women shared with the other women in the home-care sample (Porter, in press) and other older widows (Porter, 1994). As Mrs. B noted: "I hope I live to be 100, but I don't want to if I'm gonna be in bad shape, be a problem, have to go to a rest home, all of that jazz. I don't want that. I have asked that the Lord just let me go to sleep here in this house." Because the women were counting on their standbys to help them live at home, the context of the experience was structured in part by keeping my helpers' circumstances in mind. The women reported anticipatory needs for relief and supply associated with these intentions: (a) getting a good ride to the doctor's office, (b) staying in touch with the doctor through the home-care nurses, (c) limiting the load for my mainstay, (d) getting up there to the emergency room (ER) without taking an ambulance, and (e) keeping a regular home-care nurse. These intentions were parts of the phenomenon of securing the help that I might need down the road. In the ensuing overview of each woman's unique situation, her needs for accessibility are considered relative to residence location, helper network, and duration of residence in the community. In data excerpts, the interviewer's remarks are in brackets.

The Urban, Black Women

Mrs. A, aged 90, who had insulin-dependent diabetes and marked mobility impairment, had ongoing needs for relief from the perception that her freedom within her own home was jeopardized by some of her in-home providers. She felt controlled by the diabetes regimen and by some of the actions of the "sitters" who provided 24-h care.

I want to do as I please. One afternoon, I said, 'I think I'll walk now'. And she said, 'No, you're not feeling well enough to walk now'. And she took the walker away from me and wouldn't let me walk. And I said to her, in a very ugly tone of voice, 'I'm not paying you to tell me what I can do or what I can't do. I'm paying you to assist me with what I think I can do'.

These data reveal that Mrs. A had clear expectations of the sitters. In spite of her repeated efforts to influence the helpers, they were not sensitive to her expectations. She perceived a lack of accessibility to minds and hearts of those helpers. Her intention, getting help with what I think I can do, was part of the phenomenon of mobilizing her helper.

Mrs. B, aged 89, who had painful arthritis in her knees, no longer drove her unreliable car to the grocery store, believing that she might have to abandon it and walk for help in an unsafe neighborhood like hers. Sally, Mrs. B's volunteer from the Council on Aging, took her grocery shopping; over time, Mrs. B referred to Sally as "my caregiver" and "my mainstay." Characteristic of RHs who became mainstays, Sally had taken on other duties, such as bringing in hot meals and taking Mrs. B to some physician appointments.

But there may come a time, I'll need to go when she can't, because she's got a regular job. Now I notice OATS have got some little cars. And I said, 'I think I'll call and ask them what is the deal there'. It was a bus before, and you had to call way ahead, maybe 2–3 weeks, and be sure that they had, and all. And you get there and the doctor's finished and you'd have to just wait forever (for the bus). And maybe you're so tired and you want to get home and get rested. So if they've got a better deal going, I would like to know about it. Also, there is a transportation that they charge a dollar to go. And I have been trying hard to get that number, so I could call 'em or write and ask and fill out a blank or something, because I'd just be happy if I could get some place. I need now to be going to my podiatrist and to the eye doctor and so forth and so on. And Sally, she's working during the day. She couldn't take me everywhere, and I don't expect her to do it. [You thought of checking about these little cars.] Right. [And also . . .] The transit. [Paratransit?] Is that what it is? Paratransit. I knew it was trans-something. [Paratransit; they charge one dollar.] So, yes, that is the idea I wanted to check. So I will have this to go on. See, you never know when you might just really need it.

Thus, Mrs. B had anticipatory needs and two interlocking intentions. She was trying to get a good ride to appointments (compared to the OATS bus) and to limit the load on her mainstay.

Mrs. C, who was 87 years old, had arthritis and diabetes. Her data reveal the development of a linked cascade of presenting and future needs. Prior to Interview #1, she had been taking insulin injections; she had bi-weekly visits from a home-care nurse who set up medications, monitored vital signs, and reported to the physician. At Interview #1, the nurse was still coming, but

Mrs. C was no longer on insulin. At Interview #2, she said: "They have turned me loose; the nurse doesn't come anymore. You have to be on that needle for them to come out." At Interview #3, Mrs. C said that the first agency had gone out of business but that the nurses "at this other home place got it straightened out." Indeed, a nurse from another agency had come, explaining that she would be "the regular nurse," but at Interview #4, Mrs. C reported, "The nurse hadn't been here for 3 weeks." Because the nurse ceased visits without an explanation, Mrs. C had to concern herself with getting in touch with the missing nurse. Her presenting needs underscored the intentions of keeping a regular home-care nurse (the need for supply), reaching the home-care nurse (the need for relief), and reaching the doctor quickly (the need for relief).

For Mrs. C, the anticipatory need for supply was to have accessibility to her doctor through a home-care nurse. "If the nurses call in, they know it's something really wrong with me. And I can call in, and they'll put me on wait timing." She felt that she needed the nurse as an intermediary. Indeed, during a period when a nurse was not visiting, she had not been able to reach her physician by telephone for an entire afternoon when she was in great pain from arthritis. After her son took her to the hospital, where she was admitted, she reported this conversation with her physician.

> He asked me why didn't I call him before I go. I told him, 'I had been tryin' to get you all the afternoon, and all I could get was put on hold.' And he said, 'Well, I'm gonna have to kinda look into that, because there's been some others that have said the same thing'. [So if the nurse didn't return would you miss the fact that she gets a-hold of the doctor?] Yes, I would. Because I would just wonder how I'm going to get in touch with him. By puttin' me on hold all the time, and by the nurse being able to get through, well, that would affect me quite a bit. Because I feel that I didn't have anybody that could call in and get through for me.

The anticipatory intentions of Mrs. C, then, were keeping a regular nurse and staying in touch with the doctor through the home-care nurses.

The Rural, White Women

Mrs. D, aged 82, had recently relocated to Bixford to live next door to her younger sister, who was her mainstay. Mrs. D had fallen repeatedly; she could not get up without help, and her usual helpers were her mainstay sister and another sister (CWD) and brother-in-law (OCH). As a relative newcomer, she did not know her home-care nurses, and "generally always," a different nurse came. "Don't ask me their names," she said. Mrs. D had found a physician in Bixford in the same way that she found a housekeeper – through her sisters, who as licensed practical nurses, had worked for the physician. She said that the doctor had no explanation for her falls; she did not mention that she had undergone any diagnostic tests, and she had not traveled to Clarkton for health care. Mrs. D said this about one of her falls.

> I fell Sunday. I just laid there. Couldn't do nothin' else, until my sister came. I had this thing on [points to her LifeLine button], so I called and told them to call Betty (next-door sister). And she did. She came over. Then she called our other sister and brother-in-law, and they came in. They can get me up in no time. But I just can't get myself out of the floor. I hit my head, split it here. It bled quite a little. Betty tried to call the nurse from up at the place. [Your home care nurses?] Yes. She said they were supposed to be on 24-hour duty, but she couldn't get anything out of 'em at all. No answer. So they taped me together theirself. [Did you go to the doctor then?] Not until yesterday. Not very well gettin' in Sunday. We put ice packs on it. And he says, "You're doing all you can do".

Thus, her presenting need was to have immediate help from the on-call home-care nurse.

Unlike Mrs. D, Mrs. E, aged 91, was not concerned about accessibility to the home-care nurses, who had visited her three times after a recent hospitalization to monitor her status.

> They left their phone number on the receiver over there. But they told me if I needed them to call. Of course, they all knew me anyway. [Did you know them?] Yeah, I knew all of 'em. [How many different ones came?] Oh, different one ever' day, ever' time.

Mrs. E emphasized that the nurses were going to "keep my record," indicating a perception of continued accessibility to them in the event of need.

Mrs. E was under the care of a cardiologist affiliated with the public hospital in Clarkton; every 6 months he came to the clinic in Bixford that was affiliated with the public hospital.

> He comes here to the clinic. I don't go over there (to Clarkton). See, we don't have a hospital. We've got one here, but it's not running. We just have a clinic built over here (within six blocks). That's where I go now if I don't go to Clarkton.

However, Mrs. E reported a presenting need to get in touch with a doctor quickly. Once, she sought quick care from the local clinic, but she was told that she could not be seen.

> I blacked out last week when my son was here. He carried me in here and laid me down. I guess my pressure went too high. We called the doctor at the clinic. Susie called. My son got a-hold of Susie (a CWD, friend, and aide at a nursing home). But they didn't have time to see me that day. And that really made me mad. It's a wonder I didn't have a heart attack. Because the doctor had never turned me down in their lives, and that just hurt me. Said they could make it two-three weeks from now. Susie said, 'The woman could be dead in two-three weeks'. But they wouldn't see me that day. [What did you do?] Just stayed here at the house. Laid in bed the rest of the day.

Friends of Mrs. E had told her previously to go to the ER in Clarkton on
such occasions.

> I said, 'I can't, don't even get up there (to Clarkton) unless somebody takes me'. If
> someone had taken me, I would have went on to the emergency room. They have to see
> you then. I found that out in the old hospital over here. If you want a doctor, you go to
> the emergency room.

Indeed, Mrs. E had gone to the Clarkton public hospital by ambulance in
the past, but the recent introduction of 911 in Bixford had caused uncertainty; when she dialed the ambulance number, as usual, she reached "911."
The feasibility of traveling by private car was limited, because her son, who
was homeless and occasionally stayed with her, did not have a vehicle.
Furthermore, Susie, her CWD friend and most consistent helper, was not
comfortable driving in Clarkton.

> I know more about Clarkton than Susie does, I think. But she went to the hospital to
> pick up somebody, and I went with her. She's good driver, but she just don't like it. We
> ought to go get used to it, to get her used to Clarkton. I used to know Clarkton
> backwards, when I was about 17.

Mrs. E was planning to suggest pleasure trips to Clarkton to increase Susie's
comfort level in the event she would need to ask Susie to take her to the ER
there. Thus, her anticipatory need was getting a ride to the ER in Clarkton
without using an ambulance.

Unlike Mrs. E, Mrs. F, aged 93, was not concerned about reaching her
physician. After falling on her back porch, she crawled through her house
until she could pull up on a sturdy chair and reach a telephone. She called a
friend, who urged her to call her doctor, a female and an old friend. The
physician's office was at the old hospital, but Mrs. F did not go to the office.
Instead, she had an overnight house call. "Dr. Claven slept on the divan the
night I had my bad spell." Mrs. F also had good accessibility to her heart
specialist in Clarkton; a retired nurse and former neighbor, another long-
time friend in Bixford, drove her to Clarkton for her appointments.

However, Mrs. F had an anticipatory need for relief and supply; she was
very worried about losing her home-care nurses. Mrs. F had no mainstay, so
she had come to rely upon her RHs, the nurses and aides, for help with
chronic wound care, medications, and bathing, as well as daily interpersonal
contact. At Interview #5, she reported that the nurses had just closed the
case of her dearest friend.

> Then, my friend, Edith, she got a bad fall, and she was in the hospital for awhile. She
> says they're [nurses] not coming down like they were. I said, 'Well, I don't know why.
> They come here ever' day'. [Are you concerned that your nurses might stop coming?]

> Yes, I think they will. See, I've had this same thing (a wound) before, and as soon as it heals, why, they stop. [Have they said anything to you about it?] No, they haven't. But they're making a few changes up there though. Edith told me that. She's kind of up on everything. She's 95. So, no, I'm not sure how long I'll be here, just whenever they tell me. I don't try to interfere with, you know, anything, any of them. [Are you concerned that if the nurses weren't coming anymore that you wouldn't be able to stay here?] Well, I don't know. Because they're helping me a lot. I told the girl that came today, 'Well, honey, I'll just have to stay until you all tell me when you're stopping'.

Thus, Mrs. F was speculating that the nurses would close her case, just as they had done for her friend, and that the nurses' departure would spell the end of her life at home.

Thus, these six frail women, who were living in rural and urban MUAs, experienced either presenting needs, anticipatory needs, or both, about accessibility to health services. However, they did not refer to their health problems as direct causes of those needs. Instead, they referred to underlying issues such as uncertainty about the identity of the provider, inadequate interpersonal communication with providers, the loss of local health-care facilities, and dependence upon providers of unknown tenure.

DISCUSSION

Rather than understanding home-care need in the usual manner, as the "most immediate cause of health service use" (Andersen, 1968, p. 17), a different approach was taken in this study. I sought to discern the intentions of women who were receiving home-care services, but reported presenting or anticipatory needs for accessibility to providers and health services. In relation to those needs, certain intentions of the women were discerned from the data. The intentions pertained to mobilizing or retaining standby helpers at home, whereas other intentions pertained to communicating with health professionals in the community or obtaining health-related community services. Those intentions were linked to the overall goal to continue living at home alone, so they were understood as empirical facets of the experience of home care.

As is evident from the data, each woman's home-care experience was unique in many ways, just as each woman was unique. Accordingly, such studies are not designed to enable generalization of the findings; the six women are not viewed as representative of all older women residing in urban and rural places. However, with regard to understanding the complexity of the home-care experience, the importance of their inter-individual differences cannot be overstated. Even within the ANM tradition, scholars have noted that differences among older persons can transcend variables such as ethnic identity (Skinner, 1995) or residence location (Nyman, Sen, Chan, & Commins, 1991). Accordingly, researchers have been advised to compare rural people, for instance, rather than to compare urban and rural people (Cutler & Coward, 1989; Salmon, Nelson, & Rous, 1993). However, to more fully explore the theme of heterogeneity (Dannefer, 1988) in this small sample, the intentions of these six women are compared within and across categories of residence location and considered relative to residence in an MUA. Then new insights about accessibility are discussed, and a new parameter of access is proposed.

Rural–Urban Differences and Similarities

Transportation has been cited as a critical service need for all older persons, but particularly for those living in rural areas, where emergency transportation might be inadequate or non-existent. Rural volunteers have traditionally provided most of the passenger transportation. Accordingly, problems have arisen when there are few available volunteer drivers (Schauer & Weaver, 1994). The rural women in this study did not drive, and they each had a different situation with regard to emergency transportation and transportation to the city for health care. Mrs. D reported no need for transportation to the city; her doctor had not referred her, and she had not sought specialty care there. Mrs. F had a standing arrangement with her OCH to drive her to the city for specialty appointments. Mrs. F had received a flyer advising that a local person would provide transportation, but she did not know the family, so she had not inquired. Finally, Mrs. E expressed interest in securing the help of her CWD to provide emergency transportation to the city rather than taking an ambulance. Thus, Mrs. E and Mrs. F preferred to turn to standbys rather than seeking information about or using public transportation. None of the three rural women noted that the OATS bus was available in their rural town for transportation to appointments.

Compared to rural residents, "residents of urban areas can exercise more choice in meeting similar needs through a wider variety of resources" (Salmon et al., 1993, p. 665). Indeed, Mrs. B was aware of two options for transportation in the city, and due to her past problems with one option (the OATS bus), she was inclined to pursue the other. However, the simple fact of having a choice did not ameliorate her need for improved accessibility to Paratransit. Her perceptions of accessibility were influenced by the interlacing factors of awareness, knowledge, cost, and risk of burdening the mainstay, among others.

Like some other older persons, Mrs. B knew that a service was available, but she did not know whom to contact about the service (Capitman, 2003). For Mrs. B this gap in accessibility was particularly compelling, because as a former volunteer with the local Council on Aging, she had remained in contact with that agency. If familiarity with a clearinghouse is an indicator of potential access to service (Yeatts et al., 1992), then one might have expected that Mrs. B would have pursued her hunch about "transit" earlier. Her data reveal the contextual interface between awareness of a service, essential knowledge about it, and intent to seek assistance from it – an interface that is difficult to tap in quantitative studies of health services use.

Another issue for Mrs. B was the cost of transportation; in part because she had obtained rides for no cost, a dollar per ride was not a small sum. The desire to continue getting free rides from her mainstay was interwoven with worries about a potentially greater cost in the end. That is, by continuing to ask Sally for rides to the doctor, she risked adversely affecting Sally's willingness to help her with grocery shopping. Thus, in addition to cost, the contextual feature of keeping the helpers' circumstances in mind must be taken into account when health professionals encourage older persons to consider using a service. Few studies about elders' service use have incorporated appropriate measures of social support (Wolinsky & Johnson, 1991; Stoddart, Whitley, Harvey, & Sharp, 2002). This study shows that researchers should seek data about standby helpers in association with data about presenting and anticipatory needs for services.

In this small sample, keeping a regular home-care nurse was the only intention linked to both a presenting need and an anticipatory need. As a component of the phenomenon, keeping my helper, it was characteristic of women in both residence locations. Yet, within and across the residence groups, the women had quite different experiences in this regard. For one urban woman, Mrs. C, keeping a regular nurse was both an ongoing concern and as a future worry. Although there were a number of home-care agencies in the city, she did not reveal any knowledge of that situation, and she did not report a perception of being advantaged due to her urban location. When one home-care agency closed and ceased visits to her and another agency picked up the slack, Mrs. C was left wondering what had become of her "regular nurse." In contrast, Mrs. F, a rural woman, anticipated that she would experience a need for relief and supply once her regular home-care nurses ceased their visits. She knew that there was no other home-care agency in her rural town; if she lost those nurses; there was no one else to whom she could turn. However, although Mrs. F anticipated the loss of the nurses from the rural agency, Mrs. E expected that those very nurses would return when she needed them. Thus, Mrs. E and Mrs. F had different perceptions about the accessibility of nurses from the same rural agency.

There were also distinctions across the sample in perceptions that might be labeled interpersonal accessibility to the provider. Compared to Mrs. C (an urban woman) and Mrs. D (a rural woman who had relocated), Mrs. E had an immediate interpersonal connection to her home-care nurses. She had aged in place in her rural town, and she knew all of the nurses who visited her. In contrast, Mrs. C had been "jumping from nurse to nurse" and agency to agency, but at least she had a "regular" nurse, albeit a different "regular" nurse when the urban agencies changed the guard. Compared to Mrs. C and Mrs. E, Mrs. D was disadvantaged in interpersonal accessibility to the nurses. She did not know any of the home-care nurses, and different nurses visited her at random, making it less likely that she would get to know them. Although rural communities "may comprise people who know one another quite well" (McKinley & Netting, 1994, p. 39), older persons like Mrs. D who relocate, even to their communities of origin, are not necessarily acquainted. Factors that dampened her interpersonal accessibility to the nurses might have adversely influenced her accessibility to the on-call nurse when she fell and cut her head.

Thus, although researchers have used the dichotomy of formal–informal care to compare the home-care use of older adults living in rural and urban areas (Coward & Dwyer, 1991; Krout, 1988), this study reveals that such comparisons are inherently problematic. There are nuances of informality tangled within the "formal" care provided by an agency; such nuances vary for individuals in the same community, and they change or remain static over time. Home-care nursing is provided out of the same agency by the same nurses to persons who know the nurses as friends and to persons who think of the nurses as strangers. Leaving aside the formal–informal dichotomy, researchers should further explore how differences in interpersonal accessibility influence expectations of and satisfaction with care among individuals in a geographic area who have providers from the same agency.

Possible Influences of Residence in an MUA

Some presenting and anticipatory needs of the women might have been linked to their residence in an MUA. For instance, Mrs. C tried to reach the doctor quickly only to spend an afternoon on "wait-timing," while she was in terrible pain. Her residence in an urban MUA might have been contextual to this concern; on any given day, many clients in an urban MUA might seek advice by telephone from a limited number of physicians. Her physician told her directly that other clients had experienced similar problems. However, findings of a recent study suggest that such problems are not limited to older persons residing in MUAs. Among other indicators of declining quality of primary care from 1998 to 2000, older persons insured by Medicare reported decreased access to the doctor when they were ill or when they sought advice by telephone (Montgomery et al., 2004). In the case of Mrs. C, the physician mentioned that the problem should be investigated. Beyond that, practitioners should work to ensure that it does not occur. In addition to analyzing changes in survey data over time (Montgomery et al., 2004), researchers could conduct focus groups with older persons to explore issues of interpersonal accessibility to primary care providers. Improving clients' perceptions of accessibility is important; favorable perceptions of "interpersonal aspects of care" (Montgomery et al., 2004, p. 996) have been linked to improved clinical outcomes (Stewart, 1995).

Although there was little evidence that the needs and associated intentions of the urban women were influenced by their residence in an MUA, the situations of the rural women were more compelling in this regard. Like other older rural women, the three rural women in this study conveyed the idea that "staying close to shore" (Porter, 1998b, p. 25) for health care appealed to them. Each woman reported a situation when she might have accessed an ER in Bixford, had one been available. Instead, the women were monitored and tended at home. The standby helpers of Mrs. D and Mrs. E stood in for the health-care providers that they might have accessed at a local hospital. Compared to Mrs. D and Mrs. E (and to the majority of Medicare recipients whose data were analyzed by Montgomery et al., 2004, Mrs. F had more direct interpersonal accessibility to her primary provider. Without the resource of a local hospital, where Mrs. F might have been observed overnight, her physician devised a very personal way to monitor her.

The interaction between Mrs. F and her friend, the physician, should not be the sole focus in this incident, however. As related earlier, the first call that Mrs. F made after her fall was to an older female friend, an OCH who often advised Mrs. F when she had questions. Mrs. F credited that conversation as a factor in her decision to contact the physician. When older persons confer with family or friends about whether a health event warrants medical care, they are twice as likely to contact a physician (Hurwicz & Berkanovic, 2002). Thus, although the rural women lost the opportunity to have local hospital care, they obtained voluntary help from their standbys during health-related crises. It is noteworthy that some standbys had some training in health care.

There is little information about how citizens of rural communities change their patterns of interaction around health matters when rural hospitals close. As Redford and Severns (1994) observed, it is necessary to consider the influence of characteristics of rural residents and rural communities upon patterns of access to services. Ethnographic studies are needed to describe changes in the provision of local health care in small rural towns where hospitals have closed. Researchers should explore situations in which rural persons call upon local health care workers, including nursing home aides, nurses, and physicians, because there are no other options.

Need as Presenting and Need as Anticipatory

This longitudinal study afforded a new prospective, subjective view of need for health services. Need was understood relative to perceived accessibility to services, and it was captured in both presenting and anticipatory frames of time. This bi-tonal perspective on need is akin to the distinction drawn by McKinley and Netting (1994), within a discussion of information and referral for older rural adults, on "inreach" versus "outreach" (p. 30). They defined inreach as "people calling for help in a situation of immediate importance for 'fixing'" (p. 30). In contrast, outreach was viewed as "people receiving information for planning before a need arises" (p. 30). As McKinley and Netting (1994) emphasized, practitioners must discern whether the needs of any one older person, at any given time, are relevant to inreach, outreach, or both. However, the accessibility of many older persons, including the six women in this study, to the persons and agencies who might provide inreach and outreach information, is a fundamental problem (Capitman, 2003; McKinley & Netting, 1994; Yeatts et al., 1992).

Understanding the need for health services from ongoing and prospective postures, as well as from a retrospective stance, has potential utility for both research and practice. Researchers can work forward to discern the aides and barriers older persons encounter as they to achieve their intentions. Providers can ask older persons to consider the problems that they might face for which they might need additional help. To tap this information, older women can be asked to share their worries about being able to continue living alone. Practitioners can then work alongside older persons, ascertaining the perceived barriers to obtaining help and enabling the intentions of older persons to use services that might benefit them.

However, the design and conduct of this study suggests a model whereby persons other than home-care practitioners could be helpful to older women who face presenting and anticipatory needs for services. During this longitudinal study with one-on-one contacts over time, considerable rapport developed, and participants felt comfortable revealing some needs. For instance, as noted earlier, I explored what Mrs. B knew about her second option for transportation. Realizing then that she knew part of the name of the resource, but not all of it, I felt compelled to fill in the blank. Then she affirmed that she had some information "to go on." From a policy perspective it would be useful to initiate a program, free to older recipients of Medicaid, in which trained lay visitors "sit and visit" on regular occasions with older women with no strings attached, to explore their needs for health services and to offer information.

A New Parameter of Access

This study afforded the opportunity to explore in depth and reveal some concerns of six frail women about their personal accessibility to providers and to health services. The situations of these women were quite complex; they defy categorization in a schema such as "no barriers, not aware of service, and other barriers" (Lun, 2004, p. 128).

However, throughout the presentation and discussion of findings, I mentioned evidence that participants were weighing the feasibility of a particular intention. This notion has not appeared elsewhere in the literature, to my knowledge. In their conceptual model, Yeatts et al. (1992) proposed that access is associated with convenience of a service with regard to time or place; earlier, Aday and Andersen (1974) had mentioned convenience as a parameter of access. However, in this study, the perception of accessibility was not so much a matter of personal convenience as it was a matter of what seemed feasible for the older woman (with or without her standby helpers) to manage in a given situation.

Thus, I suggest that underlying transportation, affordability, and availability of services – the three parameters of access specified by Yeatts et al. (1992) – there is a contextual, personally graduated parameter of feasibility. The underlying need of Mrs. B for enhanced accessibility to a transportation service (one that would provide relatively quick, inexpensive, and attentive help akin to a personal driver) would have to be met before she could meet her need for transportation and lighten the load for her mainstay. She had to consider the feasibility of the new option relative to all of those other factors. Personal perceptions of accessibility, including presenting concerns and worries about future access to health services, are delimited, in part, by what seems feasible to the older woman. More exploratory study is needed of how older women come to understand whether it is feasible to use a health service. Clearly, the presenting and anticipatory needs for accessibility to health services reported by the women in this small study were associated with their perceptions of what might be feasible for their stand-bys. Exploration of interfaces between the feasibilities for service use perceived by older persons and those perceived by their key helpers is a fertile and necessary realm for further descriptive research.

In conclusion, it is not claimed that residence in an MUA was an evident influence upon the phenomena of mobilizing my helper or keeping my helper; for the rural women, living in an MUA might have been an influence on the phenomenon of securing the help that I might need down the road. Comparative studies should be done of the presenting and anticipated health service needs for older women who live in MUAs and those who do not live in MUAs to determine if certain presenting and future needs for accessibility are directly relevant to residence in an MUA.

However, presenting and anticipatory needs for accessibility to health services are surely not unique to older women who reside in MUAs. As noted earlier, two factors associated with designation of an MUA, old age and low income (Bureau of Health Professions, n.d.), are particularly relevant to older women without regard to residence location. More women live longer than men, and older women are more likely to live alone on marginal incomes (Katz et al., 2000). In fact, Wright, Andres, and Davidson (1996) observed that in a service area, the "percentage of elders with Medicare and Medicaid insurance may be a good proxy for potential underservice" (p. 306). The circumstances that might be associated with being underserved, then, are more likely to be part of the personal–social context for old, poor women, regardless of whether they live in an MUA. Qualitative researchers must continue exploring the nature of those circumstances to offer new insights about the unique experiences of those women, to suggest new approaches for practitioners, and to raise new questions for further research.

ACKNOWLEDGMENTS

This research was funded by NIH/NINR 5 R29 NR04364-02, awarded to Dr. Eileen J. Porter.

REFERENCES

Aday, L. A., & Andersen, R. (1974). A framework for the study of access to medical care. *Health Services Research, 9*, 208–220.

Andersen, R. (1968). *A behavioral model of families use of health services Research Series 25.* Chicago, IL: The University of Chicago Center for Health Administration Studies.

Andersen, R. M., & Newman, J. (1973). Societal and individual determinants of medical care utilization in the United States. *Milbank Memorial Fund Quarterly, 51*, 95–124.

Arfken, C. L., Lach, H. W., Birge, S. J., & Miller, J. P. (1994). The prevalence and correlates of fear of falling in elderly persons living in the community. *American Journal of Public Health, 84*, 565–570.

Auchincloss, A. H., Van Nostrand, J. F., & Ronsaville, D. (2001). Access to health care for older persons in the United States: Personal structural and neighborhood characteristics. *Journal of Aging & Health, 13*, 329–354.

Barusch, A. S. (1994). *Older women in poverty: Private lives and public policies.* New York: Springer.

Benjamin, A. E. (1992). An overview of in-home health and supportive services for older persons. In: M. G. Ory & A. P. Duncker (Eds), *In-home care for older people* (pp. 9–52). Newbury Park, CA: Sage.

Branch, L. G., Wettle, T. T., Scherr, P. H., Cook, N. R., Evans, D. H., Hebert, L. E., Masland, E. N., Keough, M. E., & Taylor, J. O. (1988). A prospective study of incident comprehensive medical home use among the elderly. *American Journal of Public Health, 78*, 255–259.

Bureau of Health Professions, Health Resources and Services Administration, U.S. Department of Health and Human Services. (n.d.). *Guidelines for medically underserved area and population designation.* Retrieved March 5, 2005 from http://www.bphc.hrsa.gov/databases/newmua/

Bureau of Primary Health Care, Health Resources and Services Administration, U.S. Department of Health and Human Services. (n.d.). MUA/MUP: Medically underserved areas/medically underserved populations. Retrieved March 5, 2005 from http://bhpr.hrsa.gov/shortage/muaguide.htm

Calsyn, R. J., & Winter, J. P. (2000). Predicting different types of service use by the elderly: The strength of the behavioral model and the value of interaction terms. *Journal of Applied Gerontology, 19*, 284–303.

Capitman, J. (2003). Effective coordination of medical and supportive services. *Journal of Aging and Health, 15*, 124–164.

Chappell, N. L. (1994). Home care research: What does it tell us? *The Gerontologist, 34*, 116–120.

Choi, N. G. (1994). Patterns and determinants of social service utilization: Comparison of the childless elderly and elderly parents living with or apart from their children. *The Gerontologist, 34*, 353–362.

Comer, J., & Mueller, K. (1995). Access to health care: Urban–rural comparisons from a Midwestern agricultural state. *The Journal of Rural Health, 11*, 128–136.

Coward, R. T., & Dwyer, J. W. (1991). A longitudinal study of residential differences in the composition of the helping networks of impaired elders. *Journal of Aging Studies, 5*, 391–407.

Coward, R. T., McLaughlin, D. K., Duncan, R. P., & Bull, C. N. (1994). An overview of health and aging in rural America. In: R. T. Coward, C. N. Bull, G. Kukulka & J. M. Galliher (Eds), *Health services for rural elders* (pp. 1–32). New York: Springer.

Cutler, R. T., & Coward, S. J. (1989). Informal and formal health care systems for the rural old. *Health Services Research, 23*, 785–806.

Dannefer, D. (1988). What's in a name: An account of the neglect of variability in the study of aging. In: J. E. Birren & V. L. Bengtson (Eds), *Emergent theories of aging* (pp. 356–384). New York, NY: Springer.

Ettner, S. L. (1994). The effect of the Medicaid home care benefit on long-term care choices of the elderly. *Economic Inquiry, 32*, 103–127.

Forbes, S., & Hoffart, N. (1998). Elders' decision-making regarding the use of long-term care services: A precarious balance. *Qualitative Health Research, 8*, 736–750.

Gillanders, W. R., & Buss, T. F. (1993). Access to medical care among the elderly in rural Northeastern Ohio. *The Journal of Family Practice, 37*, 349–355.

Grabbe, L., Demi, A. S., Whittington, F., Jones, J. M., Branch, L. G., & Lambert, R. (1995). Functional status and the use of formal home care in the year before death. *Journal of Aging and Health, 7*, 339–364.

Gubrium, J. A., & Sankar, A. (1990). Introduction. In: J. A. Gubrium & A. Sankar (Eds), *The home care experience: Ethnography and policy* (pp. 7–15). Newbury Park, CA: Sage.

Hobbs, F. B., & (with Damon, B. L. (1996). *65+ in the United States*. U.S. Department of Commerce, Economics and Statistics Administration, Bureau of the Census. Current population reports, Series no. P23–190). Washington, DC: US Government Printing Office.

Hurwicz, M.-L., & Berkanovic, E. (2002). *Do elderly Medicare recipients contact physicians appropriately? Journal of Gerontology: Social Sciences, 57B*, S187–S194.

Husserl, E. (1962). In: W.R.B. Gibson (Trans.), *Ideas: General introduction to pure phenomenology*. London: Collier–Macmillan (Original work published 1913).

Jenkins, C. L., & Laditka, S. B. (2003). A comparative analysis of disability measures and their relation to home health care use. *Home Health Care Services Quarterly, 22*(1), 21–37.

Kane, R. A., & Kane, R. L. (1987). *Long-term care: Principles, programs and policies*. New York: Springer.

Kart, C. S. (1991). Variation in long-term care service use by aged Blacks. *Journal of Aging and Health, 3*, 511–526.

Katz, S. J., Kabeto, M., & Langa, K. M. (2000). Gender disparities in the receipt of home care for elderly people with disability in the United States. *Journal of the American Medical Association, 284*, 3022–3027.

Krout, J. A. (1988). Rural versus urban differences in elderly parents' in-person contact with their children. *The Gerontologist, 28*, 198–203.

Love, D., & Lindquist, P. (1995). The geographical accessibility of hospitals to the aged: A geographic information systems analysis within Illinois. *HSR: Health Services Research, 29*, 629–651.

Luborsky, M. R., & Rubinstein, R. L. (1995). Sampling in qualitative research: Rationale, issues, and methods. *Research on Aging, 17*, 89–113.

Lun, M. W. A. (2004). The effects of race and gender on predicting in-home and community-based service use by older adults. In: J.J. Kroenfeld (Ed.), *Chronic care, health* care systems, and services integration: Vol. 4. Research in the sociology of health care (pp. 121–139). Oxford, UK: Elsevier.

McKinley, A. H., & Netting, F. E. (1994). Information and referral: Targeting the rural elderly. In: J. A. Krout (Ed.), *Providing community-based services to the rural elderly* (pp. 23–41). Thousand Oaks, CA: Sage.

Miner, S. (1995). Racial differences in family support and formal service utilization among older persons: A nonrecursive model. *Journal of Gerontology: Social Sciences, 50B*, 143–153.

Mitchell, J., & Krout, J. A. (1998). Discretion and service use among older adults: The behavioral model revisited. *The Gerontologist, 38*, 159–168.

Montgomery, J. E., Irish, J. T., Wilson, I. B., Chang, H., Li, A. C., Rogers, W. H., & Safran, D. G. (2004). Primary care experiences of Medicare beneficiaries, 1998 to 2000. *Journal of General Internal Medicine, 19*, 991–998.

Mui, A. C., Choi, N. G., & Monk, A. (1998). *Long-term care and ethnicity*. Westport, CT: Auburn House.

Neufeldt, V. (Ed.) (1997). *Webster's new world college dictionary*, (3rd ed). New York: Macmillan.

Nyman, J. A., Sen, A., Chan, B. Y., & Commins, P. P. (1991). Urban/rural differences in home health patients and services. *The Gerontologist, 31*, 457–466.

Penrod, J. D., Harris, K. M., & Kane, R. L. (1994). Informal care substitution: What we don't know can hurt us. *Journal of Aging and Social Policy, 6*(4), 21–33.

Porter, E. J. (1994). Older widows' experience of living alone at home. *Image: Journal of Nursing Scholarship, 26*, 19–24.

Porter, E. J. (1995a). The life-world of older widows: The context of lived experience. *Journal of Women & Aging, 7*(4), 31–46.

Porter, E. J. (1995b). A phenomenological alternative to the 'ADL Research Tradition'. *Journal of Aging and Health, 7*, 24–45.

Porter, E. J. (1998a). On 'being inspired' by Husserl's phenomenology: Reflections on Omery's exposition of phenomenology as a method for nursing research. *Advances in Nursing Science, 21*(1), 16–28.

Porter, E. J. (1998b). "Staying close to shore": A context for older rural widows' use of health care. *Journal of Women & Aging, 10*(4), 25–39.

Porter, E. J. (1999). Defining the accessible population for a phenomenological study. *Western Journal of Nursing Research, 21*, 796–804.

Porter, E. J. (2000). Research on home care utilization: A critical analysis of the preeminent approach. *Journal of Aging Studies, 14*(1), 25–38.

Porter, E.J. (in press). Older widows' experience of home care. *Nursing Research*.

Porter, E. J., Ganong, L. H., Drew, N., & Lanes, T. I. (2004). A new typology of home care helpers. *The Gerontologist, 44*, 750–759.

Redford, L. J., & Severns, A. B. (1994). Home health services in rural America. In: J. A. Krout (Ed.), *Providing community-based services to the rural elderly* (pp. 221–242). Thousand Oaks, CA: Sage.

Rubinstein, R. L., Lubben, J. E., & Mintzer, J. E. (1994). Social isolation and social support: An applied perspective. *Journal of Applied Gerontology, 13*, 58–72.

Salmon, M. A. P., Nelson, G. M., & Rous, S. G. (1993). The continuum of care revisited: A rural perspective. *The Gerontologist, 33*, 658–666.

Sandelowski, M. (1995). Sample size in qualitative research. *Research in Nursing & Health, 18*, 179–183.

Schauer, P. M., & Weaver, P. (1994). Rural elder transportation. In: J. A. Krout (Ed.), *Providing community-based services to the rural elderly* (pp. 42–64). Thousand Oaks, CA: Sage.

Schutz, A., & Luckmann, T. (1973). In: R.M. Zaner, & H.T. Engelhardt, Jr., (Trans.), *The structures of the life-world.* Evanston, IL: Northwestern University Press.

Skinner, J. H. (1995). Ethnic/racial diversity in long-term care use and services. In: Z. Harel & R. E. Dunkle (Eds), *Matching people with services in long-term care* (pp. 49–71). New York: Springer.

Soldo, B. J. (1985). In-home services for the dependent elderly: Determinants of current use and implications for future demand. *Research on Aging, 7,* 281–304.

Spiegelberg, H. (1994). *The phenomenological movement: A historical introduction* (3rd revised and enlarged ed.). Dordrecht, The Netherlands: Kluwer Academic Press.

Stewart, M. A. (1995). Effective physician–patient communication and health outcomes: A review. *Canadian Medical Association Journal, 152,* 1423–1433.

Stoddart, H., Whitley, E., Harvey, I., & Sharp, D. (2002). *What determines the use of home care services by elderly people? Health and Social Care in the Community, 10,* 348–360.

U.S. Department of Commerce, Bureau of the Census (1992). *Census of population, 1990: Summary of social, economic, and housing characteristics: Missouri* (GPO 1990 CPH-5-27). Washington, DC: Government Printing Office.

Wallace, S. P., Levy-Storm, L., Kington, R. S., & Andersen, R. M. (1998). The persistence of race and ethnicity in the use of long-term care. *Journal of Gerontology: Social Sciences, 49,* 253–263.

White-Means, S. I., & Rubin, R. M. (2004). Is there equity in the home health care market? Understanding racial patterns in the use of formal home health care. *Journal of Gerontology: Social Sciences, 59B,* S200–S229.

Wolinsky, F. D. (1994). Health services utilization among older adults: Conceptual, measurement, and modeling issues in secondary analysis. *The Gerontologist, 34,* 470–475.

Wolinsky, F. D., & Johnson, R. J. (1991). The use of health services by older adults. *Journal of Gerontology, 46*(6, S3), 45–57.

Wolinsky, F. D., & Johnson, R. J. (1992). Widowhood, health status, and use of health services by older adults: A cross-sectional and prospective approach. *Journal of Gerontology: Social Sciences, 47,* S8–S16.

Wright, R. A., Andres, T. L., & Davidson, A. J. (1996). Finding the medically underserved: A need to revise the federal definition. *Journal of Health Care for the Poor & Underserved, 7,* 296–307.

Yeatts, D., Crow, T., & Folts, E. (1992). Service use among low-income minority elderly: Strategies for overcoming barriers. *The Gerontologist, 32,* 24–32.

EFFECTS OF MANAGED HEALTH INSURANCE ON PHYSICAL AND EMOTIONAL WELL-BEING

D. Clayton Smith, James W. Grimm and
Zachary W. Brewster

ABSTRACT

A random sample of insured adults (n = 134) tests the effects of insurance on respondents' emotional and physical health. Results showed that being married and being widowed improved physical health while having no religious identification heralded less emotional distress. Preferred Provider Organization services satisfaction was related to better physical health. Respondents in households that restructured themselves to acquire or maintain health coverage also reported more emotional distress than those in households without such problems. Implications of our results regarding improving insurance programs and the effects of marital status and the lack of religious affiliation upon adults' health are discussed.

INTRODUCTION

Assertions that the U.S. health care system is in a state of crisis have become ubiquitous. The sources of such concerns are founded in rising medical

Health Care Services, Racial and Ethnic Minorities and Underserved Populations: Patient and Provider Perspectives
Research in the Sociology of Health Care, Volume 23, 133–155
ISSN: 0275-4959/doi:10.1016/S0275-4959(05)23007-7

costs, increasing insurance premiums, increasing out-of-pocket medical expenditures, and the growing number of uninsured or underinsured individuals in the United States (Gould, 2004; Holahan & Wang, 2004; Mechanic, 2004; Morton, 2004; Shearer, 1998). Confusion and concern about health care in the United States are further exacerbated by scholarly reports that both support (Sullivan, 1999) and negate (Miller & Luft, 2002) anecdotal views that the quality of health care provided by managed care plans is, at best, equivalent and often inferior to care provided under traditional indemnity or fee-for-service plans. While these debates concerning various aspects of health care in the United States are ongoing, disparities in access to health insurance and variation in adequacy of coverage have been identified as key factors in contributing to health care inequalities in the U.S. (Comer & Mueller, 1992; Morton, 2004; Plichta & Weisman, 1995).

According to a recent report released by the U.S. Census Bureau (2003), an estimated 43.6 million individuals were living without insurance in 2002. Among the uninsured the economically deprived and racial/ethnic minorities continue to be over-represented. When considering the effects of insurance on health behavior, studies have shown that compared *with* insured individuals, those who lack such coverage are less likely to consult a physician when ill, use outpatient health services, receive preventive health services, and follow through with recommended treatment plans (McLeer, Anwar, Herman, & Maquiling, 1989; Taylor, Cohen, & Machlin, 2001). While few would argue against the health enhancements that health insurance provides the effects of health insurance alone on health outcomes remain uncertain.

For instance, previous studies concerning the effects of private health insurance on health outcomes have focused upon aggregate comparisons between insured and uninsured people (Donelan et al., 1996; Ross & Mirowsky, 2000; Seccombe & Amey, 1995). Such research has found more support for insurance reducing a household's health care payment problems than for insurance improving health (Ross & Mirowsky, 2000). Even with insurance, the degree to which household's health payment problems are alleviated varies considerably from one plan to the next. A nonprofit consumers union report indicated that in addition to those without insurance, an estimated 31 million individuals are annually underinsured, spending more than 10% of their annual income on health care and risking financial disaster if major illness strikes (Shearer, 1998; Weitz, 2004). Thus, when researchers controlled for socioeconomic status and other health enhancing resources, such as education, they found few positive private health insurance net effects upon health (Franks, Clancy, Gold, & Nutting, 1993;

Rogers, Hummer, & Nam, 1999; Ross & Mirowsky, 2000). While studies focusing upon aggregate comparisons between insured and uninsured are important, they do not address the impediments to health care that individuals *with* insurance encounter under managed care, nor do these studies speak to the consequences of such impediments on health outcomes among the underinsured or precariously insured. Specifically, several methodological problems exist concerning private health insurance effects by aggregate comparisons of the insured and the uninsured.

First, economic resources, education, and lifestyle confound the effects of private health insurance and personal health (Ross & Mirowsky, 2000). Second, prior research suggests that managed insurance programs provide better services for preventive care than for chronic or advanced illness (Bodenheimer, 1996; Chin & Harrigill, 1999; Friedman, 1997; Kerr, Hays, Mitchinson, Lee, & Siu, 1999; Wyn, Collins, & Brown, 1997). Third, recent research on health resource mobilization highlights the importance of examining the intersection of insurance, health-related resources, and household needs (Grimm & Brewster, 2002; Lin, 2001; Ross & Mirowsky, 2000). This step isolates the effects of private health insurance on health outcomes. Fourth, private health insurance effects are not fully accessible when individuals are the units of analysis. The full range of households' health needs must be taken into account to assess if and how well health-related resources, including those provided by health insurance, enable households to obtain necessary care (Grimm & Brewster, 2002; Lin, 2001; Ross & Mirowsky, 2000; Seccombe & Amey, 1995).

This study works to isolate the effects of managed private health insurance upon people's physical and emotional health. We will attempt to avoid previous methodological problems in several ways. First, the confounding effects of household socioeconomic status and composition will be controlled, as will respondent characteristics, such as educational attainment, age, and gender. Second, we will control for households' health status and health needs for the previous year by controlling for preventive measures, such as taking part in health screenings as well as usage of health services such as rehabilitative services and home health care. In particular, we will control for this wide range of service needs to assess the potential threshold effects of managed health insurance suggested by recent studies. Third, we will disaggregate insurance effects by considering separately problems in the past year that households' have experienced with respect to insurance services, out-of-pocket expenses in paying for services, administrative problems in arranging and obtaining health care from physicians, and household adaptation strategies used to cope with insufficient insurance resources.

BACKGROUND

Previous studies have found that people with private health insurance report fewer problems in paying for health care than do uninsured people (Donelan et al., 1996; Ross & Mirowsky, 2000; Seccombe & Amey, 1995). While insurance undoubtedly plays a major role in this difference, efforts to measure insurance effects are confounded by the fact that the poor and near poor have more numerous and more serious health problems (Seccombe & Amey, 1995). This reality is particularly problematic for the working poor who lack access to Medicare. These economically disadvantaged people are unlikely to have private health insurance even if they qualify for it. Moreover, Medicaid provisions for those living in poverty are insufficient to address adequately their longer-term health problems (Ross & Mirowsky, 2000; Ross & Wu, 1995, 1996). Thus, the economically disadvantaged are more likely to pay for their medical care out of their own pocket and more likely to put off seeking medical attention until conditions become serious.

For those above the poverty line, health insurance comes as a benefit of employment. Thus, access to work-sponsored insurance plans makes more difference in resolving health care payment problems than increases in income, once the poverty line is crossed (Mirowsky & Hu, 1996). Still, among people with private managed health insurance, there is increasing evidence that people with multiple and longer-term health problems, including the elderly, are served less well than those healthier people with few needs beyond an annual checkup (Kerr et al., 1999; Schlesinger, Gray, & Perreira, 1997; Ware, Bayliss, Rogers, Kosinski, & Tarlov, 1996; Wyn et al., 1997; Young & Lowe, 1997; Zautcke, Fraker, Hart, & Stevens, 1997). Recent studies also have shown that annual private managed health insurance contracting involves cost-based competition, and that renegotiations may suddenly disrupt and/or prohibit patients' relationships with their primary care providers as well as other health care professionals. These disruptions in service continuity may prohibit individuals from obtaining necessary care, including treatment for serious or chronic illnesses (Furlong & Wilken, 2001; Kronenfeld, 2001; Ware et al., 1996; Young & Lowe, 1997; Zautcke et al., 1997).

While uninsured people statistically are more likely to report problems in paying for health care, previous studies have established that most people who report problems in paying for health care services are privately insured (Donelan et al., 1996; Marshall, 2001; Seccombe & Amey, 1995). Increasingly, formerly insured workers experience disruptions in employment due to layoffs, job loss, insufficient tenure for coverage, and cutbacks in health care coverage. These factors lead to interruptions and suspensions of health insurance and access to affordable health care (Furlong & Wilken, 2001; Kronenfeld, 2001; Marshall, 2001). For many insured and formerly insured households, difficulties in paying for health care involve the usual illnesses and injuries among children, the ailments that develop as household members age, and the additional physical and emotional problems that household members experience due to their own caregiving efforts (Marshall, 2001). The physical and emotional health of household caregivers is especially jeopardized when an elderly family member is disabled and unable to provide basic self-care (Chumbler, Grimm, Cody, & Beck, 2003; Marshall, 2001; Young & Lowe, 1997; Zautcke et al., 1997). Increasingly, households with elderly members will face mounting problems in paying for coverage and services (Furlong & Wilken, 2001; Marshall, 2001). These are some specific patterns of needs and strained resources among the precariously insured.

Recent trends in the managerial strategies and structural organization of managed private health insurance have increasingly delimited, or rationed, the health care services available to subscribers (Furlong & Wilken, 2001; Kronenfeld, 2001). Annual renegotiations now include the types of services available (or excluded) for common ailments, and the range of providers accessible to patients/consumers (Kronenfeld, 2001). For example, managed care services are often provided based on statistically developed health outcome protocols indicating the most cost-effective ways of treating various ailments and illnesses. Such standardized treatment plans often exclude considerations of alternative procedures, or at a minimum, make these alternative considerations too costly to pursue (Vandenburgh, 2001). This type of rationing has considerably reduced physicians' discretion in providing treatment options that have traditionally been available to patients seeking health care (Kronenfeld, 2001). Annual health care contracting increasingly occurs primarily under competition for pricing that may unexpectedly alter and disrupt both doctor/patient relationships and treatment plans (Kronenfeld, 2001; Vandenburgh, 2001). In response to these trends in health care provision, an active patients/consumers' rights movement has resulted in many states passing legislation to regulate various aspects of managed care, especially the rights of patients to choose their treatment options and their primary care providers, and to create state offices to handle consumers' complaints (Kronenfeld, 2001).

The trends have increased the number of complaints from both patients and physicians (Kronenfeld, 2001). These complaints fall into four basic types: coverage and provider services problems, dissatisfaction with out-of-pocket expenses and pricing, household problems in paying for health care, administrative delays, and other problems related to physicians' services (Bodenheimer, 1996; Chin & Harrigill, 1999; Friedman, 1997; Kerr et al., 1999; Wyn et al., 1997; Young & Lowe, 1997; Zautcke et al., 1997). Both patients and physicians are less satisfied when they perceive that their choices of treatment and providers, especially primary care physicians, are restricted (Bodenheimer, 1996; Friedman, 1997; Kerr et al., 1999). Moreover, health care consumers, who are given more delimited options, increasingly complain about the higher costs of health insurance including premiums, deductibles, and other charges (Bodenheimer, 1996; Friedman, 1997). In addition, various types of treatment delays have been the focus of increasing complaints, especially with respect to common health needs such as annual screens (Chin & Harrigill, 1999). Research on health-related communication has also shown increasing complaints by both patients and providers involved with managed care plans (Kerr et al., 1999; Schlesinger et al., 1997). In this study, we attempt to address the potential effects of some experiential contexts behind such complaints upon physical and emotional health.

HYPOTHESES

In this study, we test the relationship between type of insurance and physical impairment and emotional difficulties. However, our study is unique in that we test four potential mediating effects that represent aspects of households' problems with managed care in relation to health needs: coverage and service problems, consumer cost problems, administrative and communication problems, and the adaptive actions of household members, which are necessitated by major household budgetary problems in paying for health care. While we do not expect that being privately insured will be related to health outcomes, when precursors are controlled we expect that each of the four types of managed care problems will be negatively related to health outcomes. We test the following hypotheses, controlling for health status, health resources, household composition, and respondents' education, age, and gender.

1. Being privately insured in a Preferred Provider Organization (PPO) or Health Maintenance Organization (HMO) is not related to physical impairment or to self-reported emotional distress.
2. People who in the past year have experienced more private insurance coverage and service-related problems (consumers cost problems,

administrative and communication problems, and household budgetary difficulties requiring adaptive efforts to get and keep health insurance) will have more physical impairments and higher self-reported emotional distress than people who have not experienced such service problems.

METHODS

Research Context

Our community health survey data were obtained from a randomly selected sample of households ($n = 182$) in Warren County, Kentucky. The county has a population of about 100,000, less than half of which reside in Bowling Green, the regional, cultural, and economic center. Such a county is ideal for assessing managed care effects without the confounding problem of having fewer physicians available under any circumstances (AMA, 2001). Random digit dialing (RDD) was used by the WKU Social Research Laboratory to select the households in the Warren County Health Survey (WCHS). Randomized variation without substitution was used to select respondents within households.

Interviewers who were thoroughly familiar with the survey instrument and the follow-up specifications used standardized contact and follow-up scripts when contacting respondents and completing interviews that lasted an average of 20 min. Interviews were conducted between 6:30 and 8:30 p.m., Monday through Thursday, from mid-October through mid-November 1998. Up to six callbacks were made to reach desired respondents. An overall response rate of 48% is in the range of RDD procedures (Council for Marketing and Opinion Research, 1998). Remembering, however, that randomization of numbers and random selection of respondents were used for the entire sample is important for it ensures that the sample is representative despite its small size. Our sample represented the Warren County population based on comparisons with the 2000 U.S. Census data. There were no significant differences between our sample demographics and the demographics of the county with respect to age, marital status, ethnicity (i.e., proportion white), and gender.

Dependent Measures

Physical Impairment
Respondents' physical impairments were indexed by using a subset of physical functioning items in the Medical Outcomes Study's 36-item short form.

These measures have been widely used to assess physical health (Ware & Sherbourne, 1992). Items that made up this composite measure included how often in the last month the respondent's own health problems limited them in climbing stairs, bending or stooping, walking one block, walking several blocks, bathing or dressing, lifting or carrying groceries, moderate activities like moving a table or pushing a vacuum, heavy lifting or running, or doing normal work outside the home. Each component item was measured on a 5-point scale ranging from never (0) to every day (4). The WCHS respondents' answers had very high internal consistency ($\alpha = 0.94$). A little over half (56%) of the members of the sample had no impairments and half of those who did scored below seven. Therefore, the index is measuring moderate physical impairments. This limited number of physical impairments reported by WCHS respondents was expected since the sample mostly consisted of working aged adults 18 through 65.

Emotional Difficulties

Respondents' emotional difficulties were measured using self-reported answers to 10 items reflecting respondents' emotional states and general well-being during the month before their interview. The composite included both symptoms of depression and indicators of emotional well-being often used to measure people's general emotional states (Pugliesi, 1995). Using the same response categories as the physical impairments index, the emotional difficulties index reflected increased emotional distress. Index items included measures of unhappiness, lack of energy, nervousness, exhaustion, not being calm, tiredness, insomnia, self-reported stress, not being able to sleep well, and not being relaxed. The internal consistency of respondents' answers to these items was also very high ($\alpha = 0.83$).

Independent Measures

Type of Insurance

Using one question, "What type of plan do you have?", we obtained a measure of the respondents' managed health insurance program. Response categories included: Indemnity, PPO, HMO, Point of Service (POS) plan, Other, and Don't Know. Sixteen respondents (8.8%) did not have any type of health insurance and were dropped from the analysis. A significant minority (31.1%) said they had insurance but did not know what type of insurance currently covered them. The two most frequently reported managed care types, HMO (held by 28.0% of the respondents) and PPO (held by

24.8%), were developed into dummy variables in the analysis. These dummy variables allowed us to examine if HMO and PPO participants' health significantly differs from those who have other types of insurance.

Managed Health Care Experiences
The four measures of the households' managed health care experiences we use in this study were derived using a principal components factor analysis of items reflecting reports of household health care-related problems in the last year. The first, satisfaction with coverage and provider services (referred to as the Insurance Satisfaction Scale), included seven items. These items included satisfaction with health care coverage, service representatives, physicians in the plan, explanation of benefits, customer service personnel who answered questions about insurance, and the overall health insurance services in the plan. Respondents indicated their satisfaction on a 5-point scale running from 0, very dissatisfied, to 4, very satisfied. This measure corresponds closely to the physician and patient satisfaction with coverage and providers' services found in previous studies. This item also had a high degree of internal consistency ($\alpha = 0.88$).

The second measure of households' managed health care experiences dealt with respondents' specific dissatisfaction with the costs of managed health care including the deductible, monthly premium, and out-of-pocket expenses. This index of dissatisfaction with the cost of managed care services (referred to as the Fiscal Cost of Insurance Scale) was a factor-weighted scale consisting of having had what they considered an unreasonable deductible in the past year, being dissatisfied with the amount of deductibles, excessively high monthly premiums, and being dissatisfied with the out-of-pocket expenses. Although this second index is less internally consistent ($\alpha = 0.60$), it corresponds well to the complaints about the costs and pricing of managed health insurance found in previous research.

Eight indicators of dissatisfaction with various aspects of office visits with physicians over the last year comprised the third measure of household health care experiences with managed care. This index (referred to as the Insurance Alienation Scale) is used to indicate common problems household members face that alienate them from their health care professionals and is included to represent the administrative and communication complaints found in previous studies (Chin & Harrigill, 1999). This measure was a factor-weighted scale consisting of dissatisfaction with arranging and paying for physician's services that included office visits being too costly, difficult to schedule, taking too long to see physicians, being dissatisfied with patient/doctor relationships, leaving the doctors office without understanding the medications prescribed, being unable to see specialists because insurance would not cover the visits, and vagueness in what was covered by insurance. This index had considerable internal consistency ($\alpha = 0.72$).

A fourth factor emerged, that was composed of four items, that indicate the lengths that households are going to acquire and maintain adequate insurance. While previous research has not dealt with such problems, these are the sorts of issues that have been found in previous studies of disadvantaged households (Fitchen, 1981; Ross & Mirowsky, 2000). This factor-weighted index (referred to as the Insurance Adaptation Scale) included indicators of household efforts to restructure themselves to get and keep health insurance: someone taking a job for health benefits, someone taking a second job to pay for health care expenses, moving due to health issues, and costs preventing someone from seeing a doctor when they were ill ($\alpha = 0.48$). As a residual factor, the lower internal consistency was expected.

Control Variables

Individual Characteristics

Precursor variables in the present analyses included demographic traits of respondents such as educational attainment, age, gender, race, marital status, and employment status (see Table 1). Educational attainment was measured with five levels extending from less than high school up to postgraduate degree. Western Kentucky University is located in the county, and its influence is reflected by the fact that 48.8% of the respondents had completed at least 4 years of higher education.

Age was measured as a continuous variable. Over three-quarters of the sample were adults aged 25 through 64, and only 7.1% of the respondents were over the age of 65. The average age was 41.6 years. Race was coded white (1) and nonwhite (0). Gender was coded male (0) and female (1). Information in Table 1 shows that the sample was primarily white and consisted of more women than men.

Respondents' marital status was operationalized with a series of dummy variables including being married or cohabiting, being divorced or separated, and being widowed. Significant results for any of these categories will demonstrate that individuals falling into the category are significantly different from single respondents. Most of the respondents in the sample were married (61%).

Religious preferences were indicated by dummy variables including being Catholic, and being nonreligious. The comparison category for this variable

Table 1. Descriptive Statistics for Select Demographic and Household
Variables.

Variable	Categories	Percentage or Mean
Education	Less than high school	3.0%
	High school or GED	21.1%
	Junior college or trade school	27.1%
	Four-year college	34.3%
	Graduate school	14.5%
Age (mean)		41.6 years
Percentage female		57.1%
Percentage white		88.0%
Marital status	Married or cohabiting	61.2%
	Divorced or separated	10.9%
	Single	20.0%
	Widowed	7.9%
Religion	Catholic	10.3%
	No religion	5.5%
	Protestant or other religion	84.2%
Employment Status	Full-time or self-employed	69.3%
	Retired	12.0%
Household size (mean)		2.61 persons
Children in household (mean)		0.62 children
Household income	Less than $10,000	5.9%
	$10,000–$19,999	11.8%
	$20,000–$29,999	13.7%
	$30,000–$39,999	24.8%
	$40,000–$49,999	12.4%
	$50,000–$69,999	15.0%
	$70,000–$89,999	13.1%
	$90,000 or more	3.3%

is Protestant or another religion. Four out of five respondents were reportedly Protestant and only 4.2% of the sample indicated another religious
faith besides Protestant or Catholic.

Dummy variables, which included being employed full-time or being self-
employed, or being retired, were used to measure respondents' employment
status. Most respondents (69.3%) were full-time or self-employed. Only
12% of the sample was retired.

Household Characteristics
Additional precursors reflected household contextual variables that included
number of children less than 18 years of age, the number of people in the
household, and the annual household income, which was measured on an
8-point scale. Information in Table 1 indicates that nearly 69% of households reported annual family incomes of $30,000 or more.

Three measures of household health-related needs in the past year were
used. First, was a 7-item summated index of health screens that included
people getting blood pressure checks, cholesterol screens, physical exams,
eye exams, prostate checks, mammograms, and attending wellness seminars
($\alpha = 0.72$). Second, was a 3-item index of home health care activity that
included caring for a family member in the home for more than 2 weeks,
someone being treated in the home by health care professionals, and someone receiving occupational therapy ($\alpha = 0.36$). Rehabilitation services were
indexed by someone in the house being treated by a chiropractor, a message
therapist, or physical therapist ($\alpha = 0.49$). Finally, respondents' health-
related lifestyles were measured by a summated index consisting of daily
activity in the month before interviewing regarding one-half hour of exercise, not smoking, driving below the speed limit, and drinking moderately if
at all ($\alpha = 0.46$). These multiple measures were expected to differ because of
the scope of health problems across the adult life cycle. All were used in the
analyses to allow for such variation in drawing conclusions about the effects
of health insurance on health outcomes.

Analyses

To test our hypotheses we used multivariate regression analyses. As for the
multivariate analyses, the physical impairment and emotional difficulties
indices were regressed on all the precursors and the four measures of
household difficulties with managed care in a set of nested regression models. These nested regression models successively added: (1) household and
individual respondent demographic characteristics, the household health
screens index, the healthy behaviors index, and the insurance dummy variables; (2) the four indexes representing types of household difficulties with
managed care services; and (3) the home health care and the rehabilitation
services scales. In addition we checked for significant curvilinear effects and
interaction terms, using the forward entry procedure as suggested by
Cortina (1993) and Ganzach (1998). These interaction terms tested for potential differences in health care problems between insurance types.

As an additional exploratory check, a final regression model was run in which all the variables were entered into the equation and stepwise regression procedures were used to eliminate the consideration of predictors that successively were not statistically significant. The outcome of this final sequence of analysis included only those predictors that were statistically significant in explaining variation in impairment scores and self-reported well-being.

RESULTS

Results of the regression analyses used in the development of models of the variation in WCHS respondents' health outcomes appear in Tables 2 and 3. Concerning variation in physical impairments (Table 2), very few changes in the β coefficients were observed as new nests of variables were entered into regression model. In the full model, Model 4, differences in physical impairments among the WCHS respondents were contingent upon being widowed (-0.30), age (0.35), being female (0.18), households needing home health services (0.18), and the interaction between enrollment in PPOs and satisfaction with health insurance services (-0.20). In the stepwise-reduced model Model 5, a second marital status effect emerged. Respondents who were married or cohabiting (-0.21) and widowed respondents (-0.32) were both significantly less likely than single respondents to have physical impairments. The effect of age (0.43), being female (0.18), and households receiving home health services (0.20) remained statistically significant. While the full model (Model 4) explained 22% of the variation in physical impairments, the reduced model explained nearly a third of the variation in physical impairments with just one-fourth of the variables (adjusted $R^2 = 0.28$).

As predicted, we did not find a relationship between private insurance and physical impairments. There was some support for the second hypothesis in the full model, being satisfied with the service of PPOs (-0.20) was related to variation in impairments. That this insurance effect declined in the reduced model may reflect the importance of marital status and widowhood in relation to being enrolled in and receiving the services of insurance programs. Results also clearly show that private insurance effects are independent of the increased impairments that accompany aging and being female. Again the decline of this insurance effect in the final model supports the idea that such problems are fewer among married and formerly married

Table 2. Betas and Coefficients of Determination for Physical Impairments Scale Regressed upon Select Independent Variables ($n = 134$).

	Model 1	Model 2	Model 3	Model 4	Model 5
No. in household	−0.01	−0.01	−0.03	−0.01	
Household income	−0.06	−0.04	−0.03	−0.03	
Married	−0.06	−0.08	−0.12	−0.16	−0.21**
Divorced	0.08	0.08	0.06	0.04	
Widowed	−0.26*	−0.26*	−0.27**	−0.30**	−0.32***
Education	−0.09	−0.10	−0.08	−0.08	
Age	0.33**	0.32**	0.32**	0.35**	0.43***
Sex	0.16	0.17	0.16	0.18*	0.18*
No. of children	−0.13	−0.13	−0.09	−0.06	
White	−0.06	−0.03	−0.01	−0.00	
Catholic	−0.08	−0.07	−0.08	−0.08	
No religion	0.01	0.01	0.00	0.02	
Fully employed	0.00	0.01	0.03	0.05	
Retired	0.22	0.25*	0.23	0.22	0.16
Standard checkups scale	0.05	0.05	0.05	0.07	
Health behaviors scale	−0.09	−0.07	−0.06	−0.06	
PPO	0.06	0.07	0.07	0.12	
HMO	−0.03	−0.02	−0.01	−0.02	
Insurance satisfaction scale		−0.02	−0.02	0.03	
Fiscal cost of insurance scale		0.05	0.05	0.04	
Insurance alienation scale		0.03	0.01	−0.01	
Insurance adaptation scale		0.06	0.07	0.04	
Home care scale			0.13	0.18*	0.20*
Rehabilitation services scale			−0.07	−0.12	
PPO∗Insurance satisfaction scale				−0.20*	−0.17*
Adjusted R^2	0.21	0.20	0.20	0.22	0.28
F	2.99***	2.47***	2.40***	2.52***	7.93***

*$p < 0.05$.
**$p < 0.01$.
***$p < 0.001$.

respondents who appear to have greater encouragement and access to health-related resources necessary to prevent some disabilities.

In Table 3, the full model (Model 3) regarding the variance in WCHS respondents' distress levels suggests that emotional distress scores are positively related to being female (0.20) are negatively related to no religious affiliation (−0.27) and to being satisfied with health insurance services (−0.37). In the backward-reduced model (Model 4) insurance effects are much more important. The negative effect of satisfaction with insurance

Table 3. Betas and Coefficients of Determination for Emotional Difficulties Scale Regressed upon Select Independent Variables ($n = 134$).

	Model 1	Model 2	Model 3	Model 4
No. in household	0.23	0.24	0.22	
Household income	−0.11	−0.04	−0.03	
Married	−0.09	−0.13	−0.15	
Divorced	−0.09	−0.13	−0.14	
Widowed	0.07	0.05	0.03	
Education	−0.12	−0.18	−0.17	−0.17*
Age	−0.01	0.01	0.01	
Sex	0.18	0.20*	0.20*	0.18*
No. of children	−0.20	−0.18	−0.15	
White	0.09	0.13	0.14	
Catholic	−0.18	−0.13	−0.14	
No religion	−0.21*	−0.27**	−0.27**	−0.22**
Fully employed	0.00	−0.02	−0.02	
Retired	−0.16	−0.09	−0.11	
Standard checkups scale	0.07	0.08	0.07	
Healthy behaviors scale	−0.19*	−0.16	−0.15	−0.16*
PPO	0.04	0.16	0.15	
HMO	−0.01	0.07	0.07	
Insurance satisfaction scale		−0.37***	−0.37***	−0.32***
Fiscal cost of insurance scale		−0.07	−0.07	
Insurance alienation scale		0.06	0.05	
Insurance adaptation scale		0.16	0.16	0.17*
Home care scale			0.09	
Rehabilitation services scale			−0.02	
Adjusted R^2	0.07	0.20	0.19	0.22
F	1.60	2.47***	2.29**	7.11***

*$p < 0.05$.
**$p < 0.01$.
***$p < 0.001$.

services remains (−0.32), while household adaptive efforts to acquire and maintain health care coverage increased self-reported emotional distress (0.17).

Independent of insurance effects, the stepwise-reduced model shows that higher emotional distress totals are negatively related to education (−0.17), positively related to being female (0.18), and negatively related to more healthful and lower risk patterns of living (−0.16). While these effects are consistent with traditional demographic patterns in well-being, the effect of not being religiously affiliated (−0.22) was unexpected and inconsistent with the traditional role of religiosity in enhancing emotional well-being (Dwyer, Clarke, & Miller, 1990; Idler, 1987; Jarvis & Northcott, 1987; Musick, 1996). Overall, the effects of education, gender, and health lifestyle are less important in relation to divergence in distress levels among the WCHS respondents than are insurance effects and the effect of not being associated with a religion.

Findings regarding distress scores support the first hypothesis since being privately insured was not related to physical and emotional well-being. Clear support was also found for the second hypothesis regarding the negative relationship between satisfaction with insurance services and distress totals, and the positive relationship between distress scores and households' adaptive efforts to obtain or maintain health care coverage. Overall, the results show clear insurance effects in relation to variation in WCHS respondents' levels of emotional distress.

While the additional effects upon distress of education and healthy lifestyles were expected, the effect of not having a religious affiliation was not. The lack of affiliation may represent other elements in health-related resources and lifestyle rather than the absence of religiosity per se. It is possible, for example, that the relative absence of elderly respondents in the WCHS explains why religiosity is not more important in comparison to previous studies of elders' health (Idler, 1987; Musick, 1996).

DISCUSSION

Prior studies of insurance effects on physical health have interpreted the absence of such effects as resulting from the confounding influences of health resources and health lifestyles/beliefs (Franks et al., 1993; Ross & Mirowsky, 2000; Rogers et al., 1999). Our results suggest that additional factors may help in understanding how insurance effects relate to physical health. We found that physical impairments increase with age and with being female, independent of insurance effects, health resources, and lifestyles. While our results do not necessarily mean that managed insurance programs are less able to deal with the scope of health needs of females and the elderly (Chin & Harrigill, 1999; Ware et al., 1996), our findings do suggest the need for better adapting services to enrollees with increased health needs.

While access to private insurance coverage in the U.S. continues to be driven primarily by employer-provided benefits (Seccombe & Amey, 1995), our results show that being married and being widowed are important in reducing physical impairments. Previous research has shown that married people are more likely to be in better physical and mental health than unmarried people (Thoits, 1995). In addition, the married and widowed may have access to the benefits of health insurance plans of spouses as well as access to survivor benefits including those attainable from Social Security. Future research therefore should pay increased attention to the role of private and public insurance programs in providing benefits for spouses and survivors. These sorts of studies will be quite important in relation to better understanding of the generally higher impairments among females, especially in relation to the delimited options of Medicare. In addition, our results also suggest the payoffs of private insurance coverage for partners.

Our results showed that households' use of home health care services in the past year was related to increased impairments, independent of the effects of age, gender, and insurance exigencies. Home health care needs increasingly reflect the work-related illness and injuries people suffer and the increasing needs of elderly household members (Marshall, 2001). In particular, more American households include impaired elders who receive home health care from family members and health care professionals (Chumbler et al., 2003). Our results clearly call for additional research that will better specify the role of managed health care insurance in addressing these home health care needs, especially among the working poor (Marshall, 2001). Our results also showed that household health care needs and household problems in paying for care were both related to significantly more impairments.

We found clear statistical evidence of important insurance effects upon physical impairments. WCHS respondents in PPOs, which enrollees felt provided satisfactory services, reported significantly less physical impairments compared with their counterparts who were dissatisfied with services. Although our survey data do not enable us to decipher causal ordering, these results are still informative. PPOs with more satisfied enrollees may be in fact the managed insurance plans that better addresses the needs of enrollees (Chin & Harrigill, 1999). With our controls on household health needs, health-related resources, and other potentially confounding factors, it seems unlikely that fewer needs among such enrollees could explain our results.

Present findings support the results of previous studies in that we found educational attainment and healthful lifestyles were related to better emotional health (Mirowsky & Ross, 1998; Ross & Mirowsky, 2000; Ross & Wu, 1995, 1996). Unexpectedly, however, we found that lack of religious affiliation was related to less emotional distress. This effect may be the result of very well-educated people in the WCHS sample. Several studies have found that the higher levels of personal control and well-being found among the well educated and their greater interest in and motivation for healthful living may help explain the possible effect of the absence of religious affiliation on distress (Lewis & Ross, 1999; Mirowsky & Ross, 1998; Ross & Mirowsky, 2000; Ross & Wu, 1995, 1996). While educational level was not significantly correlated with religious affiliation in our data, previous studies have shown educational attainment to be negatively related to church attendance (Musick, House, & Williams, 2004). Owing to the nature of the WCHS sample, we were not able to determine time order effects. Thus, it is also possible that individuals who suffer from emotional and physical distress also seek the support of religion to alleviate this distress (Ko, Kua, & Fones, 1999; Musick et al., 2004; Pargament, Koenig, & Perez, 2000). Further research is needed to tease out this relationship. In addition, to provide a better understanding of life orientations and personal control in relation to emotional health, future research must extend the study of such effects beyond physical health (Mirowsky & Ross, 1998) to emotional well-being. It may also be that marital status, work-related injuries in relation to managed care coverage, and other factors are more important in explaining the working aged people that predominate in our sample, as compared with the role of religion in studies of elders (Idler, 1987; Musick, 1996).

Contrary to previous studies (Franks et al., 1993; Ross & Mirowsky, 2000; Rogers et al., 1999), we found insurance effects to be among the most important factors in explaining divergent emotional distress among the WCHS respondents. In particular, we found satisfaction with insurance services was related to greatly reduced levels of distress. Thus, beyond the study of insurance services as to patients/customers satisfaction (Kerr et al., 1999; Kronenfeld, 2001), our study suggests the need for assessing how service satisfaction may be related to stress. Ironically, insurance companies' customer service, the presumed means for giving people peace of mind concerning their health coverage, may actually contribute to increased stress and less certainty about the control of health (Grimm, Brewster, & Smith, 2003). Our results clearly suggest the need for better identifying the causes of stress in the patterns of daily living among working aged adults.

Our most disconcerting finding regarding emotional distress was that the increased efforts by households to restructure and adapt their activities to acquire and maintain health care were related to increased emotional distress. This result clearly shows that these household efforts to keep access to health care can undermine emotional well-being. Instead of merely assuming that economic deprivation is a longer-term cause of poor health, it is time that researchers took a better look at the shorter-term effects of being unable to acquire and maintain health care, especially upon emotional well-being and the deleterious effects of greatly increased stress. The alarming implication of our study is that more than 40 million Americans without any health insurance and the millions more working poor who have problems in accessing and maintaining coverage are being exposed to very high levels of stress (Seccombe & Amey, 1995). Leaving the needs of the precariously insured unaddressed may exacerbate these stressful circumstances and might greatly increase the future costs of health care as the population ages (Marshall, 2001). Alemayehu and Warner (2004) estimate that the lifetime health care expenditures in the United States are currently $316,600 per person and by the year 2030 this figure is likely to increase by one-fifth due to population aging alone. In fact, problems in paying for health care may be enough to offset and reverse the recent improvement in the general health status of the elderly in the U.S. Delimiting Medicare options and increasing out-of-pocket components of it will only exacerbate such problems.

CONCLUSION

The findings in this study suggest a need for better adapting managed health care insurance services for various types of enrollees and their households. First, we have found that the health needs of women and older adults (not necessarily those over 65) may be better addressed by expanded provisions related both to impairments and emotional distress. In particular, our results show that improving insurance services for households with problems in paying for health care is imperative. Second, we have found that households needing home health services, because of the increased disabilities among their members, should be provided the broader set of insurance services that will help them avoid the negative effects of not being able to afford necessary health care. Third, households that have encountered recent troubles in maintaining health care access include home members who are expressing very high levels of stress. Consequently, it is vitally important that managed health programs develop services to help households with more health problems avoid the additional complications of much greater stress because they are having serious problems in mobilizing needed health resources. Thus, the health patterns of the future may not simply reflect physical problems related to aging but also the effects of stress because of precarious insurance coverage. For these reasons we believe that it is essential that new programs create ways for helping households that are ineligible for public insurance deal with their unmet health needs. A variety of means such as tax credits, discounted services, flexible premiums, and increasing the availability public health programs are all viable possibilities.

ACKNOWLEDGMENTS

The authors would like to thank Jerry Daday, Tamela Maxwell, and the editor, Jennie Kronenfeld, for their reactions to earlier versions of this paper.

REFERENCES

Alemayehu, B., & Warner, K. E. (2004). The lifetime distribution of health care costs. *Health Services Research*, *39*(3), 627–642.
AMA Department of Physician Data Sources. (2001). *Physicians characteristics and distribution in the United States*. Chicago, IL: American Medical Association.
Bodenheimer, T. (1996). The HMO backlash – righteous or reactionary. *The New England Journal of Medicine*, *335*(21), 1601–1604.
Chin, S., & Harrigill, K. M. (1999). Delay in gynecologic surgical treatment: A comparison of patients in managed care and fee-for-service plans. *Obstetrics and Gynecology*, *93*(6), 922–927.
Chumbler, N. R., Grimm, J. W., Cody, M., & Beck, C. (2003). Gender, Kinship, and caregiver burden: The case of community-dwelling memory impaired seniors. *International Journal of Geriatric Psychiatry*, *18*, 722–732.
Comer, J., & Mueller, K. (1992). Correlates of health insurance coverage: Evidence from the Midwest. *Journal of Health Care for the Poor and Underserved*, *3*(2), 305–320.
Cortina, J. M. (1993). Interaction, nonlinearity, and multicollinearity: Implications for multiple-regression. *Journal of Management*, *19*(4), 915–922.
Council for Marketing and Opinion Research. (1998). *Industry watch*. Port Jefferson: NCMOR. Reprinted by Permission (1999) in Industry survey: CMOR's respondent cooperation audit. In: *Sawtooth news: News from Sawtooth Technologies in computer interviewing and analysis* (Vol. 15, p. 4).
Donelan, K., Blendon, R. J., Hill, C. A., Frankel, M., Hoffman, C., Rowland, D., & Altman, D. (1996). Whatever happened to the health insurance crisis in the United States? Voices from a national survey. *Journal of the American Medical Association*, *276*(16), 1346–1350.
Dwyer, J. W., Clarke, L. L., & Miller, M. K. (1990). The effect of religious concentration and affiliation on county cancer mortality rates. *Journal of Health and Social Behavior*, *31*(2), 185–202.
Fitchen, J. (1981). *Poverty in rural America*. Prospect Heights, IL: Waveland.
Franks, P., Clancy, C. M., Gold, M. R., & Nutting, P. A. (1993). Health insurance and subjective health status: Data from the 1987 National Medical Expenditure survey. *American Journal of Public Health*, *83*(9), 1295–1299.
Friedman, E. (1997). Managed care, rationing, and quality: A tangled relationship. *Health Affairs*, *16*(3), 174–182.

Furlong, B., & Wilken, M. (2001). Managed care: The changing environment for consumers and health care providers. *Research in the Sociology of Health Care, 19,* 3–20.

Ganzach, Y. (1998). Nonlinearity, multicollinearity and the probability of Type II error in detecting interaction. *Journal of Management, 24*(5), 615–622.

Gould, E. (2004). *The chronic problem of declining health coverage: Employer-provided health insurance falls for third consecutive year.* EPI Issue Brief #202. Washington, DC: Economic Policy Institute.

Grimm, J. W., & Brewster, Z. W. (2002). Explaining health-related inequalities with a social capital model. *Research in the Sociology of Health Care, 20,* 3–27.

Grimm, J. W., Brewster, Z. W., & Smith, D. C. (2003). Education, managed health care experiences and health outcomes. *Research in the Sociology of Health Care, 21,* 39–61.

Holahan, J., & Wang, M. (2004). Changes in health insurance coverage during the economic downturn: 2000–2002. *Health Affairs: The Policy Journal of the Health Sphere.* Web exclusive available online at http://content.healthaffairs.org/webexclusives/index.dtl?year = 2004

Idler, E. L. (1987). Religious involvement and the health of the elderly: Some hypotheses and an initial text. *Sociological Focus, 66*(1), 226–238.

Jarvis, G. K., & Northcott, H. C. (1987). Religion and differences in morbidity and mortality. *Social Science and Medicine, 25*(7), 813–824.

Kerr, E. A., Hays, R. D., Mitchinson, A., Lee, M., & Siu, A. (1999). The influence of gatekeeping and utilization review on patient satisfaction. *Journal of General Internal Medicine, 14*(5), 287–296.

Ko, S. M., Kua, E. H., & Fones, C. S. (1999). Stress and the undergraduates. *Singapore Medical Journal, 40*(10), 627–630.

Kronenfeld, J. J. (2001). New trends in the doctor–patient relationships: Impacts of managed care on the growth of a consumer protections model. *Sociological Spectrum, 21*(3), 293–317.

Lewis, S. K., & Ross, C. E. (1999). Establishing a sense of personal control in the transition to adulthood. *Social Forces, 77*(4), 1573–1599.

Lin, N. (2001). Building a network theory of social capital. In: N. Lin, K. Cook & R. S. Burt (Eds), *Social capital theory and research* (pp. 3–29). Hawthorne, NY: Aldine de Gruyter.

Marshall, N. L. (2001). Health and illness issues facing an aging workforce in the new millennium. *Sociological Spectrum, 21*(3), 431–439.

McLeer, S., Anwar, R., Herman, S., & Maquiling, K. (1989). Education is not enough: A systems failure in protecting battered women. *Annals of Emergency Medicine, 18,* 651.

Mechanic, D. (2004). Targeting HMOs: Stalemate in the U.S. health care debate. *Context, 3*(2), 27–34.

Miller, R. H., & Luft, H. S. (2002). HMO plan performance update: An analysis of the literature, 1997–2001. *Health Affairs: The Policy Journal of the Health Sphere, 21*(4), 63–86.

Mirowsky, J., & Hu, P. N. (1996). Physical impairment and the diminishing effects of income. *Social Forces, 74*(3), 1073–1096.

Mirowsky, J., & Ross, C. E. (1998). Education, personal control, lifestyle, and health: A human capital hypothesis. *Research in Aging, 20*(4), 415–449.

Morton, L. W. (2004). Rural health policy. In: D. L. Brown & L. E. Swanson (Eds), *Challenges for rural America in the twenty-first century* (pp. 290–304). University Park, PA: Penn State Press.

Musick, M. A. (1996). Religion and subjective health among black and white elders. *Journal of Health and Social Behavior, 37*(3), 221–237.

Musick, M. A.; House, J. S., & Williams, D. R. (2004). Attendance at religious services and mortality in a national sample. *Journal of Health and Social Behavior, 45*(2), 198–213.

Pargament, K. I., Koenig, H. G., & Perez, L. M. (2000). The many methods of religious coping: Development and initial validation of the RCOPE. *Journal of Clinical Psychology, 56*(4), 519–543.

Plichta, S. B., & Weisman, C. S. (1995). Spouse or partner, abuse use of health services, and unmet need for medical care in U.S. women. *Journal of Women's Health, 4*(1), 45–53.

Pugliesi, K. (1995). Work and well being: Gender differences in the psychological consequences of employment. *Journal of Health and Social Behavior, 36*(1), 57–71.

Rogers, R. G., Hummer, R. A., & Nam, C. B. (1999). *Living and dying in the USA: Behavioral, health, and social differentials of adult mortality*. New York: Academic Press.

Ross, C. E., & Mirowsky, J. (2000). Does medical insurance contribute to socioeconomic differentials in health? *Milbank Quarterly, 78*(2), 291–321.

Ross, C. E., & Wu, C. L. (1995). The links between education and health. *American Sociological Review, 60*(5), 719–745.

Ross, C. E., & Wu, C. L. (1996). Education, age, and the cumulative advantage in health. *Journal of Health and Social Behavior, 37*(1), 104–120.

Schlesinger, M. J., Gray, B. H., & Perreira, K. M. (1997). Medical professionalism under managed care: The pros and cons of utilization review. *Health Affairs, 16*(1), 106–124.

Seccombe, K., & Amey, C. (1995). Playing by the rules and losing: Health insurance and the working poor. *Journal of Health and Social Behavior, 36*(2), 168–181.

Shearer, G. (1998). *Hidden from view: The growing burden of health care costs*. Washington, DC: Consumers Union.

Sullivan, K. (1999). Managed care plan performance since 1980: Another look at 2 literature reviews. *American Journal of Public Health, 89*(7), 1003–1008.

Taylor, A. K., Cohen, J. W., & Machlin, S. R. (2001). Being uninsured in 1996 compared to 1987: How has the experience of the uninsured changed over time? *Health Services Research, 36*(6), 16–30.

Thoits, P. A. (1995). Stress, coping, and social support processes: Where are we? What next? *Journal of Health and Social Behavior, 36*(extra issue), 53–79.

U.S. Census Bureau. (2003). Health insurance coverage in the United States: 2002. Available online at http://www.census.gov/prod/2003pubs/p60-223.pdf

Vandenburgh, H. (2001). Emerging trends in the provision and consumption of health services. *Sociological Spectrum, 21*(3), 279–291.

Ware, J. E., Bayliss, M. S., Rogers, W. H., Kosinski, M., & Tarlov, A. R. (1996). Differences in 4-year health outcomes for elderly and poor, chronically ill patients treated in HMO and fee-for-service systems: Results from the medical outcomes study. *Journal of the American Medical Association, 276*(13), 1039–1047.

Ware, J. E., & Sherbourne, C. D. (1992). The MOS 36-item short form health survey (SF-36). I. Conceptual framework and item selection. *Medical Care, 30*(6), 473–483.

Weitz, R. (2004). *The sociology of health, illness, and health care*. Belmont, CA: Wadsworth, Thompson Learning.

Wyn, R., Collins, K. S., & Brown, E. R. (1997). Women and managed care: Satisfaction with provider choice, access to care, plan costs and coverage. *Journal of American Medical Women's Association, 52*(2), 60–64.

Young, G. P., & Lowe, R. A. (1997). Adverse outcomes of managed care gatekeeping. *Academic Emergency Medicine, 4*(12), 1129–1136.

Zautcke, J. L., Fraker, L. D., Hart, R. G., & Stevens, J. S. (1997). Denial of emergency department authorization of potentially high-risk patients by managed care. *Journal of Emergency Medicine, 15*(5), 605–609.

SECTION 4:
TREATMENT DISPARITIES AND
PROVIDERS OF CARE

'NOTHING HAPPENS IN MEDICAL SCHOOL THAT PREPARES YOU FOR WORKING WITH ANYONE WHO'S DIFFERENT:' INFORMAL LEARNING AND SOCIO-CLINICAL KNOWLEDGE AMONGST FAMILY PHYSICIANS

Eric Mykhalovskiy and Karen Farrell

ABSTRACT

This paper investigates the informal learning processes through which family physicians develop an understanding of the social context shaping the health of marginalized patients. The paper is based on the results of a qualitative study, informed by institutional ethnography, involving individual interviews with 10 family physicians working in and around Halifax, Nova Scotia, Canada. The analysis explores what knowledge of social context is for family physicians, emphasizing its hybrid, socio-clinical character. We also explore key aspects of the informal processes through which this knowledge is developed including learning about 'the other,' the

Health Care Services, Racial and Ethnic Minorities and Underserved Populations: Patient and Provider Perspectives
Research in the Sociology of Health Care, Volume 23, 159–181
ISSN: 0275-4959/doi:10.1016/S0275-4959(05)23008-9

reflexive unlearning of medical school training, and learning from clinical doing where we discuss patient-based epiphanies and learning from other health care providers.

The recent consolidation of population health research in Canada and elsewhere has occasioned a renewed interest in the social determinants of health. Early statements of the population health perspective argued that the health status of social groups and populations is shaped by broad social and economic circumstances and not primarily by health service use (Evans, Barer, & Marmor, 1994; Evans & Stoddart, 1990). In elaboration of this perspective, an interdisciplinary and heterogeneous programme of research has emerged that seeks to understand how features of organized social life, lying outside the scope of individual control, shape people's health.

One strand of this research has seized upon the notion of context to explore relationships between health and social structure. Intended largely as a corrective to the risk factor emphasis of traditional epidemiology, studies of the "context of health" have tried to explore the social processes that underlie population-based health differences. Some researchers have explored family and peer contexts (Kobus, 2003; Faith, Scanlon, Birch, Francis, & Sherry, 2004), and others the context of health policy (Liang, Chaloupka, Nichter & Clayton, 2003). One particularly popular approach focuses on neighbourhood context in studies regarding civic participation, community resources, and other features of local social organization that support health (Frohlich, Potvin, Chabot, & Corin, 2002; Chavez, Kemp, & Harris, 2004; Lochner, Kwachi, Brennan, & Buka, 2003).

This paper seeks to contribute to emerging work on social context and health. However, it does so from a perspective rather different from that found in the established literature. Most of the discussion of the "context" of health orients to the term as an analytic concept for thinking about relations external to health care that shape health status. Context is treated by this work as something that explains population-based patterns of health. By contrast, our approach treats context as an indigenous concept, that is, as a constituent of family physicians' practical reasoning drawn upon in providing care to marginalized patients. Our interest is in how practicing family physicians themselves develop an understanding of the context of health and how such an understanding enters into the care they provide to marginalized patients.

The paper has two specific objectives. First, we want to describe what knowledge of context is for physicians. Drawing on interviews with family doctors, we make a distinction between knowledge of context and forms of biomedical knowledge about marginalized groups. We emphasize that for family physicians, knowledge of context is a hybrid, socio-clinical knowledge through which aspects of the general life circumstances of marginalized patients are made clinically relevant. Second, we explore how this form of socio-clinical knowledge is developed. Our account emphasizes a process of informal learning about how to work with marginalized patients that physicians engage in after they have graduated from medical school. We outline key aspects of this learning process as suggested by our interviews, namely, learning about 'the other,' challenging the physician self, learning from other health care providers, and learning from patients. The paper also puts forward an analysis of the social organization of clinical practice that facilitates this learning, drawing attention to such relations as physician payment, multidisciplinary care, and the connection between clinic time and doctor–patient interaction.

LOCATING THE STUDY

This paper is written at the interface of research on meeting the health needs of marginalized social groups, the sociology of medical education, and the growing body of work on adult informal learning. The health circumstances of poor people, racial and ethnic minorities, those living in rural areas and other disenfranchised groups, have been a longstanding research concern in Canada. In recent years, however, a strategic problematization of the health status of individuals who have come to be collectively known as "marginalized groups" has emerged, largely as a function of the priority setting activities of national health research funding agencies (Dault, Lomas, & Barer, 2004).

This problematization is fuelled by the now unequivocal results of epidemiological and related research, demonstrating the poorer relative health status of disadvantaged Canadians (e.g. Raphael, 2004; Veenstra, 2003; MacMillan, MacMillan, Offord, & Dingle, 1996). In one study representative of this genre of research, Veugelers and Guernsey (1999) report that life expectancy in an isolated region of Nova Scotia is 5 years less than the national average. Most population health researchers interpret health inequalities of this sort in terms of nonmedical determinants of health such as income, employment, and social support. Others, however, maintain that there is a need to continue exploring the relationship between formal health services and health status (Poland, Coburn, Robertson, & Eakin, 1998; Coburn et al., 2003).

This latter suggestion is supported by a wealth of research demonstrating troubling patterns of access to health services for marginalized social groups. Like their counterparts in the United States and elsewhere, Canadian researchers have shown that when compared to national averages, marginalized patients are less likely to have regular physicians, have less access to preventive health services, and experience poorer continuity of care (Menec, Roos, Black, & Bogdanovic, 2001; Talbot, Fuller-Thomson, Tudiver, Habib, & McIsaac, 2001; Mustard, Mayer, Black, & Postl, 1996). These study results have been elaborated by qualitative research with ethnic and racial minorities, poor people, people suffering from mental illnesses, and other marginalized groups in Canada that points to linguistic, poverty-related, socio-cultural, and other barriers of access to primary health care services (Anderson, 1998; Amaratunga, 2002; Weerasinghe, 2003).

Despite the efforts of many progressive educators, the health circumstances and issues faced by vulnerable patients remain underrepresented in medical school training (Pottie, Masi, Watson, Heyding, & Roberts, 2000; Makoul, 2003). At the same time, family physicians remain key points of access to health services for marginalized patients, and reports in the medical literature testify to the challenges practitioners continue to face when working with marginalized groups (Pottie et al., 2000). This combination of factors has occasioned a call from social scientists, health researchers, and others for research that might help family physicians improve health care delivery to marginalized people (Watson, Wetzel, & Devanesen, 1991; Stewart, 1990). We offer this paper as one response.

Our central contribution to research on developing health services that better meet the needs of marginalized people lies in a careful analysis of the informal learning that family physicians engage in. We want to gather together physicians' tacit knowledge about caring for marginalized patients and give it a broader social presence than it currently has. At our most hopeful moments, we imagine our discussion of physicians' informal learning processes entering into the institutional corridors of medical schools and influencing how medical pedagogy is practiced.

In addition to this applied effort, our work contributes to the sociology of medical education. From the classic early works (Fox, 1957; Becker, Geer, Hughes, & Strauss, 1961) to more recent research (Good & Good, 1993; Beagan, 2001), most sociology of medical learning focuses on formal educational settings. Sociologists have been particularly concerned with processes of professional socialization, drawing their attention to how student culture influences learning, how scientific knowledge is represented and learned in medical schools and the role that uncertainty plays in medical practice and education (Fox, 1980; Atkinson, 1984; Lingard, Garwood, Schryer, & Spafford, 2003).

Rather than reproducing the sociological literature's characteristic emphasis on the skills and knowledge medical students gain in order to become "competent" practitioners, our study focuses on knowledge they do not typically acquire during formal training and emphasizes sites and forms of learning external to formal medical education. Our work contributes to a small but important body of work on lifelong learning among family physicians who care for marginalized patients, a particularly powerful example of which is West's (2001) study of inner-city London physicians. In doing so, we highlight discontinuities between training and practice and help to develop a broader understanding of the full range of processes through which doctors learn what is relevant to providing primary medical care to vulnerable patients.

To help explore and better bring into view these processes, we draw on contemporary social science research on informal learning. The origins of this field trace back to changes in the study of adult education in the 1970s, when researchers began recognizing the important role that self-directed, independent learning played in the reproduction of knowledge-based societies (Tough, 1979). We draw on the current work of Livingstone (in press) in approaching informal learning as "any activity involving the pursuit of understanding, knowledge or skill which occurs without the presence of externally imposed curricular criteria." Our work also engages with recent trends in the study of informal learning developed out of the work of Church, Bascia, and Shragge (2004) and Church, Fontan, Ng, and Shragge (2000). These include an emphasis on the relational character of informal learning (in the present context, how physicians learn through interactions with patients and health care providers), an interest in the tacit character of informal learning that is "continuous with doing" (Percy, Burton, & Withnall, 1994, p. 37) (how physicians' informal learning is embedded in and a part of clinical activity) and a concern for how informal learning is shaped by institutional relations (funding, clinic settings, and other factors shaping medical work).

THE STUDY

This study is informed by an approach to sociological investigation called institutional ethnography (IE), developed by the Canadian sociologist, Dorothy E. Smith (1987). IE is an approach to inquiry that explores the social determinants of everyday experience. Institutional ethnographers begin their research by identifying and describing the experiences of actual people – for example, the experiences family physicians have of providing care to marginalized patients – then seek to examine how those experiences are shaped by broad social and institutional factors. From an IE perspective, "experience" is tied to a generous notion of "work," understood broadly as people's actual activities or what they know how to do on a day-to-day basis (Devault & McCoy, 2002). IE research seeks to generate detailed analytic descriptions of people's everyday "work" or activity as it is shaped by multiple social, institutional, professional, economic, and other relations.

In the sphere of health care, IE studies have been conducted on such topics as transformations in nursing and home care work (Campbell, 2000a; Rankin, 2001; Diamond, 1992), evidence-based medicine and the reform of health care (Mykhalovskiy, 2001, 2003), the management of treatment for people with HIV (Smith, 1990; Mykhalovskiy & McCoy, 2002; McCoy, 2005), and disabled people's experiences with health care providers (Campbell, 2000b). This project builds on IE research on the work of health professionals but breaks new ground by exploring the experiences of physicians – a group that has not been well represented in IE research.

Our study is based on 11 in-depth interviews conducted with 10 physicians from March to October 2004. All physicians were family doctors working in and around Halifax, the urban centre of the Maritimes with a population of approximately 370,000 individuals. We used a process of chain sampling to select only those physicians who had at least 2 years of experience working with patients who they understood to belong to a socially or economically marginalized group. In practice, we spoke with physicians who worked closely with chronically poor people, Black Nova Scotians, people with mental illness, injection drug users, Aboriginals, homeless people, and gay men. All the physicians we interviewed worked either in solo practice or in a community health clinic setting. The physicians ranged in age from 38 to 67 years and seven of them were female. Interviews lasted between 60 and 90 min and were tape-recorded and transcribed.

CLINICAL PRACTICE, CONTEXT AND SOCIO-CLINICAL KNOWLEDGE

We did not intend to produce a study of social context and informal learning amongst family physicians. While context is a popular analytic concept in health research, we did not introduce the term into our interviews at the outset of our inquiry. Rather, talk of context arose spontaneously as participants in the study described how they learned to provide care to marginalized patients.

Much of this conversation mirrored everyday uses of the word "context." Thus, physicians spoke about context in terms that evoked a particular set of social and economic circumstances unique to any given individual. As one person put it, "each person comes with their own background, their own sort of context." In interviews we typically spoke about context as part of discussions about physicians' experiences of working with particular patients. Some participants spoke about learning to "get to know the context that [their patients] were living in," while others spoke about the challenges of working with biomedical and, particularly, evidence-based medical approaches to health which they understood "take people out of their context." Still others recognized the specificity of "a marginalized context" as against the circumstances of a middle-class life, while others emphasized the multiple contexts of their patients' lives including a "working class context," the context of immigration to Canada, and an "on welfare context."

All of these uses share with popular approaches, an understanding of context that suggests a peculiar relation of self to non-self, one in which context defines and is interior to a person while at the same time gesturing to broad external social and historical circumstances, processes, and relations. Of course, what makes these uses unique is their discursive rendering as part of interview commentary by family physicians on providing clinical care to marginalized patients.

The knowledge of context expressed by physicians in this study is not simply an understanding of the broad circumstances within which people make their lives. Nor is it a biomedical or population-based knowledge of diseases or health risks associated with particular marginalized groups as in Black Nova Scotians' greater risk for hypertension, or the typical fungal infections of homeless people. Rather, it is a uniquely hybrid knowledge in which understandings of social context are tied to the relevancies and practicalities of clinical work. We thus designate it "socio-clinical" emphasizing how, through it, physicians come to understand the way family situations, employment histories, housing circumstances, racial discrimination, homophobia, sexual abuse, and other processes shape people's health circumstances in ways that change how physicians communicate with and provide care to their patients. One physician expressed the specific interface of contextual and clinical knowledge that is involved, in the following way:

> Issues of social justice, racism, social economic inequalities, you know, prejudice, whatever. Inadequate housing, issues that are, you know, predominant in the world, really, but also exist in our societies, that create inequalities. Those kinds of issues were, I sort of had them in my mind but I hadn't related them to medicine in general. (Interview 6)

For many of the physicians we spoke with, a knowledge of context was made relevant to medical practice through changes in their approaches to communicating with their patients. We heard about how slowly, over the course of many visits, physicians tailored how and what they spoke about with their patients as they developed an emerging sense of the full circumstances of their patients' daily lives. Such changes were part of a broader organization of clinical work wherein medicine is practiced "within the constraints and priorities of patients' lives" (McCoy, 2005) rather than in ways that impose requirements ill fitted to patient's realities. In this study, providing clinical care in this fashion was not simply a matter of physicians' intentions but was enabled by a knowledge of social context. It involved a particular acknowledgement of the realities of people's lives by, for example, tempering rigid adherence expectations or working within the day-to-day limitations of a patient's drug use. In some instances it involved relocating the site of clinical delivery to the level of the community or street or, as in the case of the speaker below, tempering medical interventions.

> Well a woman came in the other day... For financial reasons she's been living with her father for the past year. She's an adult woman with two children. Has had chronic, you know, working poor... She didn't understand why she was bursting into tears and she didn't know what that was about. And then you connect it to all the other things and then she goes, 'well, oh yea, it makes kinda sense.' But many times it's stomach problems, it's headaches, it's sleep problems, it's low back pain, I mean all of those things are aggravated by you know, stress in your life... I mean there's, I think for me... I probably investigate way less than some physicians in part because I've learned over the years that when people come in with these physical complaints, you've got to dig a little bit deeper and find out what's going on. (Interview 4)

The above account expresses a particular relationship of organic phenomena and social determinants of health as socio-clinical knowledge, activated in clinical work through a specific change in practice style. The speaker begins with the circumstances of a particular patient then moves, through the language of stress, to discuss a more general formulation of the body's connection to social circumstances. We would emphasize that like others with whom we spoke, social context for this physician does not represent a facile disavowal of the organic basis of disease. Rather, it involves recognizing the interrelationship of the body and social context and working with it clinically, often through complex questions about how best to approach patients' physical complaints. In our study, socio-clinical knowledge involved a constant tension over how best to respond to patients' concerns and on what terrain of action – counselling, medical care, advocacy – from a stance that recognizes how social, economic, and other circumstances can lie at the root of medical problems.

By referring to knowledge of social context as socio-clinical, we do not mean to somehow suggest that this is the only medically oriented knowledge that is social. Foucault's (1994/1963) historical research has emphasized how clinical rationality has been fundamental to the very establishment of modern notions of the individual, while anthropological work such as Martin's (1994) on the gendered tropes of immunology sheds light upon the many cultural influences on medical knowledge. Through the designation "socio-clinical," we have instead sought to make visible a particular form of hybridity, a particular way in which biomedical knowledge of bodily phenomena is intermixed with an understanding of the individual as socially, economically, and otherwise situated.

We have come to think of this knowledge as a kind of clinician's political economy of health. In this sense it is something different or broader than a knowledge of the values and cultures of ethnically and racially diverse communities, the dominant discursive rendering of marginalized people within biomedical reasoning (Taylor, 2003a, b). Socio-clinical knowledge as made known to us in this research does not have its primary conceptual organization in diversity discourse. Rather, it is a clinician's view of how health and disease are shaped by the broad structural conditions of society. As the quote below suggests, knowledge of context harkens back to the best traditions of social medicine and opens up physicians' work onto parameters of action that extend beyond the established confines of the medical encounter.

> P: And another situation was…a patient of mine who was an alcoholic. She was about 50, or 45, I guess, living with a man who used to beat her constantly… She'd come in with terrible scalp lacerations and we were…very involved in legal proceedings. So that's the kind of thing that you inevitably get involved in. And you can't stop, you know…
>
> I: Why can't you stop?
>
> P: Well, then you're not being consistent. You're not fulfilling your obligation, really, to that patient. That woman would have kept on being beaten and would have probably been killed by this man…you have to do everything possible, everything within your ability, to assist that patient with regard to health, health being very broad, and because so many of the contexts of the people's lives impacted on their health you couldn't stop. You had to go beyond just giving the pills… I mean if you're in family medicine you have to look at all the aspects of a person's life and try to do something. (Interview 9)

LEARNING ABOUT SOCIAL CONTEXT

How do physicians learn about the social context of marginalized patients' lives? How do they develop socio-clinical knowledge of the sort we have described above? From the physicians we interviewed, knowledge about how to respond clinically to the health contexts faced by marginalized people does not circulate widely within medical school training. Rather, it develops through clinical experience, through doing and reflecting on clinical work. Interestingly, this "continuous" nature of physicians' learning – its organization as internal to clinical work rather than as a discrete activity with definite boundaries – made it something difficult for doctors to speak about. "It just happened" was a common refrain. Still, their accounts provide an empirical basis for an analytic description of how such learning takes place and is socially organized.

Learning about 'the Other'

The physicians interviewed for this study were all white and middle class. Given their social location, developing socio-clinical knowledge involved for them a process of learning about 'the other.' A prerequisite of this form of knowledge is some recognition of social diversity, a basic understanding of the specificity and difference of the lives of those who are not white and privileged. To the extent that their lives were organized within middle-class relations, such forms of awareness were not always available to the physicians we spoke with. Still, some sourced a developing understanding of this sort well before their medical school training and later clinical experiences with vulnerable patients.

One participant spoke about how her decision to enter medicine was partly shaped by her experiences of growing up in a family that "fostered a lot of kids." In her account, growing up under these circumstances helped her to develop an inchoate understanding of the connections between health and social circumstances. As she put it, early on she and her siblings "saw a lot of people with difficulties who had trouble in life and needed caring." Another participant, whose father was a physician who worked in what she described as a "low socio-economic" area, spoke about a familiarity with the lives and health of poor people and racial minorities that she developed as a child:

> I was exposed to this from way, way years ago. Ok. One of Dad's partners was a Black
> physician from Trinidad, alright? But dad already had a lot of Blacks in the population

from [a nearby town]. So…it was our norm. How can I say? It was, because the Black population was quite isolated and for dad to do house calls, and I would go with him. It wasn't, you get what I mean… It was just normal. (Interview 3)

Of course, most of the physicians we interviewed lacked such early experiences and were thus confronted with a more distinct need to better understand the life circumstances of marginalized patients once they began practicing medicine. In speaking about his experiences working with Aboriginal communities, one respondent commented,

When you go into a community hall with 800 people and you're the only three white people, you have the sense that you're not in charge anymore… You don't understand how the culture works… It makes you realize that your values aren't the predominant values in the community and that you really are kind of an outsider. And if you want to be effective you've got to understand their values. (Interview 5)

Like others we interviewed, this physician expresses learning about 'the other' as a cultural matter. His account mobilizes a terminology and form of reasoning popularized by cultural competency training programmes that have recently been established in medical schools throughout North America (Flores, Gee, & Kastner, 2000; Champaneria & Axtell, 2004). From the perspective of cultural competence, what is at issue in working successfully with marginalized groups is better communication skills. Such skills are understood to be enabled by overcoming stereotypical judgements about minorities and becoming more sensitive to their distinct beliefs, values, and cultural issues.

An important feature of this research is how liberal discourses of cultural diversity were tied with an understanding of the social and economic circumstances shaping patients' lives. This integration meant that knowing 'the other' involved bridging cultural knowledge with an understanding of structural relations of inequality. For example, many of the physicians we interviewed who worked with Black Nova Scotians spoke about adjusting their clinical work to acknowledge that they were not simply treating individuals, but families and communities. One physician contrasted this situation with working with middle class, white patients whose siblings, parents, cousins and broader family connections were not always well known to him. Participants partly accounted for the shift from treating individuals to treating families and communities in the context of race in terms of the values of "closely knit" Black Nova Scotian communities. But they also spoke in ways that recognized a history of racial discrimination in Nova Scotia and an appreciation of gendered economic disadvantage. As one participant pointed out, when mothers come in "with a lot of children...because one is looking after several, like maybe her sister's kids, her neighbour's kids, even though the appointment is just for one of them" what begins as an appointment for one child or mother is easily transformed into a group affair – with all the attendant challenges to clinic time and billing practices.

Reflexive Learning

Developing a knowledge of social context takes more than understanding 'the other,' it involves confronting social difference through processes of reflexive learning that can be profoundly self-transformative. Throughout our research, we heard poignant stories from physicians about how working with marginalized patients was an unsettling process through which a number of assumptions they had not previously confronted were called into question, often with considerable personal consequences. Such "self-work" was reflexive in the sense that it focused on practices that form part of the relations of oppression faced by marginalized people.

> Ah, being you know a white person. Recognizing my own unconscious prejudices, which includes language. I mean 'black as the ace of spades,' I mean I used to say that and never thought about it. (Interview 4)

A particularly salient feature of physicians' reflexive learning is how it was institutionally focused – it typically involved challenging or unlearning what was learned in medical school. In her research on formal medical education, Beagan (2001) argues that medical students who are working class, gay, lesbian, or members of race or ethnic minorities are more likely than others to resist the requirements of professional socialization. Our research adds to this analysis by demonstrating how white, middle-class physicians – who have already *completed* medical training – actively challenge and refuse aspects of what they have learned. Their experiences suggest that not only does medical training fail to adequately address the question of working with marginalized patients, but what is offered as part of regular medical education can be counterproductive to such clinical work. For example, a number of the physicians we spoke with emphasized how working successfully with marginalized patients required them to jettison or rethink concepts that they had encountered as part of medical training.

> Someone quite close to my colleague...began to see me as a patient. And this person had *a lot* of health care issues. And my knee jerk reaction, which would have arisen in me, and also encouraged in some of my training was 'malingerer.' You know, 'get over it and move on.' (Interview 1)

For one particular physician, the figure of the patient-as-malingerer seemed to arise as part of the so-called "hidden curriculum" in medicine (Sinclair, 1997; Cribb & Bignold, 1999) through which students cultivate a professional identity. By working with poor patients over time and learning about the realities of their day-to-day lives, she was able to recognize the conceptual damage posed by "the malingerer" and the ways it shifted her clinical activity into forms of judgement of the poor that she no longer wished to undertake.

> There's an undercurrent, I think, in medical school, in internship and stuff, that people that are off on disability especially if it's for something that's a little more difficult to diagnose or characterize, like low back pain... Um, there's a fairly negative view about those kinds of people in the medical world – that they're malingering or trying to milk the system. So I kind of just took a step back I guess and just thought, 'well, I have to say that people, the majority of people are just simply telling me the way that they see it, and this is it. And I'm not going to play the judge... I thought that's not my place, that's the insurance company's place.' (Interview 2)

In addition to unlearning concepts, the physicians we interviewed suggested how working with marginalized patients required fundamental challenges to the forms of physician subjectivity cultivated by medical school training. A number of participants, including the one quoted below, generally lamented the absence of opportunities within their formal education to consider how they might become implicated in power relations at the point of the medical encounter.

> You're training comes from a position of power and influence and doesn't acknowledge any of that stuff... We don't do any personal work in medical school. It's all looking outwards. And it's not saying 'how do you as a person, what are your strengths and weaknesses? You know, what are your prejudices? What do you come to this doctor–patient relationship, what do you bring to it?' It's always what does the patient bring. Not what does the doctor bring. (Interview 4)

For many participants, questions about what the doctor brings to the medical encounter were only posed in a serious way once they had begun ongoing clinical work with patients. It was also the case that the particular experience of working with marginalized patients typically led to answers that disrupted the subject position of the authoritative physician. We heard a number of stories, often told with some humour, about how clinical work with disadvantaged patients encouraged and required a re-imagination of the physician self. One participant expressed this as jettisoning a sense of the physician as a "fixer." Another described a gradual shift from being a "rescuer" to being a "healer." The following, broader account, from a physician who works largely with homeless men and injection drug users suggests a sentiment common to many of the physicians we spoke with.

> As a family physician we are taught to believe that we can do everything, and we know everything, as cliché as that might be. There's a very strong powerful force as you go through, particularly as a resident, to develop that persona. In fact, my belief is that's what actually makes a doctor. It's not the knowledge at all, it's the persona that you're almost forced to adopt as you go through the system. If you're going to do this kind of work, you have to get rid of that altogether. (Interview 6)

Developing a knowledge of social context requires a movement beyond traditional parameters of biomedical action or "diagnosing and fixing" as well as a more general questioning of physician authority over patients. This latter move seemed most provoked by the overwhelming feelings that physicians experience after repeated exposure to the burdens of life faced by marginalized patients. Participants described how difficult this form of clinical work can be and how doing it over the long term requires a certain "letting go," a certain recognition of their own limitations. As one physician put it, "I don't take ownership for people's problems."

For some participants, questioning physician authority also arose as an internal feature of learning about social context. For example, one physician explained how, over time she came to recognize how marginalized people have a generalized experience of not being listened to by figures of authority. Recognizing a homology between the stance of the authoritative physician and such state authorities as welfare offices, which in her view negate marginalized people, she learned to cultivate a physician self that treats disadvantaged patients as competent knowers of their own circumstances.

The descriptions of levelling the doctor–patient relationship provided in this study bear a close resemblance to the proposals for shared decision-making in the medical encounter advanced in recent health research (Charles, Gafni, & Whelan, 1997, 1999). The physicians we interviewed generally linked a refusal of medical authority with encouraging patients to become more active in decision-making. While in our research, unlearning the authoritative physician is clearly central to developing socio-clinical knowledge, we caution that it is no escape hatch from the exercise of power in clinical care. Shared decision-making does not absent power from the clinical encounter, it merely recasts it in terms that enjoin patients to take on new forms of responsibility for their health. Patient refusal of proven treatments and actions that place themselves or others at risk represented limits to the forms of shared decision-making sought after by physicians in our research. It is also the case that when working with marginalized patients, working against physician authority by cultivating the active patient can present peculiar contradictions.

> That doesn't mean they'll accept it. It's different for them to say "oh okay I'll start making decisions." There's a whole big step there that doesn't necessarily happen. Because I can say to people "well I'm here to help you, I'm not here to make your decisions for you". People will understand that, it doesn't mean they'll do it. Because most people aren't used to doing that, right? Okay, so sometimes there's a process of, um, of helping people come to the point where they can start to actually direct their own lives, specifically around health. (Interview 6)

Learning through Others: Patients and Health Care Workers

Developing a knowledge of social context is not a solo accomplishment of the individual physician, it is a process produced through interaction with others. Most obviously, physicians learn about the social context of marginalization through their relationships with patients.

In analysing our interviews, we came to recognize that physicians represent socio-clinical learning through a particular narrative strategy, one which we call "patient-based epiphanies." When pressed beyond accounts of the "it just happens" sort, physicians represented how they learned by talking about their experiences with particular patients from whom generalized changes in practice followed. One participant spoke about how her approach to reproductive health counselling changed when a patient who requested birth control shifted her understanding of the needs and lives of some Muslim women.

> She had three children and they were living on a pretty frugal income and she didn't want to have any more children. But, you know, she wasn't supposed to take birth control. So we organized for her to have an IUD, cut the strings really short so nobody would know. (Interview 7)

Another physician spoke at length about how working over the course of a number of years with a particular patient led her to fundamentally question the individually centred, lifestyle approach to health promotion to which she had been committed.

> I sort of went through a process where I kind of flipped my attitude... And there were certain patients that, ah, sort of triggered that off, you sort of, as you got to know them. I had one woman, who was diabetic, she was Black, whole family diabetic, and she had a terrible time. Her sugars were never controlled. And as I got to know the family and everything, you realized 'wait a minute, this is a heck of a lot harder than I think it is. It's not that easy for this woman to eat properly and get out and get some exercise.' I mean, where does she live? She lives out in the country. There's no sidewalk, there's no

streetlights. And when is she supposed to go for a walk? She's got two small kids. She's got very little money. (Interview 2)

More broadly, our interviews suggest that while learning about social context arises out of doctor–patient interaction, not any form of clinical encounter will do. Our research points to a distinct relationship between physician remuneration, the organization of clinical time and particular forms of doctor–patient dialogue from which knowledge about context can arise. Learning about the context of marginalized people's lives requires intimate forms of patient disclosure across considerable social distance. Openness, careful listening, and the building of trust are accomplished slowly. Socio-clinical knowledge, then, is best facilitated by an organization of clinical activity that permits extended patients visits over a lengthy duration. These conditions are not easily secured or promoted through the standard organization of primary clinical practice in Canada through fee for service billing.

> If I see somebody in five or ten minutes, they can leave and I can feel safe and comfortable because I don't know anything about them. I don't know that they're walking out the door and getting beaten by their spouse. I don't know that they're social, their welfare has been, you know held back…and they don't get their cheque for a month and food for their kids falls apart, their housing falls apart, If you walk into a [walk-in clinic] you'll get five minute treatment and they won't know anything about the context of their patients in five. It's 'get them in, get them out.' (Interview 7)

We do not mean to suggest that the physicians we interviewed who are remunerated through fee for service payment are not working successfully with marginalized patients. Our point is that they work under less favourable conditions of clinical time than their salaried counterparts. As one salaried physician suggested, "Now we book people every 15 minutes, but if I need to take 45 minutes, I do…somebody comes in in crisis, we'll sit there for 45 minutes until we get to the bottom of what's going on."

Beyond duration within the clinical visit, learning about social context requires regular contact with patients over time. One physician we interviewed who described working with large Afro-Canadian and Middle-East populations spoke about working for years to reach a point where his patients felt comfortable sharing intimacies about their family and work lives, the discriminations they faced and other aspects of their daily social circumstances. Generous clinical time and continuity of care and the organization of funding that permits them are central to generating the forms of dialogue that facilitate informal learning about the context of marginalized patients' lives.

Informal learning about social context is also intersubjective at the point of family physicians' relationships with other health care workers. Those physicians who worked in settings where other health care providers also practice had opportunities to gain knowledge about the context of marginalized patients' lives that solo practitioners did not. We heard, in particular, from physicians working in community health clinic settings about how they learned about the various social and economic circumstances faced by disadvantaged patients through their work interactions with nurses, social workers, nurse practitioners, nutritionists, and others. Their accounts point to how developing socio-clinical knowledge is facilitated by a multidisciplinary organization of clinical work that brings various practitioners into ongoing, face-to-face relationship with one another at the point of care. These relations of clinical work organize informal learning about context as a process of bringing together different forms of information from multiple sources into a composite picture of the broad circumstances that shape the health of marginalized patients.

In some instances, the sources of information drawn upon by physicians to learn about context extend beyond the limits of professional discourse. In a particularly salient example, a physician working with homeless men spoke about how he combined information about patients from a worker in a soup kitchen with other sources of information in formulating his response to patients.

> He would give me a description of the difficulties that someone's having…from a lay person's perspective, okay. So it would be issues around, behaviour difficulties that he's noticed, you know at breakfast time when we're there. Information that he gets from outside, what he's hearing about what is going on with the person, whether they be behavioural, or issues that they might be having with housing, or any number of things, right? But they're a description of the problems from a different perspective… And it provides me with a context of what's going on with that individual, right…and I have to then turn it around and sort of re-synthesize it into…my skill set. And so, I take his information and integrate with what I get from the individual which often takes a long time to get, because they don't access services, right? And sort of use both perspectives to kind of formulate a plan. (Interview 6)

Here is a striking account that underscores the complexities of working with marginalized patients. It speaks to circumstances of extreme marginalization in which, for varied reasons, people do not access conventionally organized health services. How then do physicians learn about how to work with them? Clearly, it can be more involved than initially anticipated. The account above underscores the complex and careful "work" of informal learning that goes into producing socio-clinical knowledge in all its hybridity. It points to the delicate and prolonged work of piecing together information from, at times, unexpected sources as part of responding to the health problems produced or aggravated by marginalization.

CLOSING REMARKS

In recent decades, in Canada, the health needs of marginalized people have emerged as a concern within medical education. This paper extends proposals for changing formal medical education to better address the context shaping marginalized people's health (Phillips, 1995; Watson et al., 1991), by offering a detailed exploration of informal learning processes amongst practicing family physicians. The title of our paper notwithstanding, our intention is not primarily a critique of formal medical education. There is much good work happening on the ground in medical schools in Canada and elsewhere focused on making the health needs of marginalized populations more visible to emerging physicians. We wish neither to efface such efforts nor to create, by default, a straw version of medical school training. The critical spirit of the title and, indeed, of the paper as a whole, is rather, that more work needs to be done.

Our analysis emphasizes how knowledge of social context is created experientially through physician's interaction with patients and health care providers and is supported institutionally through forms of physician remuneration that create "generous" clinical time. The questioning of physician authority that is part of providing care to marginalized patients and the development of knowledge of context as an internal feature of providing clinical care might both be read as support for the current emphasis on reflective, practice-based learning approaches within medical training. Our emphasis on the hybrid character of socio-clinical knowledge, our likening of it to a clinician's political economy of health, further suggests the potential value of deepening cultural competence training in formal medical education with population health perspectives emphasizing the social, political, and economic factors shaping health.

At the same time we recognize the limits of transferring the results of our study to the site of formal medical training. An important message arising out of our research is that formal education can never fully prepare or equip medical students to successfully work with marginalized patients. There always will and should be informal learning at the site of clinical care. At best, medical students can be prepared for its necessity.

Yet herein lies an important tension. While knowledge of social context tends to be devalued in medical schools and does not circulate widely as part of formal medical training, it is at the same time not easily produced outside of medical school settings. Socio-clinical knowledge is organizationally vulnerable. In the context of physician shortages, the imperatives of fee for service billing, and general calls for greater efficiency in health care, the time pressures placed on clinical care are considerable. A general concern expressed in our interviews is the pressure to clinically "process" patients in as timely a fashion as possible. Yet knowledge of the health contexts of marginalized people's lives is gleaned over years and is produced interactively through dialogue that requires intimacy and takes time. Working with marginalized patients in ways informed by social context will require challenges to the organizational restrictions on clinical care if it is to become a broad possibility of family medicine.

It is also the case that socio-clinical knowledge can be difficult to create at the site of physician/patient and interprofessional dialogue. Developing a practical, clinically oriented knowledge of social context requires that marginalized patients make intimate disclosures to physicians and other health care providers. Typically understood as a part of the liberal tradition of humanistic medicine (Mykhalovskiy & Weir, 2004) the forms of interaction producing such disclosure have their own power dynamic. There are obvious potential privacy concerns at work, the possibility for intrusion, and for aggravation of cultural differences over the public value of intimate knowledge. Health care providers can also be reticent to talk with one another about the details of patient's day-to-day lives. What details of social context are relevant to clinical work? How much knowledge of social context is enough? When have things gone too far?

While we offer no quick answers, we hope our paper might contribute to dialogue on such questions. Our research suggests how working with marginalized patients and embracing knowledge of context involves recognizing and working with health as embedded in broad social, political, and economic determinants. Wrestling with the institutional relations that might facilitate knowledge of social context and with the power dynamics internal to its production and use are fundamental to strengthening forms of medical care that meet the health needs of marginalized people.

ACKNOWLEDGMENTS

This research was supported through an Intramural Faculty of Medicine Grant, Dalhousie University. We would like to thank all the physicians with whom we spoke for their generosity and willingness to share their experiences with us. An earlier version of this paper was presented at the Visiting Speakers Series at the Division of Community Health, Faculty of Medicine, Memorial University of Newfoundland. We thank Natalie Beausoleil for organizing this opportunity. We also thank Fern Brunger, Diana Gustafson, Natalie Beausoleil, and others in attendance at the seminar for their helpful comments.

REFERENCES

Amaratunga, C. (Ed.) (2002). *Race, ethnicity and women's health.* Halifax, NS: Atlantic Centre of Excellence for Women's Health.

Anderson, J. (1998). Speaking of illness: Issues of first generation Canadian women – Implications for patient education and counseling. *Patient Education and Counseling, 33,* 197–207.

Atkinson, P. (1984). Training for certainty. *Social Science & Medicine, 19*(9), 949–956.

Beagan, B. L. (2001). "Even If I Don't Know What I'm Doing I Can Make It Look Like I Know What I'm Doing": Becoming a doctor in the 1990s. *The Canadian Review of Sociology and Anthropology, 38*(3), 275–292.

Becker, H. S., Geer, B., Hughes, E. C., & Strauss, A. L. (1961). *Boys in white.* Chicago, IL: University of Chicago Press.

Campbell, M. (2000a). Knowledge, gendered subjectivity and restructuring of health care: The case of the disappearing nurse. In: S. Neysmith (Ed.), *Restructuring caring labour: Discourse, state practice and everyday life* (pp. 186–208). Toronto, ON: Oxford University Press.

Campbell, M. (2000b). Participatory research on health care for people with disabilities: Exploring the social organization of service provision. *Research in Social Science and Disabilities, 1*(1), 131–154.

Champaneria, M., & Axtell, S. (2004). Cultural competence training in U.S. medical schools. *JAMA, 291*(17), 2141.

Charles, C., Gafni, A., & Whelan, T. (1997). Shared decision-making in the medical encounter: What does it mean? (Or it takes at least two to tango). *Social Science & Medicine, 44*(5), 681–692.

Charles, C., Gafni, A., & Whelan, T. (1999). Decision-making in the physician–patient encounter: Revisiting the shared treatment decision-making model. *Social Science & Medicine, 49*(5), 651–661.

Chavez, R., Kemp, L., & Harris, E. (2004). The social capital: Health relationship in two disadvantaged neighbourhoods. *Journal of Health Services Research and Policy, 9*(Suppl. 2), 29–34.

Church, K., Bascia, N., & Shragge, E. (Eds) (2004). *Making sense of lived experience in turbulent times: Informal learning.* Waterloo, ON: Wilfrid Laurier University Press.

Church, K., Fontan, J. M., Ng, R., & Shragge, E. (2000). *Social learning among people who are excluded from the labour market. Part one: Context and studies.* NALL Working Paper Series, Paper No.11. Retrieved March 1, 2005, from University of Toronto, The

Research Network on New Approaches to Lifelong Learning. Web Site: http://www.nall.ca/res/11sociallearning.pdf

Coburn, D., Denny, K., Mykhalovskiy, E., McDonough, P., Robertson, A., & Love, R. (2003). Population health in Canada: A brief critique. *American Journal of Public Health, 93*(3), 392–396.

Cribb, A., & Bignold, S. (1999). Towards the reflexive medical school: The hidden curriculum and medical education research. *Studies in Higher Education, 24*, 195–209.

Dault, M., Lomas, J., & Barer, M. (2004). *Listening for direction II: National consultation on health service and policy issues for 2004–2007*. Ottawa: Canadian Health Services Research Foundation.

Devault, M., & McCoy, L. (2002). Institutional ethnography: Using interviews to investigate ruling relations. In: J. F. Gubrium & J. A. Holstein (Eds), *Handbook of interview research: Context and method* (pp. 751–776). Thousand Oaks, CA: Sage.

Diamond, T. (1992). *Making gray gold: Narratives from inside nursing homes*. Chicago, IL: University of Chicago Press.

Evans, R. G., Barer, M., & Marmor, T. (Eds) (1994). *Why are some people healthy and others not?* Hawthorne, NY: Aldine de Gruyter.

Evans, R. G., & Stoddart, G. I. (1990). Producing health, consuming health care. *Social Science & Medicine, 31*, 1347–1363.

Faith, M. S., Scanlon, K. S., Birch, L. L., Francis, L. A., & Sherry, B. (2004). Parent-child feeding strategies and their relationships to child eating and weight status. *Obesity Research, 12*(11), 1711–1722.

Flores, G., Gee, D., & Kastner, B. (2000). The teaching of cultural issues in U.S. and Canadian medical schools. *Academic Medicine, 75*, 451–455.

Foucault, M. (1994/1963). *Birth of the clinic: An archaeology of medical perception*. New York: Vintage Books.

Fox, R. (1957). Training for uncertainty. In: R. K. Merton, G. Reader & P. L. Kendall (Eds), *The student physician* (pp. 207–244). Cambridge, MA: Harvard University Press.

Fox, R. (1980). The evolution of medical uncertainty. *Milbank Memorial Fund Quarterly, 58*(1), 1–49.

Frohlich, K., Potvin, L., Chabot, P., & Corin, E. (2002). A theoretical and empirical analysis of context: Neighbourhoods, smoking and youth. *Social Science & Medicine, 54*(9), 1401–1417.

Good, B. J., & Good, M.-J. (1993). 'Learning medicine': The constructing of medical knowledge at Harvard Medical School. In: S. Lindenbaum & M. Lock (Eds), *Knowledge, power and practice* (p. 81107). Berkeley, CA: University of California Press.

Kobus, K. (2003). Peers and adolescent smoking. *Addiction, 98*(S1), 37–55.

Liang, L., Chaloupka, F., Nichter, M., & Clayton, R. (2003). Prices, policies and youth smoking, May 2001. *Addiction, 98*(S1), 105–122.

Lingard, L., Garwood, K., Schryer, C. F., & Spafford, M. M. (2003). A certain art of uncertainty: Case presentation and the development of professional identity. *Social Science & Medicine, 56*(3), 603–616.

Livingstone, D. (in press). Informal learning: Conceptual distinctions and preliminary findings. In: Z. Bekerman, N. Bubules & D. Silberman (Eds), *Learning in hidden places: The informal education reader*. Bern: Peter Lang (forthcoming).

Lochner, K. A., Kwachi, I., Brennan, R. T., & Buka, S. L. (2003). Social capital and neighbourhood mortality rates in Chicago. *Social Science & Medicine, 56*(8), 1797–1805.

MacMillan, H. L., MacMillan, A. B., Offord, D. R., & Dingle, J. L. (1996). Aboriginal health. *CMAJ, 155*(11), 1569–1578.

Makoul, G. (2003). Communication skills education in medical school and beyond. *JAMA, 289*(1), 93.

Martin, E. (1994). *Flexible bodies: Tracking immunity in American culture from the days of polio to the age of AIDS.* Boston: Beacon Press.

McCoy, L. (2005). HIV+ patients and the doctor–patient relationship: Perspectives from the margins. *Qualitative Health Research, 15*(6), 791–806.

Menec, V. H., Roos, N. P., Black, C., & Bogdanovic, B. (2001). Characteristics of patients with a regular source of care. *Canadian Journal of Public Health, 92*(4), 299–303.

Mustard, C. A., Mayer, T., Black, C., & Postl, B. (1996). Continuity of pediatric ambulatory care in a universally insured population. *Pediatrics, 98*, 1028–1034.

Mykhalovskiy, E. (2001). On the uses of health services research: Troubled hearts, care pathways and the reform of hospital care. *Studies in Cultures, Organizations, and Societies, 7*(2), 269–296.

Mykhalovskiy, E. (2003). Evidence-based medicine: Ambivalent reading and the clinical recontextualization of science. *Health, 7*(3), 331–352.

Mykhalovskiy, E., & McCoy, L. (2002). Troubling ruling discourses of health: Using institutional ethnography in community-based research. *Critical Public Health, 12*(1), 17–37.

Mykhalovskiy, E., & Weir, L. (2004). The problem of evidence-based medicine: Directions for social science. *Social Science & Medicine, 59*(5), 1059–1069.

Percy, K., Burton, C., & Withnall, A. (1994). *Self-directed learning among adults: The challenge for continuing educators.* Lancaster: Association for Lifelong Learning.

Phillips, S. (1995). The social context of women's health: Goals and objectives for medical education. *Canadian Medical Association Journal, 152*(4), 507–511.

Poland, B., Coburn, D., Robertson, A., & Eakin, J. (1998). Critical Social Science Group. Wealth, equity, and health care: A critique of a 'population health' perspective on the determinants of health. *Social Science & Medicine, 46*(7), 785–798.

Pottie, K., Masi, R., Watson, B., Heyding, R., & Roberts, M. (2000). Marginalized patients: A challenge for family physicians. *Canadian Family Physician, 46*, 15–17.

Rankin, J. (2001). Texts in action: How nurses are doing the fiscal work of health care reform. *Studies in Cultures, Organisations and Societies, 7*(2), 251–267.

Raphael, D. (Ed.) (2004). *Social determinants of health: Canadian perspectives.* Toronto: Canadian Scholar's Press.

Sinclair, S. (1997). *Making doctors. An institutional apprenticeship.* Oxford: Berg.

Smith, D. E. (1987). *The everyday world as problematic. A feminist sociology.* Boston: Northeastern University Press.

Smith, G. (1990). Political activist as ethnographer. *Social Problems, 37*, 629–648.

Stewart, M. J. (1990). Access to health care for economically disadvantaged Canadians: A model. *Canadian Journal of Public Health, 81*, 450–455.

Talbot, Y., Fuller-Thomson, E., Tudiver, F., Habib, Y., & McIsaac, W. (2001). Canadians without regular medical doctors. Who are they? *Canadian Family Physician, 47*, 58–64.

Taylor, J. S. (2003a). Confronting "culture" in medicine's "culture of no culture". *Academic Medicine, 78*(6), 555–559.

Taylor, J. S. (2003b). The story catches you and you fall down: Tragedy, ethnography, and "cultural competence". *Medical Anthropology Quarterly, 17*(2), 159–181.

Tough, A. (1979). *The adult's learning projects: A fresh approach to theory and practice in adult learning.* Toronto: Ontario Institute for Studies in Education Press.

Veenstra, G. (2003). Economy, community and mortality in British Columbia, Canada. *Social Science & Medicine, 56*(8), 1807–1816.

Veugelers, P., & Guernsey, J. (1999). Health deficiencies in Cape Breton County, Nova Scotia, Canada, 1950–1995. *Epidemiology, 10*(5), 495–499.

Watson, W. J., Wetzel, W., & Devanesen, S. (1991). Working with inner-city families: An ecological approach for the family physician. *Canadian Family Physician, 37*, 2585–2592.

Weerasinghe, S. (2003). *Diversity and interaction of health, interaction of diversity.* Citizenship and Immigration Canada.

West, L. (2001). *Doctors on the edge: General practitioners, health and learning in the inner-city.* London: Free Association Books.

RAPID CLINICAL DECISIONS IN CONTEXT: A THEORETICAL MODEL TO UNDERSTAND PHYSICIANS' DECISION-MAKING WITH AN APPLICATION TO RACIAL/ETHNIC TREATMENT DISPARITIES

Joshua H. Tamayo-Sarver, Neal V. Dawson,
Susan W. Hinze, Rita K. Cydulka, Robert S. Wigton
and David W. Baker

ABSTRACT

The purpose of this paper is to draw on previous work in multiple disciplines to establish a theoretical framework for clinical decision-making that incorporates non-medical factors, such as race/ethnicity, into the way physicians make decisions in the practice of medicine. The proposed Rapid Clinical Decision in Context (RCDC) model attempts to understand the influence of various contextual elements on physicians' decision-

Health Care Services, Racial and Ethnic Minorities and Underserved Populations: Patient and
Provider Perspectives
Research in the Sociology of Health Care, Volume 23, 183–213
ISSN: 0275-4959/doi:10.1016/S0275-4959(05)23009-0

making process. The RCDC model provides a basis for future studies to move beyond documentation of areas where disparities exist to understand the causes of the disparities and designing interventions to address those causes. The paper concludes with a discussion on possible studies to test the proposed model.

INTRODUCTION

Healthy People 2010 lists the elimination of racial disparities in healthcare as one of the nation's objectives for the 21st century (Satcher, 2001). One of the more contentious areas of examination is the influence of patient race/ethnicity on physicians' decision-making (Bloche, 2001). A voluminous body of literature on racial/ethnic disparities in treatment contains many contradictory findings, as summarized in a recent Institute of Medicine report (Committee on Understanding and Eliminating Racial and Ethnic Disparities in Health Care, 2002). Studies have found racial differences in physicians' decisions about cardiac care (Fincher et al., 2004; Ibrahim et al., 2003; Sheifer, Escarce, & Schulman, 2000; Venkat et al., 2003), analgesia (Bernabei et al., 1998; Cleeland, Gonin, Baez, Loehrer, & Pandya, 1997; Ng, Dimsdale, Rollnik, & Shapiro, 1996; Tamayo-Sarver, Hinze, Cydulka, & Baker, 2003b; Todd, Samaroo, & Hoffman, 1993; Todd, Deaton, D'Adamo, & Goe, 2000), cancer treatment (Bach, Cramer, Warren, & Begg, 1999; Ball & Elixhauser, 1996), and HIV care (Moore, Stanton, Gopalan, & Chaisson, 1994; Shapiro et al., 1999). These studies suggest that physicians' treatment decisions are affected by patient race/ethnicity.

Other studies have not found a racial/ethnic difference in analgesia prescribing (Karpman, Del Mar, & Bay, 1997; Tamayo-Sarver et al., 2003a), cancer treatment (Dominitz, Samsa, Landsman, & Provenzale, 1998; McKinlay et al., 1997, 1998; Optenberg et al., 1995), diabetes treatment (Martin, Selby, & Zhang, 1995; Wisdom et al., 1997), or HIV treatment (Bennett, Horner, Aboulafia, & Weinstein, 1995), or have found no difference in disparity by physician race/ethnicity (Chen, Rathore, Radford, Wang, & Krumholz, 2001). These studies suggest that physicians' treatment decisions do not respond to patient race/ethnicity. Attributing racial/ethnic disparities in treatment to "unconscious bias" or "stereotyping" is insufficient for explaining contradictory findings, and it does not clarify how information is incorporated into the decision-making processes, and fails to inform interventions to eliminate the disparities where they exist.

The purpose of this paper is to establish a theoretical framework for clinical decision-making that incorporates non-medical factors, such as race, into the way physicians may make decisions in the practice of medicine. The proposed Rapid Clinical Decision in Context (RCDC) model attempts to elucidate the influence of various contextual elements on the physician's decision-making process. In this paper, we provide an overview of the model and discuss its components with references to illustrative examples from the racial disparities literature. We conclude with a discussion of implications for future interventions. The RCDC model provides a basis for future studies to move beyond documentation of areas where disparities exist along lines of social stratification (e.g., race/ethnicity, gender, and socioeconomic status) to understanding the causes of the disparities and designing interventions to address those causes.

DEFINING "RACE/ETHNICITY"

While we acknowledge the considerable debate about the meaning (Winant, 2000) and study of race (Bagley, 1995; Williams, 1997), this paper is primarily concerned with the effect of patient race/ethnicity on physicians' decision-making. Thus, race/ethnicity as perceived by the treating physician is the relevant meaning of race/ethnicity for this paper. This interpretation of race/ethnicity is consistent with the definition of race and ethnicity as "social or cultural constructs for categorizing people based on perceived differences in biology (physical appearance) and behavior" (AAA, 1997). Throughout this paper, we use examples involving African-American, and Latino patients because the research into treatment disparities among these two groups is the most robust. The theoretical framework, however, is intended to apply to decision-making in general, and is not limited to our application of the framework to the effects of patient race/ethnicity on physician's decision-making.

OVERVIEW OF THE RCDC MODEL

In the RCDC model (Fig. 1), we suggest that experienced physicians generally use a recognition-primed decision-making process and postulate how contextual factors may enter into physicians' cognitive processes. After a brief overview of the model, we will expand on each step in subsequent sections following Fig. 1.

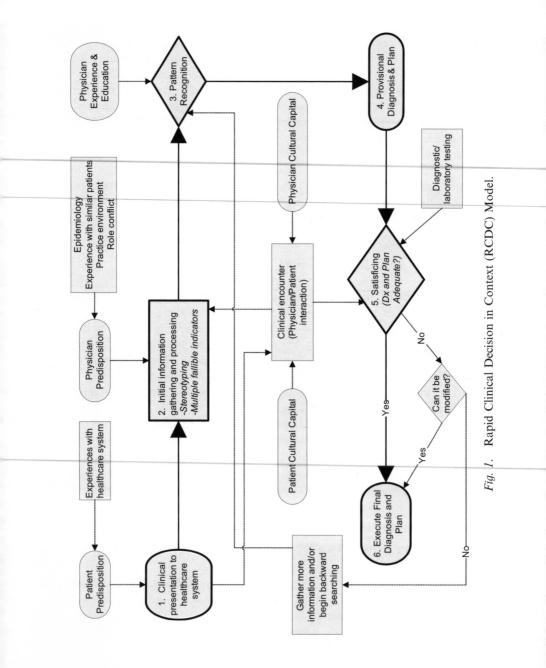

Fig. 1.   Rapid Clinical Decision in Context (RCDC) Model.

Both patients and physicians bring certain *predispositions* to the clinical encounter (Fig. 1). These predispositions are a combination of biases, opinions, and knowledge, and they influence the physician's information gathering and assessment. Often based solely on the nursing note and before seeing the patient, the physician will recognize the pattern of information presented as being similar to a mental representation of symptoms and treatment goals. The physician's provisional diagnosis and treatment plan are components of this mental representation that includes symptoms and treatment goals. The amount of information required before a pattern is recognized and the robustness of the physician's mental representations of patients depends upon the physician's education and experience. Once the provisional diagnosis and treatment plan are formulated, the physician ensures an adequate diagnosis and plan instead of searching for the ideal treatment and plan. This process, called *satisficing*, may require physician–patient interaction and/or testing to ensure a satisfactory match between the physician's mental representation and the patient's presentation. This interaction is influenced by the predispositions of the patient and the physician as well as the degree to which the physician and the patient have a shared background, experiences, beliefs, values, and tastes, i.e. *cultural capital*. When the physician must rely on information communicated by the patient, the quality of the communication and the physician's ability to determine if the provisional diagnosis and plan are satisfactory hinges upon their shared cultural capital. If the physical exam, communication, or testing fails the physician's expectations, the physician will reject the provisional diagnosis and plan and attempt to modify them. If the provisional diagnosis and plan cannot be modified to be adequate, the physician will gather more information to enable recognition of a different pattern. Once adequate, the physician will execute the diagnosis and plan. The experience of this encounter will inform the physician's future pattern recognition as well as the predispositions of both the physician and the patient.

BEFORE THE ENCOUNTER – PATIENT AND PHYSICIAN PREDISPOSITION

Neither patients nor physicians enter the medical encounter without experiences, pre-formed opinions, or expectations for that current encounter. The physician's decision-making process is activated before entering the examination room by the nurse's note, which typically includes the patient's chief complaint, vital signs, age, sex, medical conditions, and medications. To understand how patients affect physicians' decision-making requires a broader understanding of the social structure within which the encounter occurs (Waitzkin, 1991, 2000). Racial and ethnic minorities have significantly less wealth, education, occupational prestige, and political influence than Whites; racial/ethnic segregation persists in neighborhoods and schools; and discrimination continues in housing and employment (Lillie-Blanton & Laveist, 1996). While some evidence suggests that European attitudes toward racial and ethnic minorities have improved (in part due to the rise of the Black middle class), other evidence reveals that negative racial stereotyping, especially of African-Americans and Latinos, is common among European-Americans (Bobo, 1997, 2001). Like members of any dominant group, physicians act within a social structure that is gendered, raced, and classed. And while there are, undoubtedly, physicians who intentionally give preferential treatment to one race or ethnicity over another, anecdotal evidence, based upon the experiences of the co-authors, suggests that the overwhelming majority of physicians do not intentionally deliver different care based on patient race/ethnicity. Why then, do we find evidence that patient race/ethnicity is a factor in physicians' decision-making?

Physicians, like all individuals, develop an understanding, perception, and expectation of the environment common to members of their group (Bourdieu & Passeron, 1977). We will refer to the individual's understanding, perception, and expectation of a given situation as the individual's *predisposition*. Because an individual's predisposition is also influenced by unique life experiences, it is both shared with the group and unique to the individual. An individual's predisposition shapes the individual's interpretation, satisfaction with, and actions in response to a given situation. Predisposition is similar to the individual's experience that colors and informs the understanding of the present situation, except that the concept of predisposition acknowledges the role of social group in shaping the individual's experience.

Patients' predispositions influence the clinical encounter because patients' expectations and beliefs influence the information patients present, how patients present the information, and their investment in the decision-making process. Evidence suggests some racial/ethnic minority patients, based on past experiences, approach the medical encounter with little trust, low value placed on the encounter, and little legitimacy attached to the physician's opinions (LaVeist, Nickerson, & Bowie, 2000; Lillie-Blanton, Brodie, Rowland, Altman, & McIntosh, 2000).

Physicians' predisposition influences the clinical encounter and their pattern recognition. Physician pattern recognition is influenced by the information the physician has prior to evaluating the patient (Hatala, Norman, & Brooks, 1999). Most physicians are likely to have a similar predisposition due to the homogenizing effects of extensive schooling and because the majority of physicians come from European-American, upper-middle to upper-class families (Waitzkin, 1983, 2000). Physicians' predispositions may influence their understanding of patients. For example, an individual physician may expect that an African-American or Hispanic-American patient is uninsured or is unable to afford recommended therapies. These expectations may be epidemiologically correct (Ammons, 1997), but may bias the physician's treatment of the patient based on race/ethnicity. Physicians' predisposition is influenced by four main factors: (1) epidemiology/base rate, (2) experience with similar patients, (3) practice environment, and (4) role conflict. While stereotyping is assigning information based on social categorization, predisposition describes what information is likely to be assigned via stereotyping.

First, physicians' predisposition, in terms of expectations for the encounter, includes physicians' assessments of the base rate of possible problems. Pattern recognition will be influenced by factors that determine the baseline likelihood that a patient has a given disease (Hatala et al., 1999). Studies suggest that physicians use base rates rationally when in familiar situations (Bergus, Chapman, Gjerde, & Elstein, 1995; Chapman, Bergus, & Elstein, 1996), but neglect base rates in unfamiliar situations (Casscells, Schoenberger, & Graboys, 1978). Physicians' perception of the base rate of a disease given a patient's specific scenario is likely a combination of physicians' education, clinical experience, and personal background.

Second, as the physicians' repertoire of mental representations increases with experience, it is more likely that the physicians' will recognize symptoms and goals based solely on the nurse's note. The more the patient appears similar to a previous patient based on the nurse's note, the more likely physicians' predispositions will reflect the expectations of the previous encounter.

Third, practice environment shapes physicians' predispositions. When physicians and patients have a continuity of care relationship, physicians' predispositions toward patients may be increasingly based on experiences with the individual patients and decreasingly based on inferred, assumed, or stereotyped information about the patient. One would expect that physician use of stereotyped information based on predispositions developed from population characteristics, such as race/ethnicity, would decrease in strong continuity relationships. In the case of racial and ethnic disparities, however, minorities are overrepresented in settings that may compromise continuity of the physician–patient relationship. Certain racial minorities are more likely to rely on hospital outpatient clinics for ambulatory care (Lillie-Blanton, Martinez, & Salganicoff, 2001), public and major teaching hospitals for inpatient care (Gaskin, 1999), present to the emergency department with less urgent conditions (Lowe et al., 2001), and lack a regular primary care provider (Collins, Hall, & Neuhaus, 1999) compared to Whites.

Fourth, the role conflict experienced by physicians plays a part in their predisposition. The role of physicians is often conceptualized as pure patient advocate: physicians take the Hippocratic Oath and proclaim their intention to serve patients' needs, regardless of the individual attributes of patients. According to sociologist Talcott Parsons, the physician (ideally) views the patient objectively, without moral judgment, and with an emphasis on medical facts (Clark, Potter, & McKinlay, 1991). As a pure patient advocate, the physician (Parsons, 1951) does not allow personal feelings to enter into the medical decision. However, in conflict with the ideal role of patient advocate is physicians' gatekeeping position in the structure of Western medicine (Lorber, 1997)[1].

Physicians are mandated by law and policy to validate sickness so patients can: (a) qualify for services, and (b) receive work- and school-related exemptions.[2] For example, physicians regularly engage in disability assessment, and make medical decisions that influence disability-related housing, insurance eligibility, exclusion from military service, and disability-related income. Furthermore, physicians' societal gatekeeper role has expanded as healthcare practice environments have changed (Starr, 1982) and physicians must increasingly determine whether patients qualify for certain finite resources (Inui, 1992; Lorber, 1997). The U.S. healthcare environment has engendered an acute awareness of healthcare costs (Hillman, Nash, Kissick, & Martin, 1986; Pauly, Hillman, & Kerstein, 1990) with a consequent obligation to protect the healthcare system from unnecessary use (Cohen, Asch, & Ubel, 2000; Veatch, 1991). Increasingly, the physician, as gatekeeper, must ensure that the patient does not use more resources than needed.

Physicians' conflicting roles of patient advocate and societal gatekeeper may have significant effects on physicians' decision-making. If one imagines a continuum between patient advocate and societal gatekeeper, it seems reasonable that physicians will increasingly search for features to distinguish patients' levels of need as the physician adopts the role of societal gatekeeper. Thus, the physician may be more willing to spend resources on patients felt to be "deserving" or likely to benefit from such resources (Murphy-Berman, Berman, & Campbell, 1998). Patients perceived as "deserving" or likely to benefit tend to be from middle to upper class, cooperative, articulate, compliant, and not demanding (Mizrahi, 1986; Murphy-Berman et al., 1998).

If physicians do not feel a need to conserve resources, physicians may be less influenced by contextual factors in an attempt to differentiate patients' level of need. According to this hypothesis, physicians who feel little obligation to serve as a resource gatekeeper in a given patient encounter should be less influenced by race. Available evidence is consistent with this hypothesis. While Blacks are generally likely to receive less-intensive treatment for cancer (Bach et al., 1999; Mayberry, Mili, & Ofili, 2000), there is substantial racial equality in cancer treatment in universally accessible Department of Defense health system (Optenberg et al., 1995) and Veterans Administration medical centers (Dominitz et al., 1998). Alternatively, this finding may suggest that the populations served by these two health systems are relatively homogenous and (a) patient race/ethnicity is not used as a surrogate for other information, or (b) the degree to which cultural capital is shared between patient and provider is similar across races. Assuming that physicians' decisions are more influenced by race/ethnicity when fulfilling a gatekeeper role, one would expect that minorities would receive less care. This expectation is consistent with African-Americans receiving less-invasive cardiac procedures (Sheifer et al., 2000), African-Americans and Latinos receiving less analgesia (Bernabei et al., 1998; Cleeland et al., 1997; Ng et al., 1996; Todd et al., 1993, 2000; Tamayo-Sarver et al., 2003b), African-Americans receiving less aggressive cancer treatment (Bach et al., 1999; Ball & Elixhauser, 1996) and less-aggressive HIV care (Moore et al., 1994).

DURING THE ENCOUNTER

Patient's Clinical Presentation to the Healthcare System

The presenting features of illness in individual patients, regardless of contextual factors, are paramount in physician's decision-making. Physicians' decision-making processes, in terms of pattern-recognition and salient information gathering, vary when faced with a catastrophic motor vehicle accident versus an earache. While the patients' presentations are the main driving force in the pattern recognition, patients' predispositions influence the presentation. A patient might, for example, have had an experience or heard of a friend's experience where pain from a fracture was not addressed. Thus, the patient may try to exaggerate their report of pain so that the physician will address it. Typically, the patient will initially talk with a nurse who will record the patient's presentation on the chart and then pass that information to the physician. Thus, a physician's first impression of the patient is from the nurse's short description.

Information Interpreting/Gathering

It is impossible for physicians to acquire exhaustive knowledge about patients in a brief clinical encounter, so physicians focus the initial information gathering and assessment as the initial pattern is being recognized. Physicians make decisions under uncertainty and may rely on many pieces of information that approximate what they truly want to know, that is, they rely on multiple fallible indicators. Additionally, physicians may assume varying amounts of information through stereotyping. Both the fallible indicators and the stereotyped information constitute a part of the patterns that physicians recognize.

Physicians, like many decision-makers facing uncertainty, rely on multiple fallible indicators. Uncertainty is prevalent in many decision-making contexts: (i) a jury must decide the veracity of a witness's testimony, (ii) an employer must decide the competence of a job applicant, and (iii) a romantically involved couple must decide the desirability of their relationship. In each of these situations, there is no perfect indicator or set of indicators on which the decision-maker can unerringly rely: a witness looking away may indicate deception or it may not, a diploma from a prestigious college may guarantee competence or it may not, and a shared interest may be the harbinger of a long and fruitful relationship or it may not.

Hammond (1996) has reviewed the causes and consequences of decision-making under uncertainty. He demonstrates that error is inevitable when decision-makers are forced to rely on unreliable indicators. The indicators that are chosen and the errors that are tolerated determine who will suffer from the error. Physicians frequently diagnose and treat based on the recognition of a pattern of information, but this information is imperfect. For example, physicians may choose indicators to determine the accuracy of patients' reports, the physiological mechanisms occurring in patients' bodies, the psychological mechanisms occurring in patients' minds, the social context in which patients live, and the probability that a given treatment will be successful. While some indicators are better than others, none is perfect.

In medical encounters that are full of uncertainty, physicians may consciously or unconsciously use stereotyped information about social categories to infer information about individual patients (van Ryn, 2002). Using stereotypes permits physicians to feel as if they have more information and greater control over the situation (Mackie, Hamilton, Susskind, & Rosselli, 1996; Dovidio, 1999). The inferred social category is used as a surrogate variable. Thus an accessible variable (such as race or ethnicity) becomes a surrogate for inaccessible variables (such as likelihood of compliance). Using race as a surrogate variable may be inaccurate in many situations, but the process of stereotyping (i.e., classifying someone out of one social category and into another social category) engenders additional cognitive problems. The stereotyped information may be highly inaccurate about an individual patient and may cause physicians to overlook other information that does not conform with the stereotype (Fiske, 1998). In addition, assigning an individual to a social category to which the physician does not feel he or she belongs may make the physician less likely to advocate for the patient (Tajfel & Turner, 1979), have less of an emotional feeling of affiliation (Fiske, 1998; Operario & Fiske, 2001), and be more oppositional toward the patient (Mackie, Devos, & Smith, 2000).

Use of Race/Ethnicity as a Surrogate for Clinically Relevant Information may Depend on Physicians' Characteristics

Not all physicians will use race/ethnicity in the same way just as not all physicians will use any piece of information the same way (Green & Yates, 1993, 1995; Weisse, Sorum, Sanders, & Syat, 2001). The use of race as a surrogate for clinically relevant information may depend on a given physician's personal experience, background, and practice environment. A novice physician may not have been exposed to enough patients to be able to bring to mind a similar pattern of diagnosis and treatment. Without being able to use previous experience as a guide, the physician may be forced to work through the problem methodically and explicitly collect the specific information for which race would have been used as a surrogate.

A physician's background and personal attitudes toward race may shape that physician's interpretation of race and what it indicates. For example, an African-American physician may be more likely to notice that socioeconomic status is driving non-urgent emergency department use rather than patient's race. This illustrates that the use of race as a surrogate depends upon the physician's interpretation of what race indicates in that specific context. The possible information that race may represent depends on the physicians' practice environment. For example, physicians who practice within a staff-model HMO are unlikely to associate race with insurance status because all patients are insured. In contrast, physicians who practice in a suburban ED may associate race with insurance status. The use of race as a surrogate may depend on the decision-making process used by each physician, patients to whom each physician is exposed, and each physician's personal understanding of race.

Pattern Recognition and (4) Provisional Diagnosis & Plan

Studies suggest that physicians, as they gain expertise, increasingly rely on pattern recognition, while their hypothetico-deductive reasoning skills either plateau or diminish (Berwick, Fineberg, & Weinstein, 1981; Bordage, Brailovsky, Cohen, & Page, 1996; Deber & Baumann, 1992; Elstein, Shulman, & Sprafka, 1978; Elstein, 1992; Friedman, Korst, Schultz, Beatty, & Entine, 1978; Grant & Marsden, 1988; Hamm, Scheid, Smith, & Tape, 2000; McLeskey & Ward, 1978; Schmidt, Norman, & Boshuizen, 1990). Schmidt et al. (1990) discuss the development of medical knowledge as moving from understanding discrete facts to causal models of pathophysiology to recognizing the pattern of a clinical presentation. Although multiple memory organization theories have been proposed, only a memory type that includes script models can support both diagnostic reasoning and pattern recognition (Custers, Regehr, & Norman, 1996b; Hamm, 2003). Multiple authors have formulated models of decision-making that involve recognizing the pattern of a clinical presentation, testing expectations based on the pattern recognized, or backward searching (looking for signs/symptoms based on the known features of the possible disease) when the pattern of the clinical presentation is not recognized (Hamm et al., 2000; Hamm, 2003).[3] This model is referred to variously as script use (Abernathy & Hamm, 1994; Feltovich & Barrows, 1984; Schmidt et al., 1990), rule-based reasoning (Anderson, 1990, 1993), and recognition-primed decision-making (Klein, 1993). Several studies have demonstrated support for this model in expertise development (Charlin, Roy, Brailovsky, Goulet, & van der Vleuten, 2000; Lesgold, 1984), the relationship between memory and expertise (Green & Gilhooly, 1992; Schmidt & Boshuizen, 1993; van de Wiel, Schmidt, & Boshuizen, 1998), deviations from analytical use of statistical data (Norman, 2000), and practice patterns resistant to relevant information (Elstein, Christensen, Cottrell, Polson, & Ng, 1999). In short, physicians using recognition-primed decision-making recognize a pattern of patient presentation based on a mental representation of such a case, activate the diagnosis and treatment plan components of that mental representation, verify that the diagnosis and treatment plan will suffice in the present situation, and then carry out the diagnosis and plan. Essentially, the physicians are saying, "I've seen this before and treated this before. I will diagnose and treat this patient like I did similar patients in the past unless I find something that convinces me that I'm wrong".

One example of a clinical encounter according to the recognition-primed decision-making model may start with a patient presenting with a chief complaint of cough, sputum production, and fever. A physician would try to recognize the whole pattern of presentation as similar to a previously formed mental representation based on four aspects: (1) goals (e.g., relieve chest discomfort and cough), (2) cues (e.g., patient "looks" like other patients with viral bronchitis), (3) diagnosis/expectations (e.g., patient fits the diagnosis of viral bronchitis, and therefore should have signs and symptoms consistent with the diagnosis), and (4) actions/plans (e.g., treat this patient with symptomatic relief). The efficiency of this process is substantially dependent on physician's experience.

A physician must draw on experience to recognize the pattern of the clinical presentation. When physicians fail to recognize the pattern, they may begin a backward searching strategy, which entails searching for signs/symptoms based on the known features of the possible disease (Feltovich, Sprio, & Coulson, 1989; Schmidt et al., 1990). Decision-making strategies vary based on level or specialty of training (Johnson, Hassebrock, Duran, & Moller, 1982; Poses et al., 1997) or location (Tape, Heckerling, Ornato, & Wigton, 1991). More experienced decision-makers are more likely to use pattern recognition (Anderson, 1990, 1993; Custers, Boshuizen, & Schmidt, 1996a; Hobus, Schmidt, Boshuizen, & Patel, 1987; Klein, 1993). Similarly, more experienced physicians are more likely to use a patient's background and contextual factors to formulate their first provisional diagnosis and plan. Indeed, the diagnostic ability of expert clinicians is largely explained by their use of patient background and contextual factors (Custers et al., 1996a; Hobus et al., 1987; Hobus, Hofstra, Boshuizen, & Schmidt, 1988). The reliance of experienced physicians on patient's background and contextual factors was illustrated in a study by Custers et al. (1996a) who found atypical patient background and contextual factors greatly hampered experienced physicians but had little effect on the diagnostic abilities of senior medical students.

During the formative years, physicians learn what constitutes "desirable" and "deserving" patients as part of their socialization process (Mizrahi, 1986). Many physicians gain experience and build their repertoire of mental representations during residencies at teaching hospitals that care for urban, low-income, minority populations (Gabriel, 2002). Although hypothesized by this RCDC framework, the possibility that physicians' perceptions of minority patients and the mental representations prompted by a patient's race may differ depending on the environment in which residency training occurred has not been empirically evaluated.

Satisficing

Once a physician arrives at a provisional diagnosis and treatment plan, she does not perform all tests, nor does she consider every possibility to be certain that the best diagnosis and treatment plan were selected. Instead, the physician does a physical examination, laboratory testing, and communicates with the patient to ensure that the provisional diagnosis and plan are sufficient (Hamm, 1988; Klein, 1997; Payne, Bettman, & Johnson, 1993). In other words, the physician makes sure the choice of diagnosis and treatment plan *satisfy* the physician's criteria for an acceptable choice rather than searching for the absolutely best choice. This process, called "satisficing", is an important aspect of the recognition-primed decision-making model (Simon, 1956). In the satisficing step, using the above example, the physician might want to rule out pneumonia. Once the physician is satisfied that the diagnosis and plan are sufficient, the diagnosis and plan are executed unless information showing them to be inadequate arises.

It is important to keep in mind that pattern recognition involves recognizing that a patient's presentation is similar to a mental representation of the pattern of symptoms along with both the diagnosis and the treatment plan. Because the diagnosis and plan are components of the mental representation, the provisional diagnosis and plan are accepted from the beginning of the process until proven otherwise. The physician has several approaches to determine if the diagnosis and plan are adequate: (1) physical exam/laboratory testing, and (2) physician–patient interaction.

To determine the adequacy of the provisional diagnosis and treatment plan, the physician will likely perform a physical exam and diagnostic testing. Ideally, the physician's interpretation of physical exam findings and diagnostic tests would be independent pieces of information by which to judge the adequacy of the provisional diagnosis and treatment plan. However, several studies have demonstrated that the physician is most likely to recognize those features that agree with the provisional diagnosis and treatment plan, while minimizing or neglecting those features that are inconsistent with the physician's expectations (Hatala et al., 1999; Poses, Bekes, Winkler, Scott, & Copare, 1990).

Physicians often rely exclusively on interactions with the patient (e.g., obtained patient history) to determine if the diagnosis and plan are adequate. Undoubtedly, the physician–patient interaction often reveals the inadequacy of the diagnosis and plan to the physician. However, there is significant room for contextual factors, such as patient's social characteristics, to influence the decision-making process at this step. For example, there is good reason to suspect that physicians interact with certain racial and ethnic minority patients differently, with more negative feelings and less feelings of affiliation than with white patients (Spector, 2001; van Ryn & Burke, 2000). One way to examine the contextual influences on the patient–physician interactions is through predisposition and cultural capital.

The predispositions of the physician and the patient influence their interactions and, importantly, their expectations for the interaction. As discussed under patient presentation and stereotyping above, either the physician, the patient, or both, may be unreceptive or feel that certain elements must be exaggerated to be recognized. In the case of stereotyping, the patient or physician may behave in the interaction in a manner that leads the other to respond in stereotype-confirming ways (Sibicky & Dovidio, 1986).

An unexplored factor in communication that may contribute to the treatment of disparities along the lines of social categorization is cultural capital. Bourdieu describes cultural capital as a group's shared cultural background in terms of beliefs, values, language, appreciation of the arts, musical taste, and morals (Bourdieu & Passeron, 1977). Sharing cultural capital enables individuals to establish rapport and communicate with one another. According to Bourdieu and Passeron (1977), educators share more cultural capital with those from higher social classes than those from lower social classes.

Defining Cultural capital can be thought of as "dispositions which are unconsciously embodied in providers and users of health-care and which structure expectations concerning their interaction in health-care settings," (Smaje, 2000, p. 125). Smaje (1995) argues that dissonance results from a mismatch between provider and patient expectations of a "competent" patient and a "competent" provider. Notions of competence are associated with the class and racial positioning of both. Dissonance in physician–patient cultural capital may lead some physicians to view patients from some racial or ethnic groups as presenting with trivial complaints.

Shared cultural capital enables the building of rapport and effective communication. After training in a certain area (e.g., law, medicine, sociology, etc.), an individual's cultural capital expands to include that of the professional group. Humor unique to that group may be very funny to individuals who share the cultural capital, but nonsensical to those who do not (i.e., "medical humor", "lawyer humor", etc.). Since physicians tend to embody upper-middle class culture (even those few who come from lower class or working class backgrounds), there is evidence that physicians may experience anxiety in dealing with patients from lower social classes (Dungal, 1978), and may be generally biased toward middle class patients who are perceived as cleaner, more intelligent, more cooperative, and better historians than lower class patients (Mizrahi, 1986). Support of the hypothesis that minority physicians largely, but not completely, share the cultural capital of white physicians is found in a study by Cooper-Patrick et al. (1999). Cooper-Patrick et al. found that minority patients were less participatory than white patients, even when their physician was racially concordant. Interestingly, this study also supports the role of cultural capital because participation was highest within patient racial groups when the patient was racially concordant with their physician (Cooper-Patrick et al., 1999). From the patient perspective, racial minority patients may perceive physicians as insensitive to their needs (Donovan, 1986; Judge & Solomon, 1993). Furthermore, physicians may prove more competent advocates for patients who share their cultural capital (Waitzkin, 1985).

Adequacy of Diagnosis and Plan

A key feature of the RCDC model is the satisficing step. Recognition-primed decision-making is fast, uses the pattern of information, and produces an adequate, if not optimal, solution. The major difference between the rational/analytical decision model and the recognition-primed decision-making model is the point at which the decision is made. A physician operating under rational/analytical decision-making collects all information and decisions are made on the type of information collected, but diagnosis and plan are not formulated until all pertinent information has been gathered. A physician using recognition-primed decision-making, in contrast, hypothesizes the most likely diagnosis and plan at the beginning, then collects data to make sure the hypothesized diagnosis and plan will suffice, even if they are not optimal.

There is a lack of research to understand how physicians determine the threshold that a provisional diagnosis and treatment plan must meet before they are considered adequate and consequently executed. It is possible that such a threshold is influenced by stress (Hammond, 1999), unconsciously assigning the patient to a social category (see discussion of stereotyping above) (Fiske, 1998; Mackie et al., 2000; Operario & Fiske, 2001;Tajfel & Turner, 1979), the costs and benefits of additional satisficing (Arkes, 1991; Payne et al., 1993), and the degree to which physicians feel that patients' problems are amenable to medical treatment (Mizrahi, 1986).

Modification of the Provisional Diagnosis and Plan

If there is some aspect of the provisional diagnosis or treatment plan that is inadequate, that is it fails to satisfice, then the physician may attempt to modify the diagnosis or treatment plan to address the inadequacy. If it cannot be modified, then the physician may gather new information to recognize a new pattern or begin backward reasoning to attempt to identify possible diagnoses. Once the physician feels the provisional diagnosis and treatment plan are adequate, they are executed. For example, if the physician makes a provisional diagnosis of viral bronchitis and a treatment plan of symptomatic therapy, but finds radiographic evidence of pneumonia, the physician may modify the diagnosis to pneumonia and treat with an antibiotic.

AFTER THE ENCOUNTER

Interactions between physicians and patients are likely to reinforce and further develop each other's predisposition and future stereotyping behavior (Sibicky & Dovidio, 1986). Thus, patients' predisposition, physicians' predisposition, and the interactions between physicians and patients may shape patients' preferences as well as medical decisions. Therefore, attributing racial/ethnic disparities to patient preferences may fail to account for racially or ethnically based causes of differences in patient preferences (Committee on Understanding and Eliminating Racial and Ethnic Disparities in Health Care, 2002). The encounter will also serve to build the physician's mental representation of symptoms, context, diagnosis, and treatment plan, to be used for future patients (Abernathy & Hamm, 1995; Anderson, 1990).

SUMMARY AND ILLUSTRATIVE EXAMPLE OF RCDC

The RCDC framework provides a theoretical basis to begin to understand physician's decision-making (Fig. 1). An example may help demonstrate the usefulness of the framework to understand how racial/ethnic disparities in treatment may happen. Imagine that a European-American and an African-American patient present to the emergency department with an uncomplicated ankle fracture. The European-American patient is optimistic that she will be treated with respect and competence and the pain will be dealt with quickly. The physician, based on societal structure, practice environment, role conflict, and experience with similar patients has a fairly good idea of the diagnosis and treatment plan from reading the nurse's note even before entering the room. The physician expects to find a cooperative, easy to understand, likable woman in moderate to severe pain from a bad sprain or stable fracture. Upon entering the room, the physician wants to know certain salient details to make sure the provisional diagnosis, stable ankle fracture, and the provisional treatment plan, "immobilize and treat with opioid analgesic", will be sufficient. The physician and the patient interact and have a short discussion about their preferred running shoes, as they are both avid runners. The physician feels that the patient is being forthright and has little concern about the patient seeking an opioid for secondary gain. The physician quickly and easily learns enough to be satisfied that it is all adequate and leaves the room feeling like a competent healer. The patient is discharged with a splint, crutches, and an opioid analgesic.

Based on past experiences that the African-American patient either had personally or has heard about from peers, the African-American patient expects to sit in pain for a while. Based on negative past experiences, the African-American patient does not expect the physician to believe her and feels she must exaggerate her pain for it to be addressed. The physician enters the room expecting to find someone who is exaggerating their pain and unable to describe the problem using language that is helpful in making the diagnosis. The physician, because of an association between race and nonurgent emergency department use, expects to find an ankle sprain and provide the person a recommendation to purchase some ibuprofen over-the-counter. Upon entering the room, the physician has difficulty understanding the nature of the pain. Suspecting that the extent of the pain is exaggerated, the physician feels manipulated and becomes concerned that the patient may be seeking an opioid for secondary gain. Meanwhile, the patient feels that her pain is being minimized, as she expected. The physician leaves the room frustrated. Upon learning that the X-rays demonstrate a stable ankle fracture, the physician changes the provisional diagnosis to stable fracture, but feels that over-the-counter ibuprofen, immobilization with a splint, and the use of crutches will adequately control the pain.

The physician in this example did not consciously try to give the African-American patient inferior care on the basis of race. However, the physician's bias when entering the room and the chasm in cultural capital between the upper-middle class physician and the lower socioeconomic status patient allowed two different analgesic treatments to occur for the same condition.

DISTINCTIONS BETWEEN THE RCDC MODEL AND STEREOTYPING

Stereotyping is a process of assigning an individual to a social group and inferring information about the individual based on that assignment. There is no doubt that physicians, like most people, have conscious and unconscious stereotypes. But how does stereotyping lead to treatment differences? Simply attributing disparities in physician treatment decisions to "stereotyping" does not elucidate how the stereotyping process or the stereotyped information influences the cognitive decision-making process.

In contrast, our model presents a much more complex framework built on research into medical decision-making and examines how the cognitive decision-making process may be influenced by stereotyping, stereotyped information, use of multiple fallible indicators, surrogate variables, predisposition (including epidemiology, practice environment, role conflict, experience), training, communication, and cultural capital. Moreover, this model explains how stereotyping affects decisions. We hypothesize that stereotyping affects physicians' initial information processing of patients' clinical presentation, leading to different assumptions (i.e., pattern recognition) and different provisional treatments. This is important because it shows how stereotypes can *subconsciously* lead to differences in treatment plans. If stereotyping occurs *consciously* at later steps (i.e., satisficing), and leads to different treatment decisions, this can only be called racism (e.g., "This might not be the best treatment, but the Irish are so noncompliant that it's not worth it to try the more aggressive plan."). We believe subconscious use of stereotyping is probably the more common cause of racial differences in treatment, although conscious stereotyping undoubtedly occurs as well.

LIMITATIONS

The RCDC framework takes the well-studied principles of human expert decision-making in context and applies it to physicians. Although the

RCDC framework is based on general decision-making theory that includes the flexibility of the decision-making process, it is not without limitation. Indeed, the most striking limitation of the framework may be the difficulty in testing it empirically. While discrete portions of the framework can be tested, it would be very difficult to disprove the model as a whole because of its flexibility. While there is general support for the RCDC framework in the literature, research is needed to test the framework prospectively. Many current approaches addressing racial and ethnic disparities in treatment could be tailored specifically to test different pathways in the framework.

The purpose of this framework is to begin to understand how contextual information is incorporated into physician's decision-making so that the decision-making can be improved. Although understanding the root causes of physician decision-making is a critical first step toward finding solutions to eliminate racial differences in treatment patterns, the model does not point to easy solutions. The RCDC model suggests that it is very difficult to change physician's decision-making because physicians are forming provisional diagnoses and treatment plans in a fairly rigid way, as do most human decision-makers with expertise in a given area. This does not imply, however, that physicians should not be held to a high standard of quality or that they are not ultimately responsible for eliminating disparities. If physicians are not responsible for their decisions, then there is no hope of improving medical care for anyone, let alone the disadvantaged. It is important to note that humans have very poor insight into their own decision-making process and tend to believe that they consider factors that do not empirically appear to influence the decision (Hammond, 1971; Hammond & Brehmer, 1973; Slovic & Lichtenstein, 1971). Furthermore, the limited insight one has into one's own decision-making decreases with expertise (Slovic & Lichtenstein, 1971; Hammond, 1996). It is our hope that the framework will be used to target decision-making in productive ways so that physicians make better decisions for everyone.

IMPLICATIONS AND FUTURE DIRECTIONS

One approach to addressing disparities is to improve physician's decision-making through education. Viewed from within the RCDC framework, education would seek to alter the pattern recognition step of the decision-making process. Previous interventions have demonstrated that physician diagnostic accuracy can improve through computer education with cognitive feedback (Wigton, Poses, Collins, & Cebul, 1990). In this approach, physicians are asked to diagnose computer-simulated vignettes and are then told the true probability of the diagnosis. This approach could more directly follow the RCDC framework by teaching both the diagnosis and the treatment plan simultaneously. To specifically address racial and ethnic disparities, it may be effective to include racially or ethnically appropriate distracters. Physicians could be encouraged to always inquire about these factors directly and not allow race or ethnicity to be used as a surrogate for truly meaningful information.

Another approach to improving decision-making is the use of guidelines that the physician is asked to use as a decision aid. From the RCDC perspective, the physician has already formulated a provisional diagnosis and treatment by the time the physician begins assessing the information required to follow the guideline. Thus, guidelines alter physicians' decision in the satisficing step by suggesting explicit and consistent criteria for determining if the decision is satisfactory. While pattern-recognition and stereotyping may be unconscious and thus not easily amenable to educational intervention, the physician can be given explicit criteria, in the form of practice guidelines, against which to judge the adequacy of the diagnosis and plan. Indeed, the use of guidelines has been associated with a reduction in racial and ethnic treatment disparities (Owen, Szczech, & Frankenfield, 2002).

Based on the RCDC framework, it would appear that one promising approach would be to find ways to increase patient's participation in relevant ways. For example, the current recommendations to have patients rate their pain severity on a scale of 1 to 10 could open a dialogue about pain severity. Physicians could be encouraged to follow this by asking if there is a particular analgesic that the patient has found helpful in the past. In this way patient's preferences, attitudes, and concerns can be openly addressed.

Viewed from the RCDC model, cultural competence training would seek to expand physicians' cultural capital to include some overlap with their patients or alter physicians' predispositions toward patients. From this perspective, the lack of documented success of cultural competence training in improving patient outcomes (Committee on Understanding and Eliminating Racial and Ethnic Disparities in Health Care, 2002; Brach & Fraser, 2000) may be related to the difficulty in getting physicians to internalize additional cultural capital or significantly alter their developed predisposition through brief educational interventions. While a broad acquisition of cultural capital may be difficult in the setting of a brief, educational intervention, it may be that condition- or symptom-specific cultural competence training is more effective. For example, traditional African-American family dynamics may have little relevance to physicians' decisions to prescribe analgesics for an ankle fracture, but a perception that there is a need to exaggerate the expression of pain so that the pain will be addressed is highly relevant.

Viewing communication from the perspective of cultural capital implies that there are situations where physicians are unable to establish rapport and effective communication with patients when there is very little or no shared cultural capital. Improved communication skills may help physicians bridge such differences and establish trust and agreement (Levinson, Stiles, Inui, & Engle, 1993). Perhaps training physicians to better identify commonalities with patients from diverse backgrounds would improve communication in general. Additional interventions may create a system for physicians to address communication failures while they are occurring. For example, if the physician is having difficulty in establishing rapport with that patient, the physician could be trained to acknowledge the difficulty in communication and enlist a nurse or social worker trained in communication to assist with the discussion.

CONCLUSION

If the RCDC model is accurate, it becomes clear that there are no easy solutions to racial and ethnic disparities in decision-making. Altering the context of physicians' and patients' lives is a major challenge. The first step is understanding the context within which physicians' decisions unfold. Physicians and patients approach the medical encounter with perspectives and expectations based upon years of personal and group experiences. In situations where physicians subconsciously associate patients' perceived race or ethnicity with information that may alter the provisional diagnosis and plan, there will be a disparity in physicians' treatment decisions based upon their patients' race. Because patient–physician communication becomes worse as the social distance between physicians and patients increases, poor communication makes it more difficult for physicians to determine whether their provisional diagnosis and plan are satisfactory. Drawing on crossdisciplinary research, the RCDC model specifies pathways and mechanisms potentially amenable to interventions. Interventions can target physicians' predispositions (e.g., increase the accuracy of population-specific rates), patients' predispositions (e.g., provide realistic expectations), physicians' pattern recognition step (e.g., clinical education), or the satisficing step (e.g., guidelines, improved cultural competence training, or more active patient participation). However, knowing which intervention strategies will be effective requires empirical testing of the theoretical model. In short, understanding physician's decision-making in context has the potential to reduce racial disparities in clinical decision-making and that is a goal worth achieving.

NOTES

1. The role conflict experienced by physicians in the U.S. may be more extreme than in European nations given the historical split between clinical medicine and public health. Physicians in Britain, for example, have more social and behavioral science training and are schooled in a variety of public health roles (Inui, 1992).

2. There is an additional underlying concept, the sick role, described by Parsons (1951). Parson's theories have been widely researched, discussed, debated, and expanded (for example, Chalfant & Hurtz, 1971, 1978; Segall, 1976a,b; Petroni, 1969). While his theories are often criticized for failing to account for variation in health behavior and the patient–provider relationship, his conception of the role of the physician as legitimizing illness is widely accepted.

3. For a more complete discussion of the psychological aspects of medical decision-making, see Hamm (2003), Krieger (2000), and Williams (1997).

ACKNOWLEDGMENTS

Dr. Tamayo-Sarver is supported by the Agency for Healthcare Research and Quality Training Grant HS-00059-06 and the Dual Degree Program in Medicine and Health Services Research at Case Western Reserve University. This study was supported by the Agency for Healthcare Research and Quality Dissertation Grant R03 HS11948-01, the Center for Healthcare Research and Policy at Metro Health Medical Center and the Department of Epidemiology and Biostatistics at Case Western Reserve University. The authors would like to acknowledge Robert Hamm and Said Ibrahim for their contribution to the development of this manuscript, and Maritza Tamayo-Sarver and Joshua Tercheck for their editorial suggestions.

REFERENCES

Abernathy, C. M., & Hamm, R. M. (1994). *Surgical scripts*. Philadelphia, PA: Hanley and Belfus.

Abernathy, C. M., & Hamm, R. M. (1995). *Surgical intuition*. Philadelphia, PA: Hanley and Belfus.

American Anthropological Association (AAA). (1997). Race and ethnic standards for federal statistics and administrative reporting. Retrieved March 30, 2005 from http://www. aaanet.org/gvt/ombdraft.htm.

Ammons, L. (1997). Demographic profile of health-care coverage in America in 1993. *Journal of National Medical Association, 89*(11), 737–744.

Anderson, J. R. (1990). *Cognitive psychology and its implications.* New York, NY: W. H. Freeman.

Anderson, J. R. (1993). *Rules of the mind.* Hillsdale, NJ: Erlbaum.

Arkes, H. R. (1991). Costs and benefits of judgment errors: Implications for debiasing. *Psychological Bulletin, 110,* 486–498.

Bach, P. B., Cramer, L. D., Warren, J. L., & Begg, C. B. (1999). Racial differences in the treatment of early-stage lung cancer. *North England Journal of Medicine, 341*(16), 1198–1205.

Bagley, C. A. (1995). A plea for ignoring race and including insured status in American research reports on social science and medicine. *Social Science of Medicine, 40,* 1017–1019.

Ball, J. K., & Elixhauser, A. (1996). Treatment differences between blacks and whites with colorectal cancer. *Medical Care, 34*(9), 970–984.

Bennett, C. L., Horner, R. D., Aboulafia, D., & Weinstein, R. A. (1995). Patterns of care for and outcomes of Pneumocystis carinii pneumonia among persons with transfusion-acquired AIDS. *Transfusion, 35*(8), 674–678.

Bergus, G. R., Chapman, G. B., Gjerde, C., & Elstein, A. S. (1995). Clinical reasoning about new symptoms despite preexisting disease: Sources of error and order effects. *Family Medicine, 27*(5), 314–320.

Bernabei, R., Gambassi, G., Lapane, K., Landi, F., Gatsonis, C., Dunlop, R., Lipsitz, L., Steel, K., & Mor, V. (1998). Management of pain in elderly patients with cancer. SAGE study group. Systematic assessment of geriatric drug use via epidemiology. *JAMA, 279*(23), 1877–1882.

Berwick, D. M., Fineberg, H. V., & Weinstein, M. C. (1981). When doctors meet numbers. *American Journal of Medicine, 71*(6), 991–998.

Bloche, M. G. (2001). Race and discretion in American medicine. *Yale Journal of Health Policy, Law, and Ethics, 1*(1), 95–131.

Bobo, L. D. (1997). Race, public opinion, and the social sphere. *Public Opinion Quarterly, 61*(1), 1–15.

Bobo, L. D. (2001). Racial attitudes and relations at the close of the twentieth century. In: N. J. Smelser, W. J. Wilson & F. Mitchell (Eds), *America becoming: Racial trends and their consequences.* Washington, DC: National Academy Press.

Bordage, G., Brailovsky, C. A., Cohen, T., & Page, G. (1996). Maintaining and enhancing key decision-making skills from graduation into practice: An exploratory study. In: A. J. J. A. Scherpbier, C. P. M. van der Vleuten & J.-J. Rethans (Eds), *Advances in medical education* (pp. 128–130). Dordrecht, Netherlands: Kluwer Academic.

Bourdieu, P., & Passeron, J. C. (1977). *Reproduction in education, society and culture.* Beverly Hills, CA: Sage Publications.

Brach, C., & Fraser, I. (2000). Can cultural competency reduce racial and ethnic health disparities? A review and conceptual model. *Medical Care Research and Review, 57*(Suppl 1), 181–217.

Casscells, W., Schoenberger, A., & Graboys, T. B. (1978). Interpretation by physicians of clinical laboratory results. *North England Journal of Medicine, 299*(18), 999–1001.

Chalfant, H., & Hurtz, P. (1978). The alcoholic and the sick role: Dimensions of rejection by social workers (Comment on Segall, JHSB June, 1976). *Journal of Health and Social Behavior, 19*(1), 118–119.

Chalfant, H., & Kurtz, P. (1971). Alcoholics and the sick role: Assessments by social workers. *Journal of Health and Social Behavior, 12*(1), 66–72.

Chapman, G. B., Bergus, G. R., & Elstein, A. S. (1996). Order of information affects clinical judgment. *Journal of Behavioral Decision Making, 9*, 201–211.

Charlin, B., Roy, L., Brailovsky, C., Goulet, F., & van der Vleuten, C. (2000). The script concordance test: A tool to assess the reflective clinician. *Teaching and Learning in Medicine, 12*(4), 189–195.

Chen, J., Rathore, S. S., Radford, M. J., Wang, Y., & Krumholz, H. M. (2001). Racial differences in the use of cardiac catheterization after acute myocardial infarction. *North England Journal of Medicine, 344*(19), 1443–1449.

Clark, J. A., Potter, D. A., & McKinlay, J. B. (1991). Bringing social structure back into clinical decision making. *Social Science of Medicine, 32*(8), 853–866.

Cleeland, C. S., Gonin, R., Baez, L., Loehrer, P., & Pandya, K. J. (1997). Pain and treatment of pain in minority patients with cancer. The eastern cooperative oncology group minority outpatient pain study. *Annals of Internal Medicine, 127*(9), 813–816.

Cohen, J., Asch, D., & Ubel, P. (2000). Bioethics and medical decision making: What can they learn from each other? In: G. B. Chapman & F. A. Sonnenberg (Eds), *Decision making in health care: Theory, psychology, and applications* (pp. 253–266). New York, NY: Cambridge University Press.

Collins, K. S., Hall, A., & Neuhaus, C. (1999). U.S. minority health: A chartbook. New York, The Commonwealth Fund. Ref Type: Report.

Committee on understanding and eliminating racial and ethnic disparities in health care. (2002). *Unequal treatment: Confronting racial and ethnic disparities in health care.* Washington, DC: National Academy Press.

Cooper-Patrick, L., Gallo, J. J., Gonzales, J. J., Vu, H. T., Powe, N. R., Nelson, C., & Ford, D. E. (1999). Race, gender, and partnership in the patient–physician relationship. *JAMA, 282*(6), 583–589.

Custers, E. J. F. M., Boshuizen, H. P. A., & Schmidt, H. G. (1996a). The influence of medical expertise, case typicality, and illness script component on case processing and disease probability estimates. *Memory & Cognition, 24*(3), 384–399.

Custers, E. J., Regehr, G., & Norman, G. R. (1996b). Mental representations of medical diagnostic knowledge: A review. *Academy of Medicine, 71*(10 Suppl), S55–S61.

Deber, R. B., & Baumann, A. O. (1992). Clinical reasoning in medicine and nursing: Decision making versus problem solving. *Teaching and Learning in Medicine, 4*, 140–146.

Dominitz, J. A., Samsa, G. P., Landsman, P., & Provenzale, D. (1998). Race, treatment, and survival among colorectal carcinoma patients in an equal-access medical system. *Cancer, 82*(12), 2312–2320.

Donovan, J. (1986). *We don't buy sickness, it just comes: Heath, illness and health care in the lives of black people in London.* Aldershot: Gower.

Dovidio, J. F. (1999). Stereotyping. In: R. A. Wilson & F. C. Keil (Eds), *The MIT encyclopedia of the cognitive sciences.* Cambridge, MA: MIT Press.

Dungal, L. (1978). Physicians' responses to patients: a study of factors involved in the office interview. *Journal of Family Practice, 6*(5), 1065–1073.

Elstein, A. S. (1992). Paradigms for research on clinical reasoning: A researcher's commentary. *Teaching and Learning in Medicine, 4*, 147–149.

Elstein, A. S., Christensen, C., Cottrell, J. J., Polson, A., & Ng, M. (1999). Effects of prognosis, perceived benefit, and decision style on decision making and critical care on decision making in critical care. *Critical Care Medicine, 27*(1), 58–65.

Elstein, A. S., Shulman, L. S., & Sprafka, S. A. (1978). *Medical problem solving. An analysis of clinical reasoning.* Cambridge, MA: Harvard University Press.

Feltovich, P. J., & Barrows, H. S. (1984). Issues of generality in medical problem solving. In: H. G. Schmidt & M. L. de Volder (Eds), *Tutorials in problem-based learning. New directions in training for the health professions* (pp. 128–142). Assen/Maastricht: Van Gorcum.

Feltovich, P. J., Sprio, R. J., & Coulson, R. L. (1989). The nature of conceptual understanding in biomedicine: The deep structure of complex ideas and the development of misconceptions. In: D. A. Evans & V. L. Patel (Eds), *Cognitive science in medicine: Biomedical modeling* (pp. 113–172). Cambridge, MA: MIT Press.

Fincher, C., Williams, J. E., MacLean, V., Allison, J. J., Kiefe, C. I., & Canto, J. (2004). Racial disparities in coronary heart disease: A sociological view of the medical literature on physician bias. *Ethnicity & Disease, 14*(3), 360–371.

Fiske, S. T. (1998). Stereotyping, prejudice, and discrimination. In: D. T. Gilbert & S. T. Fiske (Eds), *The handbook of social psychology* (pp. 357–411). New York: McGraw-Hill.

Friedman, R. B., Korst, D. R., Schultz, J. V., Beatty, E., & Entine, S. (1978). Experience with the simulated patient–physician encounter. *Journal of Medical Education, 53*(10), 825–830.

Gabriel, B. A. (2002). Confronting "unequal treatment": The institute of medicine weighs in on health care disparities. http://www.aamc.org/newsroom/reporter/june02/unequaltreatment.htm. AAMC Reporter. 6-16-2003.

Gaskin, D. J. (1999). The hospital safety net: A study of inpatient care for non-elderly vulnerable populations. In: M. Lillie-Blanton, R. Martinez & D. Rowland (Eds), *Access to health care: Promises and prospects for low-income Americans* (p. 123). Washington, DC: Kaiser Commission on Medicaid and the Uninsured.

Grant, J., & Marsden, P. (1988). Primary knowledge, medical education and consultant expertise. *Medical Education, 22*(3), 173–179.

Green, A. J. K., & Gilhooly, K. J. (1992). Empirical advances in expertise research. In: M. T. Keane & K. J. Gilhooly (Eds), *Advances in the psychology of thinking* (pp. 45–70). Hemel Hempstead, UK: Harvester Wheatsheaf.

Green, L. A., & Yates, J. F. (1993). Influence of pseudodiagnostic information in acute chest pain admission decisions. *Medical Decision Making, 13*, 387.

Green, L. A., & Yates, J. F. (1995). Influence of pseudodiagnostic information on the evaluation of ischemic heart disease. *Annals of Emergency Medicine, 25*, 451–457.

Hamm, R. M. (1988). Moment by moment variation in experts' analytic and intuitive cognitive activity. *IEEE Transactions on Systems, Man, and Cybernetics, 18*, 757–776.

Hamm, R. M. (2003). Decision scripts: Combining cognitive scripts and judgment strategies to fully account for medical decision making. In: D. Hardman & L. Macchi (Eds), *Thinking: Psychological perspectives on reasoning, judgment, and decision making.* Cambridge, UK: Cambridge University Press.

Hamm, R. M., Scheid, D. C., Smith, W. R., & Tape, T. G. (2000). Opportunities for applying psychological theory to improve medical decision making: Two case histories. In: G. B.

Chapman & F. A. Sonnenberg (Eds), *Decision making in health care: Theory, psychology, and applications* (pp. 386–422). New York, NY: Cambridge University Press.

Hammond, K. R. (1971). Computer graphics as an aid to learning. *Science, 172,* 903–908.

Hammond, K. R. (1996). *Human judgment and social policy: Irreducible uncertainty, inevitable error, unavoidable injustice.* New York, NY: Oxford University Press.

Hammond, K. R. (1999). *Judgments under stress.* New York: Oxford University Press.

Hammond, K. R., & Brehmer, B. (1973). Quasi-rationality and distrust: Implications for international conflict. In: L. Rappoport & D. A. Summers (Eds), *Human judgment and social interaction* (pp. 338–391). New York: Holt, Rinehart, & Winston.

Hatala, R., Norman, G. R., & Brooks, L. R. (1999). Impact of a clinical scenario on accuracy of electrocardiogram interpretation. *Journal of General Internal Medicine, 14*(2), 126–129.

Hillman, A. L., Nash, D. B., Kissick, W. L., & Martin, S. P. (1986). Managing the medical-industrial complex. *North England Journal of Medicine, 315*(8), 511–513.

Hobus, P. P. M., Hofstra, M. L., Boshuizen, H. P. A., & Schmidt, H. G. (1988). De context van de klacht als diagnosticum [The context of the complaint as a diagnostic tool]. *Huisarts en Wetenschap, 31,* 261–267.

Hobus, P. P. M., Schmidt, H. G., Boshuizen, H. P. A., & Patel, V. L. (1987). Contextual factors in the activation of first diagnostic hypotheses: Expert-novice differences. *Medical Education, 21,* 471–476.

Ibrahim, S. A., Whittle, J., Bean-Mayberry, B., Kelley, M. E., Good, C., & Conigliaro, J. (2003). Racial/ethnic variations in physician recommendations for cardiac revascularization. *American Journal of Public Health, 93*(10), 1689–1693.

Inui, T. S. (1992). The social contract and the medical school's responsibilities. In: K. L. White & J. E. Connelly (Eds), *The medical school's mission and the population's health: Medical education in Canada, the United Kingdom, the United States and Australia* (pp. 23–52). New York: Springer-Verlag.

Johnson, P. E., Hassebrock, F., Duran, A. S., & Moller, J. H. (1982). Multimethod study of clinical judgment. *Organizational Behavior and Human Decision Processes, 30*(2), 201–230.

Judge, K., & Solomon, M. (1993). Public opinion and the national health service: Patterns and perspectives in consumer satisfaction. *Journal of Social Policy, 22*(3), 299–327.

Karpman, R. R., Del Mar, N., & Bay, C. (1997). Analgesia for emergency centers' orthopaedic patients: Does an ethnic bias exist? *Clin. Orthop. Relat. Res., 1*(334), 270–275.

Klein, G. A. (1993). A recognition-primed decision (RPD) model of rapid decision making. In: G. A. Klein, J. Orasanu, C. E. Calderwood & C. E. Zsambok (Eds), *Decision making in action: Models and methods* (pp. 138–147). Norwood, NJ: Ablex.

Klein, G. A. (1997). The recognition-primed decision (RPD) model: Looking back, looking forward. In: C. E. Zsambok & G. A. Klein (Eds), *Naturalistic decision making* (pp. 285–292). Mahwah, NJ: Lawrence Erlbaum Associates.

Krieger, N. (2000). Refiguring "race": Epidemiology, racialized biology, and biological expressions of race relations. *International Journal of Health Services, 30*(1), 211–216.

LaVeist, T. A., Nickerson, K. J., & Bowie, J. V. (2000). Attitudes about racism, medical mistrust, and satisfaction with care among African-American and white cardiac patients. *Medical Care Research and Review, 57*(Suppl 1), 146–161.

Lesgold, A. (1984). Human skill in a computerized society: Complex skills and their acquisition. *Behavior Research Methods, Instruments, and Computers, 16,* 79–87.

Levinson, W., Stiles, W. B., Inui, T. S., & Engle, R. (1993). Physician frustration in commu-
    nicating with patients. *Medical Care, 31*(4), 285–295.
Lillie-Blanton, M., Brodie, M., Rowland, D., Altman, D., & McIntosh, M. (2000). Race,
    ethnicity, and the health care system: Public perceptions and experiences. *Medical Care
    Research and Review, 57*(Suppl 1), 218–235.
Lillie-Blanton, M., & Laveist, T. (1996). Race/ethnicity, the social environment, and health.
    Social Science & Medicine, 43(1), 83–91.
Lillie-Blanton, M., Martinez, R. M., & Salganicoff, A. (2001). Site of medical care: Do racial
    and ethnic differences persist? *Yale Journal of Health Policy, Law, and Ethics, 1*(1), 1–17.
Lorber, J. (1997). *Gender and the social construction of illness.* Thousand Oaks: Sage Publi-
    cations.
Lowe, R. A., Chhaya, S., Nasci, K., Gavin, L. J., Shaw, K., Zwanger, M. L., Zeccardi, J. A.,
    Dalsey, W. C., Abbuhl, S. B., Feldman, H., & Berlin, J. A. (2001). Effect of ethnicity on
    denial of authorization for emergency department care by managed care gatekeepers.
    Academic Emergency Medicine, 8(3), 259–266.
Mackie, D. M., Devos, T., & Smith, E. R. (2000). Intergroup emotions: Explaining offensive
    action tendencies in an intergroup context. *Journal of Personality & Social Psychology,
    79*(4), 602–616.
Mackie, D. M., Hamilton, D. L., Susskind, J., & Rosselli, F. (1996). Social psychological
    foundations of stereotype formation. In: N. Macrae, C. Stangor & M. Hewstone (Eds),
    Stereotypes and stereotyping (pp. 41–78). New York: Guilford Press.
Martin, T. L., Selby, J. V., & Zhang, D. (1995). Physician and patient prevention practices in
    NIDDM in a large urban managed-care organization. *Diabetes Care, 18*(8), 1124–1132.
Mayberry, R. M., Mili, F., & Ofili, E. (2000). Racial and ethnic differences in access to medical
    care. *Medical Care Research and Review, 57*(Suppl 1), 108–145.
McKinlay, J. B., Burns, R. B., Durante, R., Feldman, H. A., Freund, K. M., Harrow, B. S.,
    Irish, J. T., Kasten, L. E., & Moskowitz, M. A. (1997). Patient, physician and presen-
    tational influences on clinical decision making for breast cancer: Results from a factorial
    experiment. *Journal of Evaluation in Clinical Practice, 3*(1), 23–57.
McKinlay, J. B., Burns, R. B., Feldman, H. A., Freund, K. M., Irish, J. T., Kasten, L. E.,
    Moskowitz, M. A., Potter, D. A., & Woodman, K. (1998). Physician variability and
    uncertainty in the management of breast cancer. Results from a factorial experiment.
    Medical Care, 36(3), 385–396.
McLeskey, C. H., & Ward, R. J. (1978). Validity of written examinations [letter]. *Anesthesio-
    logy, 49*(3), 224.
Mizrahi, T. (1986). *Getting rid of patients. Contradictions in the socialization of physicians.* New
    Brunswick, NJ: Rutgers University Press.
Moore, R. D., Stanton, D., Gopalan, R., & Chaisson, R. E. (1994). Racial differences in the use
    of drug therapy for HIV disease in an urban community. *North England Journal of
    Medicine, 330*(11), 763–768.
Murphy-Berman, V. A., Berman, J. J., & Campbell, E. (1998). Factors affecting health-care
    allocation decisions: A case of aversive racism? *Journal of Applied Social Psychology,
    28*(24), 2239–2253.
Ng, B., Dimsdale, J. E., Rollnik, J. D., & Shapiro, H. (1996). The effect of ethnicity on
    prescriptions for patient-controlled analgesia for post-operative pain. *Pain, 66*(1), 9–12.
Norman, G. R. (2000). The epistemology of clinical reasoning: Perspectives from philosophy,
    psychology, and neuroscience. *Academic Medicine, 75*(10, Suppl), S127–S135.

Operario, D., & Fiske, S. T. (2001). Stereotypes: Processes, structures, content, and context. In: R. Brown & S. Gaertnet (Eds), *Intergroup processes* (pp. 22–44). Cambridge, MA: Blackwell.

Optenberg, S. A., Thompson, I. M., Friedrichs, P., Wojcik, B., Stein, C. R., & Kramer, B. (1995). Race, treatment, and long-term survival from prostate cancer in an equal-access medical care delivery system. *JAMA, 274*(20), 1599–1605.

Owen, W. F., Jr., Szczech, L. A., & Frankenfield, D. L. (2002). Healthcare system interventions for inequality in quality: Corrective action through evidence-based medicine. *Journal of the National Medical Association, 94*(8, Suppl), 83S–91S.

Parsons, T. (1951). *The social system*. New York, NY: Free Press.

Pauly, M. V., Hillman, A. L., & Kerstein, J. (1990). Managing physician incentives in managed care The role of for-profit ownership. *Medical Care, 28*(11), 1013–1024.

Payne, J. W., Bettman, J. R., & Johnson, E. J. (1993). *The adaptive decision maker*. Cambridge: Cambridge University Press.

Petroni, F. A. (1969). Significant others and illness behavior: A much neglected sick role contingency. *Sociological Quarterly, 10*, 32–41.

Poses, R. M., Bekes, C., Winkler, R. L., Scott, W. E., & Copare, F. J. (1990). Are two (inexperienced) heads better than one (experienced) head? Averaging house officers' prognostic judgments for critically ill patients. *Archives of Internal Medicine, 150*(9), 1874–1878.

Poses, R. M., McClish, D. K., Smith, W. R., Chaput de Saintonge, D. M., Huber, E. C., Clemo, F. L., Schmitt, B. P., Alexander-Forti, D., Racht, E. M., Colenda, C. C., III, & Centor, R. M. (1997). Physicians' judgments of the risks of cardiac procedures. Differences between cardiologists and other internists. *Medical Care, 35 AB*(6), 603–617.

Satcher, D. (2001). Our commitment to eliminate racial and ethnic health disparities. *Yale Journal of Health Policy, Law, and Ethics, 1*(1), 1–14.

Schmidt, H. G., & Boshuizen, H. P. (1993). On the origin of intermediate effects in clinical case recall. *Memory & Cognition, 21*(3), 338–351.

Schmidt, H. G., Norman, G. R., & Boshuizen, H. P. (1990). A cognitive perspective on medical expertise: Theory and implication [published erratum appears in Academic Medicine, 1992 April, *67*(4), 287]. *Academic Medicine, 65*(10), 611–621.

Segall, A. (1976a). The sick role concept: Understanding illness behavior. *Journal of Health and Social Behavior, 17*(2), 162–169.

Segall, A. (1976b). Sociocultural variation in sick role behavioural expectations. *Social Science and Medicine, 10*(1), 47–51.

Shapiro, M. F., Morton, S. C., McCaffrey, D. F., Senterfitt, J. W., Fleishman, J. A., Perlman, J. F., Athey, L. A., Keesey, J. W., Goldman, D. P., Berry, S. H., & Bozzette, S. A. (1999). Variations in the care of HIV-infected adults in the United States: Results from the HIV cost and services utilization study. *JAMA, 281*(24), 2305–2315.

Sheifer, S. E., Escarce, J. J., & Schulman, K. A. (2000). Race and sex differences in the management of coronary artery disease. *American Heart Journal, 139*(5), 848–857.

Sibicky, M. E., & Dovidio, J. F. (1986). Stigma of psychological therapy: Stereotypes, interpersonal reactions, and the self-fulfilling prophecy. *Journal of Counseling Psychology, 33*, 148–154.

Simon, H. A. (1956). Rational choice and the structure of the environment. *Psychological Review, 63*, 129–138.

Slovic, P., & Lichtenstein, S. (1971). Comparison of Bayesian and regression approaches to the study of information processing in judgment. *Organizational Behavior and Human Performance, 6*, 649–744.

Smaje, C. (1995). *Health, "race" and ethnicity: Making sense of evidence.* London: King's Fund.

Smaje, C. (2000). Race, ethnicity and health. In: C. E. Bird, P. Conrad & A. M. Fremont (Eds), *Handbook of medical sociology* (pp. 114–128). New Jersey: Prentice Hall.

Spector, R. (2001). Is there a racial bias in clinicians' perceptions of the dangerousness of psychiatric patients? A review of the literature. *Journal of Mental Health, 10*(1), 5–15.

Starr, P. (1982). *The social transformation of American medicine.* New York, NY: Basic Books, Inc.

Tajfel, H., & Turner, J. C. (1979). An integrative theory of intergroup conflict. In: W. G. Austin & S. Worchel (Eds), *The social psychology of intergroup relations.* Monterey, CA: Brooks/Cole.

Tamayo-Sarver, J. H., Dawson, N. V., Hinze, S. W., Cydulka, R. K., Wigton, R. S., Albert, J. M., Ibrahim, S. A., & Baker, D. W. (2003a). The effect of race/ethnicity and desirable social characteristics on physicians' decisions to prescribe opioid analgesics. *Academic Emergency Medicine, 10*(11), 1239–1248.

Tamayo-Sarver, J. H., Hinze, S. W., Cydulka, R. K., & Baker, D. W. (2003b). Racial/ethnic disparities in analgesia prescribing in the emergency department. *American Journal of Public Health, 93*(12), 2067–2073.

Tape, T. G., Heckerling, P. S., Ornato, J. P., & Wigton, R. S. (1991). Use of clinical judgment analysis to explain regional variations in physicians' accuracies in diagnosing pneumonia. *Medical Decision Making, 11*(3), 189–197.

Todd, K. H., Deaton, C., D'Adamo, A. P., & Goe, L. (2000). Ethnicity and analgesic practice. *Annals of Emergency Medicine, 35*(1), 11–16.

Todd, K. H., Samaroo, N., & Hoffman, J. R. (1993). Ethnicity as a risk factor for inadequate emergency department analgesia. *JAMA, 269*(12), 1537–1539.

van de Wiel, M. W., Schmidt, H. G., & Boshuizen, H. P. (1998). A failure to reproduce the intermediate effect in clinical case recall. *Academic Medicine, 73*(8), 894–900.

van Ryn, M. (2002). Research on the provider contribution to race/ethnicity disparities in medical care, *40*(1, Suppl), I140.

van Ryn, M., & Burke, J. (2000). The effect of patient race and socio-economic status on physicians' perceptions of patients. *Social Science & Medicine, 50*(6), 813–828.

Veatch, R. M. (1991). Allocating health resources ethically: New roles for administrators and clinicians. *Frontiers in Health Service Management, 8*(1), 3–4.

Venkat, A., Hoekstra, J., Lindsell, C., Prall, D., Hollander, J. E., Pollack, C. V., Jr., Diercks, D., Kirk, J. D., Tiffany, B., Peacock, F., Storrow, A. B., & Gibler, W. B. (2003). The impact of race on the acute management of chest pain. *Academic Emergency Medicine, 10*(11), 1199–1208.

Waitzkin, H. (1983). *The second sickness.* New York, NY: The Free Press.

Waitzkin, H. (1985). Information giving in medical care. *Journal of Health and Social Behavior, 26*(2), 81–101.

Waitzkin, H. (1991). *The politics of medical encounters: How patients and doctors deal with social problems.* New Haven, CT: Yale University Press.

Waitzkin, H. (2000). The changing patient–physician relationship in the changing health-policy environment. In: C. E. Bird, P. Conrad & A. M. Fremont (Eds), *Handbook of medical sociology* (pp. 271–283). New Jersey: Prentice Hall.

Weisse, C. S., Sorum, P. C., Sanders, K. N., & Syat, B. L. (2001). Do gender and race affect decisions about pain management? *Journal of General International Medicine, 16*(4), 211–217.

Wigton, R. S., Poses, R. M., Collins, M., & Cebul, R. D. (1990). Teaching old dogs new tricks: Using cognitive feedback to improve physicians' diagnostic judgments on simulated cases. *Academic Medicine, 65*(9 Suppl), S5–S6.

Williams, D. R. (1997). Race and health: Basic questions, emerging directions. *Annals of Epidemiology, 7*(5), 322–333.

Winant, H. (2000). Race and race theory. *Annual Review of Sociology, 26*, 169–185.

Wisdom, K., Fryzek, J. P., Havstad, S. L., Anderson, R. M., Dreiling, M. C., & Tilley, B. C. (1997). Comparison of laboratory test frequency and test results between African–Americans and Caucasians with diabetes: Opportunity for improvement. Findings from a large urban health maintenance organization. *Diabetes Care, 20*(6), 971–977.

SECTION 5:
POLICY CONCERNS

THE IMPACTS OF PUBLIC POLICY IMPLEMENTATION ON TRIBAL HEALTH CARE MANAGEMENT: THE CASE OF OEO/CAP

Michèle Companion

ABSTRACT

This study examines the impact of one of President Johnson's "War on Poverty" programs on Native American control over current health care management. This program has been widely credited as a huge success – a tool that prompted tribes to increase their drive for self-determination. However, no one has ever empirically validated this claim. The results provided here do not support this contention. Participation in the program as a whole proved detrimental for tribal self-determination. The primary component within the program actively discouraged tribal development. However, another component did have the desired impact, encouraging capacity-building and supporting local input and control. This study contributes to both the international development and Native American literatures by demonstrating support for "bottom-up" development models and thereby offering a better option for self-determination and long-term sustainability.

Health Care Services, Racial and Ethnic Minorities and Underserved Populations: Patient and Provider Perspectives
Research in the Sociology of Health Care, Volume 23, 217–232
Copyright © 2005 by Elsevier Ltd.
ISSN: 0275-4959/doi:10.1016/S0275-4959(05)23010-7

INTRODUCTION

Health care is critical for the long-term cultural survival of all indigenous groups, especially for Native Americans.[1] Without combating the wide range of social and physiological pathologies that are plaguing reservations around the country, tribal survival as distinct cultural and political units is in jeopardy. Recent scholarly work suggests that the best way to improve overall health status is to increase local control over health care management, including increasing discretionary power over program design and management options.[2] The primary focus of much of this literature is the impact of self-determination policy and public programs, which expanded and created opportunities for more independent sovereign actions.

The Office of Economic Opportunity's Community Action Program (OEO/CAP) has been heavily touted as the turning point for the self-determination process. It was designed to provide tribes with their first opportunities to reclaim control over management decisions and program design since the late 1800s. However, support has always been anecdotal. This study seeks to determine the impact of tribal participation in OEO/CAP on control over health care management. Based on the literature, early participation in capacity-building programs should positively impact tribal ability to take advantage of the sovereignty expansion opportunities that became available during the period from 1975 to 1996. As a result, tribes who participated should have a greater degree of control over their current health care management systems.

BACKGROUND AND THEORETICAL FRAMEWORK

The social and economic programs in Johnson's "War on Poverty" offered a means to loosen the Bureau of Indian Affairs' (BIA) strangle hold over Native nations. Under Title II of the Economic Opportunity Act of 1964 (EOA),[3] OEO/CAP was established. These programs are hailed as the precursor to the Self-Determination Act[4] (Castile, 1998; Cohen, 1982; Levitan & Johnston, 1975). CAP was an opportunity to "relearn" sovereignty by honing capacity-building skills.[5] This includes expanding networks of resources and ties and reducing dependence on outside experts, thereby increasing overall autonomy. Greater autonomy provides the opportunity to select from a wider variety of options, improving chances of success and reducing vulnerability to administrative, policy, or economic shifts. Joe

(1986) states, "For the first time, tribes were allowed to have a voice in developing and managing their own programs. The OEO program thus indirectly rejuvenated the ideology of self-determination ..." (p. 4).

Grants awarded through this program provided many tribes with their first opportunities to create and target programs to fit the needs of their specific populations (Greenstone & Peterson, 1973; Hough, 1967; Human Services Research, Inc., 1966; Levitan, 1964, 1969; Levitan & Hetrick, 1971; Davidson & Levitan, 1968). OEO/CAP brought money onto the reservations and opened up political avenues between nations and the federal government that were not mediated by the BIA.

This is critical. Most explanations for continued reservation poverty and underdevelopment place responsibility for the current state of Native America on the federal government and its agents, particularly the BIA. The two primary models are both forms of domination arguments. Borrowing from the Weberian tradition, the first revolves around structural domination, stressing the importance of federal bureaucracies and the promotion of state interests at the expense of Native populations (Bee, 1992; Perry, 1996; Barsh, 1988). Domestic dependency[6] codified the subjugation of Native American political, social, and economic interests to those of the dominant United States system and the process was intensified by the creation of reservations (Jorgensen, 1978). The Indian Reorganization Act (IRA)[7] cemented this domination by turning tribal governments into a form of administered state (Castile, 1974) controlled by the BIA, making real sovereignty unlikely.[8]

The second is Dependency Theory, which borrows from political science, anthropology, and the international development community. This focuses on the process of interaction between societies and their environments that results in the creation and maintenance of asymmetrical power dynamics, consequently leading to the economic exploitation and political subjugation of the weaker society. Research in this area has focused on development as a process of internal colonization,[9] where resources are leeched from more peripheral areas for the primary benefit of a dominant core area. The continuing extraction of resources from these internal colonies results in increasing impoverishment and a growing dependence upon the dominant structure. This theory has been extended to Native nations by conceptualizing reservations as the periphery and American society as the dominant core (Castile & Kushner, 1981; Castile, 1974; Pommersheim, 1995).

Kardam (1993) fuses both domination and dependence models by arguing that persistent poverty among indigenous groups ultimately boils down to reliance on the State (1775). He finds that the greater the degree of resource dependency, the more insecure or unstable the funding is. This makes the recipient populations more vulnerable to factors that affect funding levels, including administrative turnovers that shift balances of power, changes in overall economic situations,[10] and changes in the laws that expand or constrict access to resources. This ties into autonomy issues.[11] In cases where there is heavier reliance on outsiders for information and other resources, there will also be greater sensitivity to external pressures to conform to certain courses of action or to support policy platforms.

The Importance of the BIA

Many scholars believe the BIA is responsible for controlling and manipulating Native affairs in harmful ways.[12] The BIA played an active role in the Native disempowerment process by monitoring and actively repressing traditional activities and mediating tribal interactions with federal representatives. Three primary explanations for these actions have been advanced. First, the agency is responsible for implementing programs that support shifting policy needs, often disadvantageous for the tribes.[13] Second, the BIA, as part of a larger bureaucratic structure, reifies a certain institutionalism. This rigid structure is imposed on Native nations in a top-down fashion, leaving little room for adaptation. It fails to map onto many traditional Native governance forms,[14] thereby increasing the professional and cultural distance between the nations and the agency that is supposed to represent their interests.

Institutional self-preservation is also cited (Deloria & Wilkins, 1999).[15] Because the reservation process created a dependant client population, the BIA's survival rests on the continued need for their intervention on behalf of Native people. With the existence of their jobs threatened by Native success, there is little incentive for Bureau personnel to put forth their best efforts (Krepps & Caves, 1994; Stull, Schultz, & Cadue, 1986).

Given the literature, participation in capacity-building programs not mediated by the BIA should have a significant, positive impact on policy advocacy and response to opportunities, leading to a testable hypothesis about the influence of participation in the OEO/CAP programs.

Hypothesis 1. Tribes who participated in CAP programming are more likely to have higher levels of control over their health care systems because of increased capacity to advocate on their own behalf and improved network ties, leading to greater independence from BIA influence and less reliance on outside experts.

It is also important to address the timing of participation. It is reasonable, given the literature, to assume that a relationship exists between early CAP participation and later willingness to take advantage of sovereignty opportunities. Early participants take the greatest amount of risk and have the steepest learning curves. Those who enter the field later benefit from the experience of the earlier tribes. They are able to avoid pitfalls and have the option to pattern themselves after those perceived as successful. This leads to the second hypothesis:

Hypothesis 2. Tribes that enter the CAP programs early are more likely to take risks in other areas. Thus, they are more likely to switch to higher levels of health care management when the opportunity presents itself.

METHODOLOGY

Reliable data on small tribes is limited. Thus, a purposive sample was constructed based on an enrolled population of 700 or greater (Cornell & Kalt, 1992, 1995), resulting in 104 tribes.[16] Using the National Indian Health Board's (1998) definitions, tribes are broken out into one of three categories based on their Indian Health Service (IHS) status for fiscal year 1997[17] to allow for a more sensitive level of analysis (p. 11). There are 52 direct service tribes, 31 contracting tribes, and 21 compacting tribes in the sample:

1. *Compacting tribes.* This represents the greatest degree of indigenous control. Every tribe has negotiated a Title III self-governance compact with the IHS, regardless of types of services.
2. *Contracting tribes.* This represents a moderate degree of indigenous control. Tribes do not have a Title III compact with the IHS, but operate at least one outpatient medical clinic through a Title I contract under P.L. 93-638.
3. *IHS direct service.* This is the lowest level of indigenous control and includes tribes that do not have a Title III compact with IHS and do not operate any outpatient medical clinics. These tribes may operate other health services under Title I, but these are not associated with ambulatory care. They include social and behavioral programs, such as outreach workers, alcohol and mental health services, and community nursing. These tribes receive outpatient medical services from an IHS-operated clinic or purchase them from the private sector.

Data on OEO/CAP participation were derived from a series of encoded files from the National Archives in Washington, DC. These data were used to identify the types of component programs participated in. This plays an important role in capacity building, because greater participation increases exposure to ideas, information, and network ties. Ideally, training in an array of skills should also reduce dependence on outsiders and allow the communities to become more self-sufficient in the long run.

Four primary components were identified. Conduct and administration (C&A) was designed to administer other components, stimulate interagency cooperation, and develop new programs. Participation is an indicator of capacity building and interaction with non-BIA government agencies.

Community-level mobilization projects focused on community empowerment by instilling pride through cultural rejuvenation and inspiring a sense of ownership in that process. Unlike the C&A program, these could take a variety of forms. Projects ranged from community beautification to establishing cultural centers and programs.

The third category is the head start program. Head start provides enhanced educational training to underprivileged children to help them catch up to others in their age group. Finally, OEO offered economic development programs.

It is logical to assume that greater time spent in the program allows the components to become established, increases the number of network ties, provides more management experience and a better opportunity to correct for approaches that are not working. This engenders a more positive overall experience and encourages long-term sustainability. Therefore, years spent in CAP are also coded. Dichotomous variables are created to capture the timing of entry into CAP. Tribes are grouped based on the first fiscal year and a grant was funded. Those who joined in 1965/1966 are earliest and 1973 or later are latest.

Two key factors are controlled for. The first is reservation population size. It can be argued that larger tribes have access to greater resources, while smaller tribes are disadvantaged (Barsh & Henderson, 1980). However, it can also be argued that smaller tribes are better able to use the resources they have because they are not spread across as wide a base.[18]

Regional variations, along with BIA influence, can also have a profound impact on resources for development. As BIA area offices serve a number of tribes in specific regional areas, these have been collapsed into five dummy variables. The variable "GRTPLNS" covers the Great Plains region and comprises the Billings and Aberdeen BIA offices. "WEST" includes the Portland and Sacramento offices. Navajo, Albuquerque, and Phoenix serve the southwest. The mid-west is served by Anadarko and Minneapolis. Finally, "EASTERN" accommodates all tribes in the eastern United States.

The data are analyzed using STATA 6.0. Multinomial logistic regression (MLOGIT) assesses the effects of independent variables on the three discrete levels of health care management. Due to case size sensitivity issues, some effects may be masked. To reinforce the MLOGIT and to help identify additional influences, all of the models are also run using maximum-likelihood logit estimation (LOGIT). To capture movement away from direct service provision, a dichotomous dependent variable has been created by collapsing the two higher levels of health care management. These results are only presented when case size masks important influences.

FINDINGS AND DISCUSSION

Hypothesis 1

The initial exploratory findings were surprising. They *disprove* the anecdotal evidence cited in the literature, demonstrating CAP participants are *more* likely to stay with IHS direct services than to switch to a higher level of control. Further analysis shows that the types of programs participated in drive this effect, rather than involvement in OEO/CAP as a whole. The results from the final models can be found in Table 1.[19]

As seen in the table, with all else being equal, tribes that participated in C&A programs are significantly *less* likely to have jumped to contracting and more likely to remain with IHS direct service provisions. Despite controlling for the number of years spent in the program (Model 2) and the time of entry into the program (Model 3), C&A participation still has a detrimental effect on moving away from BIA/IHS control. It does not statistically affect the likelihood of moving from contracts to compacts.

Tribes that participated in economic development programs, however, were significantly *more* likely to have moved away from IHS direct services and into contracting (one and half times more likely). As with C&A, this relationship remains statistically significant in all three models. Interestingly, participation decreases the likelihood of moving from contracting to compacting. This effect is significant ($p < 0.05$) in both Models 2 and 3.

Despite seeming counterintuitive, these results jibe with international development and Native American literatures and fail to disprove the hypothesis. The structural reality of programmatic elements making up OEO/CAP did not map onto the legislative framers' intent. Though designed as a training opportunity for participants, certain components did not encourage capacity building. This is especially true of C&A. Memos,

Table 1. Multinomial Logistic Regression Estimates of CAP Impact on IHS Health Care Management Status[20].

Variables	Comparison of Contracting to Direct Service Tribes			Comparison of Compacting to Direct Service Tribes		
	Model 1	Model 2	Model 3	Model 1	Model 2	Model 3
Conduct and administration	−3.02**	−2.85*	−2.72*	−1.23	−1.43	−1.59
	(1.19)	(1.24)	(1.27)	(1.08)	(1.15)	(1.21)
Economic development	2.82**	3.19***	3.50**	1.16	0.95	0.99
	(1.03)	(1.18)	(1.26)	(1.07)	(1.11)	(1.14)
Mobilization	0.95	1.11	1.07	1.62	1.53	1.76
	(0.88)	(0.96)	(0.97)	(0.99)	(1.06)	(1.09)
Head start	−1.24	−0.87	0.17	−1.50	−1.69	−1.30
	(0.92)	(1.24)	(1.41)	(0.90)	(1.18)	(1.23)
Number of years	—	−0.08	0.08	—	0.05	0.13
		(0.14)	(0.18)		(0.14)	(0.17)
Earliest	—	—	−3.62*	—	—	−1.95
			(1.87)			(1.58)
Latest	—	—	−2.07	—	—	−1.89
			(1.28)			(1.36)
Control						
1997 Population	−0.00	−0.00	−0.00	−0.00	−0.00	−0.00
	(0.00)	(0.00)	(0.00)	(0.00)	(0.00)	(0.00)

	(1)	(2)	(3)	(4)	(5)	(6)
West	4.25***	4.27***	4.90***	4.96***	5.06***	5.60***
	(1.19)	(1.22)	(1.32)	(1.46)	(1.50)	(1.56)
Midwest	3.49***	3.47***	3.82***	3.25*	3.39**	3.69**
	(1.00)	(1.02)	(1.06)	(1.36)	(1.39)	(1.40)
Great plains	0.85	0.83	0.45	1.54	1.65	1.44
	(1.39)	(1.41)	(1.42)	(1.66)	(1.68)	(1.66)
Eastern	27.50***	27.72	28.39	26.94	26.98	27.45***
	(2.02)	—	—	—	(2.12)	(2.13)
Constant	-2.84**	-2.75*	-2.45*	-3.20*	-3.37*	-3.09*
	(1.06)	(1.15)	(1.12)	(1.34)	(1.44)	(1.42)
Observations	104	104	104	104	104	104
$\chi^{2\,21}$	81.77	82.71	88.59	81.77	82.71	88.59
Degree of freedom	18	20	24	18	20	24
Pseudo R^2	0.382	0.386	0.413	0.382	0.386	0.413

* $p < 0.05$ (two-tailed tests).
** $p < 0.01$.
*** $p < 0.001$.

reports, and former participants characterize it as a highly formalized program with rigid accountability structures,[22] intrusive supervision, and
bureaucratic restrictions. Despite its promise of local control, C&A had a
very top-down/imposed structure similar to that of the BIA. As noted
above, studies find that top-down programming does not work. This type of
organizational structure does not encourage autonomy, empowerment, or
leave room for agency or self-governance. Rather, programs like C&A reinforce a "power over"/dominance model. This represents a continuation of
structural domination and may have inhibited capacity building. Therefore,
though not actively mediated by the BIA, C&A programs did not provide
opportunities for establishing and widening network ties nor for improving
self-governance capacities.

The economic development programs, however, had "bottom-up" implementation. The process was much more collaborative. Communities
participated in identifying problems that needed to be addressed and were
involved in helping to design programs that fit with their needs and cultures.
Cultural match, as Cornell and Kalt (1992) note, is an important contributing factor to successful economic development projects. Engaging the
community provides incentive for participation and local support. This ex-
poses a larger group to learning experiences thereby disseminating knowledge and skills across a wider base.

The fact that participating tribes are statistically significantly *less* likely
to compact then contract may be a function of OEO as a whole. While
the bottom-up approach encourages the establishment of various economic
development projects on the reservations, Castile (1974) reminds us
that OEO funding was intended as a catalyst not a permanent means
of support. Given the general lack of self-sufficiency on reservations at
the time, he finds this to be highly problematic. Both he and Levitan and
Johnston (1975) are critical of these programs because they encouraged
development without providing sustained funding. Longer-term economic
losses and increased debt load may have occurred when CAP was disman-
tled, especially if ventures were not yet stable enough to generate sufficient
working capital to compensate for the loss of federal contributions. As
compacting is complex and resource intensive, this could discourage tribes
from seeking this level of control over health care management.

Neither participation in mobilization projects nor Head Start proved to
be statistically significant in these models. LOGIT models do reveal a significant negative effect of Head Start participation on higher levels of health
care management ($p < 0.001$). Direct service tribes had the highest participation in Head Start programs (75%), while compacting tribes had the

lowest (29%). Fisher's exact tests indicate these differences to be highly significant ($p < 0.001$). Head Start, like C&A, is a rigidly bureaucratic, top-down program. The Perry pre-school model, the core of Head Start, is stringent. Participants are supposed to meet higher space requirements, higher teacher/student ratios, and have age-specific bathrooms. Rural and more impoverished areas are not provided with sufficient funds to meet these requirements, so they cannot implement the programs properly.

Hypothesis 2

This hypothesis accounts for the timing of response to opportunities, assuming that tribes joining CAP earliest are more willing to take risks. The timing of CAP participation does have an impact. Those who participated earliest in CAP are 58% *less* likely to contract than remain with IHS direct services. In these models, timing has no statistical impact on the likelihood of compacting over contracting. While not statistically significant, LOGIT models indicate that small case size may be masking the effect ($p < 0.05$) of entering OEO/CAP late. The consistently negative direction of effect suggests that these tribes did not have sufficient time to establish network ties or hone management and self-governance capabilities. The results of the MLOGIT runs can be found in Model 3 of Table 1.

Taken together these results fail to support Hypothesis 2. Being early risk takers in the CAP program has the opposite impact of what was predicted. It is most likely that those who entered the program earliest suffered from a combination of factors. First and foremost, they were exposed to steeper learning curves, as agencies were working out how best to enact the legislation and launch the programs, leading to implementation and funding delays and additional negotiations. Similar to interactions with the BIA, this resulted in heightened frustration. It is also likely that increased exposure to the structural restrictions of the C&A program reduced incentives to interact more with government agencies.

The effect of the economic development program also contributes to the explanation for this finding. As noted above, longer participation provides opportunity to establish a greater number of economic development projects. As funding for these projects disappeared with CAP's sudden termination, tribes were left holding the bag. Those with more projects underway and in partial states of completion or implementation were more vulnerable to failure from the sudden loss of input capital. Having to finance these ventures increased debt loads and resulted in the abandonment of many projects (see

White, 1990). This was more devastating for tribes that are also natural resource poor, as they had fewer options for economic recovery.

SUMMARY AND CONCLUSION

OEO/CAP's capacity-building opportunities do have a positive impact on moving away from IHS direct services, however, not in the manner antic-ipated. The component programs that empowered tribes to become actively involved in decision-making, design, and program implementation (eco-nomic development and mobilization) made a positive impact, as predicted. These tribes are more likely to contract for health care services rather than remain with IHS direct service provisions.

However, this study finds that these benefits can be offset by other pro-grams that do not facilitate self-governance or help to build administrative and management skills. Because the organizational structure of both the C&A and Head Start programs were reminiscent of the BIA's, participation had a negative impact on moving to higher levels of health care manage-ment. These were highly bureaucratic, rule oriented, and administratively driven top-down programs that did not encourage Native autonomy. The benefits of these programs are not sustainable over the long term because they are resistant to local input. Bureaucratic modes of organization are also less likely to fit with traditional methods and can increase feelings of dis-empowerment, lack of ownership of the project, frustration, and resentment.

While CAP participation did not provide the degree of independence from the BIA or the skill sets that it strived to impart, it did play a crucial role in the struggle for sovereignty. CAP participation and the success of some programs provided a potent symbol to the federal government, the public, and the nations themselves that they could and should be treated as gov-ernments capable of managing their own affairs and programs. It reintro-duced the viability of self-determination and self-government, despite the fact that the programs did not always foster autonomy. This paved the way for the Self-Determination Act that followed.

These findings are important for both international development and Native American studies literatures. They support more recent studies that suggest that bottom-up development models are both more effective and more sustainable over the long term. Redirecting development projects to focus on local input and collaboration can ultimately reduce the negative impact of imposed development plans that have left indigenous groups in situations worse than when they started. It can also provide a useful model for Native nations to address the array of pathologies on the reservations that are themselves the result of years of outside control and administration.

NOTES

1. For a detailed overview of this issue, please refer to Companion (2003).

2. See Bebbington and Kopp (1998), Blunt and Warren (1996), Cernea (1991, 1997), Cernea and McDowell (2000), Chambers (1983), Eade and Williams (1995), Edwards, Drews, Seaman, and Edwards (1994), Escobar (1995), Feeney (1998), Kardam (1993), Redclift (1987), and Watt (2000).

3. Pub. L. No. 88-452, 78 Stat. 508.

4. Pub. L. 93-638, 88 Stat. 2203, 25 USC. §§ 450–458 (as amended).

5. See Castile and Bee (1992), Chaudhuri (1985), Cornell (1988), Davidson and Levitan (1968), Deloria and Lytle (1984), Deloria and Wilkins (1999), Esber (1992), Holder (1967), Human Services Research, Inc. (1966), Jorgensen (1978), Levitan (1969), Levitan and Hetrick (1971), Levitan and Johnston (1975), Smith (2000), Snipp (1988), and Trosper (1996).

6. See Companion (2003) for a detailed discussion of domestic dependency.

7. Ch. 576, 48 Stat. 984 (codified as amended at 25 U.S.C. §§ 461, 462, 463, 464, 465, 466–470, 471–473,474, 475, 476–478, 479).

8. See Companion (2003) and Perry (1996) for a more detailed discussion.

9. The term is borrowed from the works of Paul Baran (1957, *The political economy of growth.* New York: Monthly Review Press) and Andre Gunder Frank (1967, *Capitalism and underdevelopment in Latin America; historical studies of Chile and Brazil.* New York: Monthly Review Press).

10. Tighter economies create greater restrictions on financial allocations to programs (Trosper, 1996; Castile, 1974).

11. Evans (1994), Weisgrau (1997), and Smith (2000) also note the importance of autonomy within the system, supporting a "bottom-up" development model. Stull et al. (1986) applied this framework to Native American nations and find that top-down planning does not work because it ignores indigenous methods of doing things (see also Jacobs, 1978), demonstrating bottom-up models to be more effective with better long-term outcomes (Cornell, 1988; Cornell & Kalt, 1992, 1998).

12. Bee (1992), Chaudhuri (1985), Esber (1992), Pommersheim (1995), Senese (1991), Shattuck and Norgren (1991), Snipp (1988), Trosper (1996), Krepps and Caves (1994), and Stull et al. (1986).

13. Albrecht's (1982) examination of energy resource leases administered by the BIA supports this. He finds a conflict of interest between executing a national energy policy based on resource exploitation and development and acting as a trustee and manager of Native resources.

14. See Cornell and Kalt (1995, 1998) for a discussion of the importance of cultural match.

15. See Companion (2005) for a discussion of government agencies as interest groups.

16. Because of comparability issues, tribes from Oklahoma and Alaska are excluded. See Cohen (1982), and Cornell and Kalt (1992,1995).

17. This cut-off date is used because major amendments were made to the Self-Determination Act in 1998 that fundamentally alters compacting abilities.

18. The Mashantucket Pequot are a prime example – see Sioux (1996). Two models of sovereignty: A comparative history of the Mashantucket Pequot tribal nation and the Navajo Nation. *American Indian Culture and Research Journal,* 20(10), 147–194.

19. Including the results for a comparison between compacting and contracting tribes in the table is redundant, as it can be derived from the other two. In that model, the only variable that impacts the likelihood of compacting over contracting is participation in the economic development program, as is discussed below.

20. Standard error in parentheses.

21. χ^2 for all models are significant at the $p < 0.001$ level.

22. See also Levitan (1969), Levitan and Hetrick (1971) and Levitan and Johnston (1975).

REFERENCES

Albrecht, S. L. (1982). Unique impacts of rapid growth on minority groups: The Native American experience. In: B. A. Weber & R. E. Howell (Eds), *Coping with rapid growth in rural communities* (pp. 171–190). Boulder: Westview Press.

Barsh, R. L. (1988). Indian resources and the national economy: Business cycles and policy cycles. *Policy Studies Journal, 16*(4), 799–825.

Bebbington, A., & Kopp, A. (1998). Networking and rural development through sustainable forest management: Frameworks for pluralistic approaches. *Unasylva, 194*(49), 11–19.

Bee, R. L. (1992). Riding the paper tiger. In: G. P. Castile & R. L. Bee (Eds), *State and reservation: New perspectives on Federal Indian Policy* (pp. 139–164). Tucson: University of Arizona Press.

Blunt, P., & Warren, D. M. (1996). *Indigenous organizations and development.* London: Intermediate Technology Publications.

Castile, G. P. (1974). Federal Indian Policy and the sustained enclave: An anthropological perspective. *Human Organization, 33*(3), 219–228.

Castile, G. P. (1998). *To show heart: Native American self-determination and Federal Indian Policy (1960–1975).* Tucson: The University of Arizona Press.

Castile, G. P., & Kushner, G. (1981). *Persistent peoples: Cultural enclaves inperspective.* Tucson: University of Arizona Press.

Castile, G. P., & Bee, R. L. (1992). *State and reservation: New perspectives on Federal Indian Policy.* Tucson: University of Arizona Press.

Cernea, M. M. (1985, 1991). Putting people first: Sociological variables in rural development. New York: Oxford University Press, published for the World Bank.

Cernea, M. M. (1997). The risks and reconstruction model for resettling displaced populations. *World Development, 25*(10), 1569–1588.

Cernea, M. M., & McDowell, C. (2000). *Risks and reconstruction: Experiences of resettlers and refugees.* Washington, DC: The World Bank.

Chambers, R. (1983). *Rural development: Putting the last first.* London: Longman.

Chaudhuri, J. (1985). American Indian Policy: An overview. In: V. Deloria Jr. (Ed.), *American Indian Policy in the twentieth century* (pp. 15–33). Norman: University of Oklahoma Press.

Cohen, F. (1982). *The handbook of Federal Indian Law.* Charlottesville, VA: Michie Co.

Companion, M. (2003). *Embracing autonomy: The impact of socio-cultural and political factors on tribal health care management levels.* Doctoral Dissertation, University of Arizona.

Companion, M. (2005). The politics of signification: A frame analysis of social movement discourse in an institutionalized setting. Unpublished paper, currently under review.

Cornell, S. (1988). *The return of the native: American Indian political resurgence.* NY: Oxford University Press.

Cornell, S., & Kalt, J. P. (1992). *What can tribes do? Strategies and institutions in American Indian economic development.* Los Angeles: American Indian Studies Center, University of California.

Cornell, S., & Kalt, J. P. (1995). Where does economic development really come from? Constitutional rule among the contemporary Sioux and Apache. *Economic Inquiry, 33,* 402–426.

Cornell, S., & Kalt, J. P. (1998). Sovereignty and nation-building: The development challenge in Indian Country today. *American Indian Culture and Research Journal, 22*(3), 187–214.

Davidson, R. H., & Levitan, S. A. (1968). *Antipoverty housekeeping: The administration of the Economic Opportunity Act.* Ann Arbor: The Institute of Labor and Industrial Relations, Policy Papers in Human Resources and Industrial Relations, No. 9.

Deloria, V., Jr., & Lytle, C. M. (1984). *The nations within: The past and future of American Indian sovereignty.* New York: Pantheon Books.

Deloria, V., Jr., & Wilkins, D. E. (1999). *Tribes, treaties, & constitutional tribulations.* Austin: University of Texas Press.

Eade, D., & Williams, S. (1995) The Oxfam handbook of development and relief (Vol. 1). Approaches, focusing on people, capacity building. UK: Oxfam.

Edwards, D. E., Drews, J., Seaman, J. R., & Edwards, M. E. (1994). Community organizing in support of self-determination within Native American communities. *Journal of Multicultural Social Work, 3*(4), 43–60.

Esber, G. S., Jr. (1992). Shortcomings of the Indian Self-Determination Policy. In: G. P. Castile & R. L. Bee (Eds), *State and reservation: New perspectives on Federal Indian Policy* (pp. 212–223). Tucson: University of Arizona Press.

Escobar, A. (1995). *Encountering development: The making and unmaking of the Third World.* New Jersey: Princeton University Press.

Evans, P. B. (1994). Predatory, developmental, and other apparatuses: A comparative political economy perspective on the Third World State. In: A. D. Kincaid & A. Portes (Eds), *Comparative national development: Society and economy in the new global order* (pp. 84–111). Chapel Hill: The University of North Carolina Press.

Feeney, P. (1998). *Accountable aid: Local participation in major projects.* UK: An Oxfam Publication.

Greenstone, J. D., & Peterson, P. E. (1973). *Race and authority in urban politics: Community participation and the war on poverty.* New York: Russell Sage Foundation.

Holder, L. E. (1967). Indian community action programs can be self-initiated. *Journal of American Indian Education, 7*(1), 1–4.

Hough, H. W. (1967). *Development of Indian resources.* Denver: World Press Inc.

Human Services Research, Inc. (1966). A comprehensive evaluation of OEO community action programs on six selected American Indian reservations. On Contract OEO- 935, McLean, Virginia.

Jacobs, S.-E. (Fall 1978). Top-down planning: Analysis of obstacles to community development in an economically poor region of the Southwestern United States. *Human Organization, 37*(3), 246–256.

Joe, J. R. (1986). Introduction. In: R. J. Jennie (Ed.), *American Indian Policy and cultural values: Conflict and accommodation* (pp. 1–6). LA: University of California Press.

Jorgensen, J. G. (1978). A century of political economic effects of American Indian Society, 1880–1980. *The Journal of Ethnic Studies, 6*(3), 1–82.

Kardam, N. (1993). Development approaches and the role of policy advocacy: The case of the World Bank. *World Development, 21*(11), 1773–1786.

Krepps, M. B., & Caves, R. E. (1994). Bureaucrats and Indians: Principal-agent relations and efficient management of tribal forest resources. *Journal of Economic Behavior and Organization, 24*, 133–151.

Levitan, S. A. (1964). *Federal aid to depressed areas: An evaluation of the area redevelopment administration.* Baltimore, MD: The Johns Hopkins Press.

Levitan, S. A. (1969). *The great society's poor law: A new approach to poverty.* Baltimore: The Johns Hopkins Press.

Levitan, S. A., & Hetrick, B. (1971). *Big brother's Indian Programs – With reservations.* New York: McGraw-Hill Book Company.

Levitan, S. A., & Johnston, W. B. (1975). *Indian giving: Federal programs for Native Americans.* Policy Studies in Employment and Welfare Series, Number 20. Baltimore: The Johns Hopkins University Press.

National Indian Health Board. (1998). Tribal perspectives on Indian self-determination and self-governance in health care management, (Vols. 2 and 3). Denver, CO: NIHB.

Perry, R. J. (1996). *From time immemorial: Indigenous peoples and state systems.* Austin: University of Texas Press.

Pommersheim, F. (1995). *Braid of feathers: American Indian Law and contemporary tribal life.* Berkeley: University of California Press.

Redclift, M. (1987). *Sustainable development: Exploring the contradictions.* London: Methuen.

Senese, G. B. (1991). The development ideology of self-determination. In: *Self-determination and the social education of Native America* (pp. 35–57). NY: Praeger Publishers.

Shattuck, P. T., & Norgen, J. (1991). *Partial justice: Federal Indian Law in a liberal constitutional system.* Providence and Oxford: Berg Publishers, Inc.

Smith, D. H. (2000). *Modern tribal development: Paths to self-sufficiency and cultural integrity in Indian Country.* Walnut Creek: Alta Mira Press.

Snipp, C. M. (1988). Public policy impacts and American Indian economic development. In: C. M. Snipp (Ed.), *Public policy impacts on American Indian economic development.* Development Series No 4 (pp. 1–22). University of New Mexico: Native American Studies Institute for Native American Development.

Stull, D. D., Schultz, J. A., & Cadue, K. (1986). Rights without resources: The rise and fall of the Kansas Kickapoo. *American Indian Culture & Research Journal, 10*(2), 41–59.

Trosper, R. L. (1996). American Indian poverty on reservations, 1969–1989. In: G. D. Sandefur, R. R. Rindfuss & B. Cohen (Eds), *Changing numbers, changing needs: American Indian demography and public health* (pp. 172–195). Washington, DC: National Academy Press.

Watt, P. (2000). *Social investment and economic growth: A strategy to eradicate poverty.* Oxford: Oxfam Publications.

Weisgrau, M. K. (1997). *Interpreting development: Local histories, local strategies.* Lanham: University Press of American, Inc.

White, R. H. (1990). *Tribal assets: The rebirth of Native America.* New York: Henry Holt and Company.

HEALTH SYSTEMS AND HEALTH PROMOTION PROGRAMS – THE NECESSITY OF CULTURAL COMPETENCE: AN ETHICAL ANALYSIS

Valda Ford and Beth Furlong

ABSTRACT

Health promotion programs in global health systems need to incorporate culturally competent care and provide linguistic access. This article describes the challenges in one country, the United States, and reports on research studies, which articulate the current gaps in meeting the above goals. Health care providers are bound by both legal and ethical standards to provide such care. Legal standards are cited. Regardless of legal standards, health care providers are also bound ethically to provide such care. An analysis of basic ethical concepts of principalism is described for the importance of these aspects of care.

The premise of this article is that one cannot have a successful health system without inclusion of culturally competent health promotion programs. And, one cannot have such health promotion programs without an understanding of the role that cultural and linguistic competence plays in

Health Care Services, Racial and Ethnic Minorities and Underserved Populations: Patient and Provider Perspectives
Research in the Sociology of Health Care, Volume 23, 233–243
Copyright © 2005 by Elsevier Ltd.
ISSN: 0275-4959/doi:10.1016/S0275-4959(05)23011-9

the provision of clinically competent and cost-effective services. Not only is there a need for culturally competent care that is legally mandated in some countries, such care is ethically necessary. The first part of this paper will address the need for culturally and linguistically appropriate care and applicable laws and standards. The latter part of the paper will provide an ethical analysis. However, before doing that, one global perspective of health care concerns for underserved populations will be presented as well as a discussion of the importance of the use of ethical frameworks.

HEALTH CARE CONCERNS FOR UNDERSERVED POPULATIONS

The poor tell us who we are,
  The prophets tell us who we could be,
  So we hide the poor,
  And kill the prophets – Phil Berrigan (Personal e-mail communication, Pat Sullivan, May 11, 2004).

People in poverty comprise one of the health care underserved populations. Their poverty may be the reason why some of the individuals, we discuss in the second half of this paper, are now living in the United States. There are 1.2 billion people globally who live in extreme poverty, i.e., living on less than one U.S. dollar daily. The International Council of Nurses (ICN) responded to this concern by focusing their theme for Nurses Day in May 2004 as "NURSES: Working with the Poor; Against Poverty." (News, 2005, p. 22). Because of their knowledge that poverty and health status and access to care are related, the ICN promoted strategies that promotes equal access to health care, fair labor practices, safe working conditions, and equal rights for women. While 23% of the world's population is living in extreme poverty, another 25% is living in poverty, i.e., living on between one and two U.S. dollars per day (Poorer people, 2004). The correlation of poverty and health are many – increased morbidity and mortality, lack of access to health care at all levels – health promotion to tertiary care, living and working in unsafe and unsanitary environments, etc. As noted earlier, it may be some of these immigrants that U.S. health providers will be caring for – and must demonstrate their cultural competence in the immigrants' care. The increasingly great disparities in global health and human rights compels one to also focus on ethical frameworks, which underscore our work as health professionals.

ETHICAL FRAMEWORKS

Every health professional and other societal professionals operate by a Code of Ethics of their profession. Because this article is about nursing providers, we are using the Code of Ethics of the American Nurses Association (ANA). Every nurse is bound professionally, ethically, and legally by this Code of Ethics. Thus, the ethical analysis we do of the premise of this paper, i.e., that one cannot have a successful health system without culturally competent health promotion programs, includes an analysis using this Code. We include the concept, legal obligation, above because in lawsuits during questioning about Standards of Care, nurses are reminded that they are to follow this Code of Ethics. A second way that we analyze the paper's premise is via the ethical framework of Principalism and we focus on distributive or social justice. Principalism includes several concepts (do no harm, do good, autonomy versus paternalism, and distributive justice). The reason we make a distributive justice argument is because this paper and this volume are concerned about the health status of population groups – not individuals. And, whenever populations are being studied, the public health ethic of social justice has to be included. For example, the ANA Code of Ethics has been critiqued because it is too individualistic and has too much emphasis on autonomy (Stanhope & Lancaster, 2000). A late 20th and early 21st century trend in the U.S. health care system is that of the use of Evidence-Based Knowledge by all health practitioners. In following these Best Practices, health professionals are focusing on patients as part of populations or aggregates and what the research demonstrates as the Best Practices for such populations to follow. Thus, all health professionals now (not just public health professionals or public/community health nurses) are using distributive and social justice ethical analysis models. Dr. Paul Farmer has said it best – "Without a social justice component, medical ethics risks becoming yet another strategy for managing inequality." (Farmer, 2005, p. 201).

While many statistics could be given on underserved populations, the above information on the global picture of poverty sets the scene for many immigrants who seek life in the United States. This is a major part of the population we are addressing in this next section of the paper. We believe that nurses and other health professionals need to be culturally competent, implement the Culturally and Linguistically Appropriate Services (CLAS) standards and Title VI of the Civil Rights Act of 1964. We will now discuss those aspects.

CULTURAL COMPETENCE

The basic cornerstone of the healthcare profession is "to do no harm" (Bosek, 2001). However, as one example, because of the phenomenal growth in the number of people who have immigrated to the United States over the past 30 years (Smidley, 2000), health care providers are challenged to provide safe, effective, and linguistically and culturally appropriate services. According to the U.S. census, one of every 10 people living in the United States was born outside of the United States with 9 of the 10 top leading countries of foreign birth being in Latin America and Asia (Smidley, 2001). Is the United States healthcare system equipped to address the needs of so diverse a society as it relates to acute care, emergency, or preventive services? The answer is a resounding "no"!

Health promotion, even for the majority of Americans, is a component of the health care delivery system that is sometimes lost in the era of "managed care". For those outside the majority – racial/ethnic minorities, those with limited-English proficiency (LEP), new immigrants, and those who are socially and economically disadvantaged, health care in general and health promotion strategies in particular, are provided at a different and lesser level than for the majority population.

As providers are encouraged to do more with less, acute care treatment regimens are taken care of, but education – to facilitate care of the present illness or to prevent future illness suffers. Developing strategies to effectively overcome barriers to health promotion stemming from language deficits between the patient and the provider and cultural disconnects are essential to improving the health of the community.

According to the Behavioral Risk Factor Surveillance System (BRFSS) reports, 40% of people who speak English as a second language stated that they felt their care would be better if they speak English (Centers for Disease Control and Prevention, 2000). A study by Wirthlin Worldwide for the Robert Wood Johnson Foundation found that 19% of Hispanics stated they never try to access care because of language/communication deficits (Robert Wood, 2002). The Wirthlin group reported that 68% of patients say that positive outcomes are made more difficult if there are no bilingual providers or interpreters (2001). Those who do seek care may obtain substandard care because of the lack of priority placed on ensuring appropriate care.

Unfortunately, many providers have failed to appropriately address the issue of care to vulnerable groups. The Wirthlin Worldwide study reveals that providers use a variety of approaches when confronted with clients who have LEP: provide no interpreter services, ask the patient to provide interpreter services, use pantomime and gestures, use providers with varying levels of language proficiency, use ancillary personnel who speak the desired language but who have no experience with medical terminology or medical procedures, or use language line services or a qualified medical language interpreter (2001). Far too often the patient's care is compromised because of the lack of well-designed and organized infrastructures within health care organizations.

This decreased ability to communicate may be considered as an inconvenience to the provider but serious, if not irreparable harm, may be the outcome for clients with cultural and linguistic differences. When other differences, i.e., culture, religion, family hierarchical structure, etc. are added to the problems of language access, safe care is almost an impossibility to assure.

CULTURALLY AND LINGUISTICALLY APPROPRIATE SERVICES STANDARDS

The Culturally and Linguistically Appropriate Services (CLAS) standards are mandates, guidelines, and recommendations issued by the Health and Human Services Office of Minority Health "intended to inform, guide, and facilitate required and recommended practices related to culturally and linguistically appropriate health services" (U.S. Department of Health and Human Services, 2001). CLAS standards were developed to provide guidance to providers who may be unsure of their legal and ethical responsibilities in providing services targeted to those who are frequently the most vulnerable among us, and have dramatically different and disparate health outcomes. According to Donna Shalala, "we as a nation cannot move ahead as long as any one of us is left behind" (Healthy People, 2010, 2002). Unfortunately, many have been and continue to be left behind. How can we consider ourselves effective when so many of our residents have health outcomes that approach or rival those of people in Third World nations?

The CLAS standards are based on the Civil Rights Act of 1964, which states that, "[n] o person in the United States shall, on the ground of race, color, or national origin, be excluded from participation in, be denied the benefits of, or be subjected to discrimination under any program or activity receiving federal financial assistance"(Civil Rights Act of 1964). The Act, and subsequent policies and statutes to provide guidance and structure, have not been acknowledged in some settings, and, even where they have, many providers may feel they are immune to the effects or fallout because they believe that new immigrants they serve are undocumented aliens and are not entitled to the same care or that the underserved are also undeserving of care. However, the Supreme Court has held that "no person" is not limited to just citizens of the United States. Because of this, health care providers and patients (actual or potential) need to be aware of their responsibilities and rights.

TITLE VI

Title VI covers any organization receiving federal financial assistance and its reach is extensive. Such agencies may receive direct federal dollars for programs and services or may provide services to those on Medicaid, Medicare, or other federally financed programs. There are two primary theories of Title VI: intentional discrimination/disparate treatment and disparate impact/effects. Under the second theory, the provider or agency uses a neutral procedure or practice that has a disparate impact on individuals of a particular race, color, or national origin, and such practice lacks a "substantial legitimate justification."(Title VI, 1964) Title VI claims may occur when disparate care is given in an intentional or unintentional fashion. This, too, is confusing for many who believe that, unless they are overtly providing different levels of care to different people, they are immune to the consequences of providing disparate care.

JOINT COMMISSION ON ACCREDITATION OF HEALTHCARE ORGANIZATIONS

The Joint Commission on Accreditation of Healthcare Organizations (JCAHO) is another accrediting agency that specifically addresses the necessity for culturally and linguistically competent care. The intent of JCAHO standard RI.1.2.2 is "the responsible licensed independent practitioner or his or her designee clearly explains the outcome of any treatments or procedures to the patient and, when appropriate, the family, whenever those outcomes differ significantly from the anticipated outcomes" (Joint Commission on Accreditation of Healthcare Organizations, 2001). Failing to understand and appreciate cultural and linguistic differences means that this standard cannot be adhered to and the patient lacks the ability to be informed about and participate in his or her care. There is a real need to educate health care providers and administrators about applicable laws and standards that guide our practice. This aspect is necessary to further the understanding that cultural and linguistic competences are critical components of clinical competence and of health promotion programs. Care given that is not culturally or linguistically appropriate creates several problems for patients and providers: the patient may be less trusting and therefore less forthcoming with a provider, patients are unable to address, verify, or explain nuances of their condition, no appropriate follow-up can be given, and there is an absence of informed consent. Current health care manpower shortages may be exacerbated as providers attempt to avoid the discomfort and frustration of poor communication and the resultant poor care. Perhaps an even worse outcome may be that the provider, forced to constantly compromise in the communication arena, becomes complacent in delivering substandard care and patient education.

> The literature indicates that recent immigration and lack of fluency in English may affect the prevalence of risks for chronic disease and injury among certain racial and ethnic groups. In 1997, 61% of the Asian or Pacific Islander portion and 38% of the Hispanic portion of the U.S. population were foreign born; in contrast, only 8% of the white portion, 6% of the black portion, and 6% of the American Indian or Alaska Native portion were foreign born. Although some immigrants are highly educated and have high incomes, lack of familiarity with the U.S. public and private health systems, different cultural attitudes about the use of traditional and U.S. conventional medicine, and lack of fluency in English pose barriers to obtaining appropriate health care (CDC, 2000).

ETHICAL ANALYSIS

The latter half of this article will articulate the ethical analysis of why cultural competence and linguistic access are of such importance in health promotion programs in health systems. Since 1960s in the United States, there has been an increasing emphasis on the education and socialization of health providers – whether they be physicians, nurses, pharmacists, health educators, dentists, physical therapists, occupational therapists, and so forth to be knowledgeable in the field of bioethics. The main model of ethical analysis that has been used is that of principalism, or the application of one of the following principles to healthcare dilemmas: (1) do no harm or non-maleficence, (2) do good or beneficence, (3) paternalism versus autonomy, and, (4) distributive justice (Zerwekh & Claborn, 2000). Other concepts such as the importance of veracity and fidelity have also been taught. While most health providers in the United States, Great Britain, Western Europe, and the Newly Independent States of the former Soviet Union are knowledge-able and experienced with this model of analysis, it is acknowledged that other theories have been introduced since the 1980s. For example, because of the broad sociological research work conducted by feminists, a new way of studying ethics has been pursued by many nurses – that of an ethics of caring model – which integrates the patient's holistic life context and re-lationships into the ethical decision-making process (Zerwekh & Claborn, 2000). Further, John Rawl's writings on ethics has developed another model (Bandman & Bandman, 1995). For purposes of this article, ethical analysis will focus on principalism and the use of a nursing Code of Ethics. However, in a parallel manner, other health providers could apply similar concepts from their professions' Codes of Ethics. We argue that changing health systems with an increased or strong focus on health promotion are only ethical when the planning of new health promotion programs have included cultural competence of the health providers and linguistic access for pa-tients. Further, we argue not only should health providers be individually culturally competent – but they also have an ethical obligation to structure a health system to have culturally competent aspects and linguistic access for patients. We expect both of these latter aspects to be the norm – and, not the exception, as is now the case. We support our arguments from two per-spectives – first, use of the Code of Ethics of the ANA, and, second, ap-plying the ethical model of principalism.

CODE OF ETHICS

As nurses, the above beliefs are supported by the Code of Ethics of the ANA (American Nurses Association, 2001). This Code, revised in June 2001, has several provisions, which address the above necessities. The first provision, "The nurse, in all professional relationships, practices with compassion and respect for the inherent dignity, worth and uniqueness of every individual, unrestricted by considerations of social or economic status, personal at-tributes, or the nature of health problems." If nurses are to meet this first provision of the Code, then quality-nursing care must reflect being culturally competent. The third provision, "The nurse promotes, advocates for, and strives to protect the health, safety, and rights of the patient" also integrates with our belief. Patients have a right not to be harmed. They have been and can be harmed when culturally competent care is not delivered. The sixth provision of the Code further discusses a nurse's responsibility in a health system – "The nurse participates in establishing, maintaining, and improving healthcare environments and conditions of employment conducive to the provision of quality health care and consistent with the values of the profession through individual and collective action." The language of the first half of this sixth provision is one of the language of obligation – the nurse is obligated to do this. One must improve the healthcare environment, i.e., the practice setting, so that patients receive quality care. Two ways of doing this are being individually culturally competent and of changing the structures of an environment so that environment is culturally competent. The last provision from the Code that will be discussed is the eighth provision – "The nurse collaborates with other health professionals and the public in promoting community, national, and international efforts to meet health needs." There has been ample evidence of health disparities among cultural groups. Nurses have a responsibility to decrease these disparities; striving for cultural competence in the practice setting with health promotion programs is one way to reduce them. Next, an analysis will be done of the major concepts of principalism.

PRINCIPALISM

Our first argument is based on the ethical principle – do no harm or non-maleficence. We agree with Bosek (2001), who states this ethical principle (of the four main principles) is the one that has the highest priority. The dilemma for health providers in implementing health care for patients is that there is often tension between two of these four ethical principles. Thus, we strongly advocate our belief – the first principle is to do no harm to patients. And, we assert – health promotion programs in a health system must be culturally competent and linguistically accessible. Otherwise, harm is being done to patients.

Our second argument is based on the ethical principle of distributive justice. We believe it to be unjust to allocate the majority of resources to dominant populations because that is where the current power structure exists. To follow the distributive justice principle means having a just allocation of resources. The research literature is replete with data on health status outcomes and the needs of many cultural groups in our society. Yet, that scientific objective research data has not translated into action in the area of cultural competence and linguistic access. A major goal of Health People 2010 is to eliminate disparities among groups in the United States.

SUMMARY

This article has addressed the role of cultural competence and ethical analysis in health systems, which emphasizes health promotion. The spirit of this article can be best summed with this quote –

> If I am not for myself, who will be for me?
> But, if I for myself alone, what am I? (Jewish proverb)

Health systems, which include a strong emphasis on health promotion programs have to include culturally competent care and have linguistic access. It is unethical to do otherwise. If we only provide competent health promotion programs for the dominant groups in a society, what are we?

REFERENCES

American Nurses Association. (2001). http://www.nursingworld.org.
Bandman, E. L., & Bandman, B. (1995). *Nursing ethics through the life span*. Norwalk, CT: Appleton & Lange.
Bosek, M. (2001). Reaffirming a primary commitment to nonmaleficence. *JONA'S Healthcare Law, Ethics, and Regulation, 3*, 31–34.
CDC. (2000). http://cdc.gov
Centers for Disease Control and Prevention. (2000). State-specific prevalence of selected health behaviors, by race and ethnicity – Behavorial risk factor surveillance system. *Morbidity and Mortality Weekly Report: Surveillance Summaries, 49*(SS02, March 24), 1–60. Available at www.cdc.gov/nnwr/preview/mmwrhtml/ss4902a1.htmon February 10, 2002.
Farmer, P. (2005). *Pathologies of power*. Berkely: University of California.
Healthy People 2010 (2002). *Partnerships for health in the new millennium – broadcast program. Opening Session*. Available at www.surgeongeneral.gov/ram/012500A.ram News (2004). *AJN, 4*(104), 22.
Joint Commission on Accreditation of Healthcare Organizations. (2001). http://www.jcaho.org
Poorer people live shorter lives and are sick more often than the well-off. (2004). http://www.icn.ch/pr05_04.htm
Robert Wood Johnson Foundation Media Release. (2002). *New study shows language barriers causing many Spanish-speaking Latinos to skip care* (February 10). Available at www.rwjf.org/app/rw_new_and_events/rw_new_media_article.jsp?id = 1008111168672

Smidley, D. A. (2000). *U.S. Census Bureau, Current Population Reports P 23–206, Profile of Foreign-born population in the United States*. U.S. Government Printing Office: Washington, DC.

Stanhope, M., & Lancaster, J. (2000). *Community and public health nursing* (5th Ed.). St. Louis: Mosby.

Title VI of the Civil Rights Act of 1964, as amended, 42 U.S.C. Section 2000d, et Seq. http://www.usdoj.gov/crt/grants_statutes/legalman.html#IntroductionAvailable 2-10-02.

U.S. Department of Health and Human Services. (2001). Office of miniority health. http://www.omhrc.gov/clas/Frclas2.htm.

Wirthlin Worldwide. (2001). *Hablamos Juntos - We speak together* (December 12). Available at www.rwjf.org/app/rw_news_and_events/Wirthlin_presentation/ppsFebruary 10, 2002.s

Zerwekh, J., & Claborn, J. C. (2000). *Nursing today*. Philadephia, PA: W.B. Saunders.

THE BIOMEDICAL LEGACY IN MINORITY HEALTH POLICY-MAKING, 1975–2002

Drew Halfmann, Jesse Rude and Kim Ebert

ABSTRACT

Through content analysis, the study traces the relative prominence of "biomedical" and "public health" approaches in congressional bills aimed at improving the health of racial and ethnic minorities over a 28-year period. It documents a surge of interest in minority health during the late 1980s and early 1990s and highlights the dominance of biomedical initiatives during this period. Drawing on historical methods and interviews with key informants, the paper explains these patterns by detailing the ways in which policy legacies shaped the interests, opportunities, and ideas of interest groups and policy-makers.

Since the mid-1980s, the United States has witnessed marked growth in policy-making on the health of racial and ethnic minorities[1]. This expansion began with the 1985 report of the U.S. Department of Health and Human Services (HHS) Task Force Report on Black and Minority Health – the first government report to deal comprehensively with the issue of racial and ethnic health disparities (U.S. Department of Health and Human Services,

Health Care Services, Racial and Ethnic Minorities and Underserved Populations: Patient and Provider Perspectives
Research in the Sociology of Health Care, Volume 23, 245–275
Copyright © 2005 by Elsevier Ltd.
ISSN: 0275-4959/doi:10.1016/S0275-4959(05)23012-0

1985). Subsequent developments included the establishment of minority health offices in the Public Health Service (PHS), the National Institutes of Health (NIH), and most states, as well as the elevation of the NIH office to center status, giving it independent grant-making authority.

In this paper, we examine proposals for improving the health of racial and ethnic minorities that reached the congressional agenda from 1975 to 2002 in the form of introduced bills. We address two questions: First, what was the relative prevalence of "biomedical" and "public health" idea packages over time? Second, what explains these patterns? We begin by describing our methods, including the identification of five minority health policy "packages" and six "sub-packages". We follow this with an overview of minority health policy-making, attending to congressional enactments that incorporated the biomedical and public health packages. We then present historical trends in the relative prevalence of these packages in congressional bills. Finally, we offer an explanation for those trends that shows how policy legacies influenced the interests, opportunities and ideas of policy-makers and interest groups, and highlights the role of events exogenous to the minority health policy domain such as the AIDS and women's health movements, and the development of the "new perspective on health".

MEASURING POLICY PACKAGES

The study combines content analysis, interview and historical methods. We conducted confidential interviews with 45 key informants – members of Congress and their staffs, federal and state officials (both appointed and non-appointed), as well as researchers and representatives of interest groups. The organizational affiliations of the informants are listed in Table 1. The study also draws on observations at the 2002 annual legislative conference of the Congressional Black Caucus Health Brain Trust and at the 2002 Department of Health and Human Services National Leadership Summit on eliminating racial and ethnic disparities in health.

For the content analysis, we first developed a list of possible policy proposals for addressing the health of racial and ethnic minorities. We based this list on several sources: the HHS *Healthy People 2000* report, congressional hearings on minority health, interviews with key informants, and selective reading of academic journals, the prestige press, and reports of major foundations. Our list contained 63 possible proposal codes. We then conducted subject searches in the U.S. Congress's THOMAS database and identified all bills ($N = 147$) that dealt with health and explicitly targeted

Table 1.   Organizational Affiliations of Informants.

9	U.S. House of Representatives (members and staff)
3	U.S. Senate (members and staff)
5	Offices of the Secretary and Assistant Secretary, Health and Human Services
7	Centers for Disease Control and Prevention (CDC)
4	Office of Minority Health, Health and Human Services
2	National Institutes of Health (NIH)
1	Health Resources and Services Administration (HRSA)
1	Substance Abuse and Mental Health Services Administration (SAMHSA)
2	State offices of minority health
3	Institute of Medicine (IOM)
2	Schools of medicine
6	Schools of public health
3	Think tanks
12	Interest groups
2	Foundations
45	TOTAL INTERVIEWS

Note: Some informants are included in more than one category.

racial and ethnic minorities from 1975 to 2002 (see Methodological Appendix for selection criteria). We then performed content analyses of the bill summaries using our proposal codes.

Gamson and Modigliani (1987, 1989) argue that policy ideas on particular issues are "organized and clustered" into "packages". Through our reading of a wide variety of works on minority health and the bills themselves, we arrived at five main proposal packages that encompassed the 63 proposal codes: *Biomedical, Public Health, Non-Health Social Welfare, Government Capacity and Accountability, and Community Participation.* Below, we provide a brief description of the five packages and offer a more detailed description in Table 2.

Biomedical Package

Lavis (2000, p. 314) contrasts the Biomedical and Public Health packages as follows:

> The public health model adopts a multicausal and ecological perspective that allows for reciprocal associations among variables. Its focus is groups of people, usually communities, and its goal is health promotion and disease prevention.

Table 2.   Minority Health Proposal Packages.

Package	Position	Summary of Proposals	Sample Signature Elements
Biomedical	Policy proposals should focus on curative medicine and individuals.	See biomedical sub-packages	See biomedical sub-packages
Public health	Policies should focus on groups of people (i.e., communities) and the overall goal should be health promotion and disease prevention.	See public health sub-packages	See public health sub-packages
Non-health social welfare	The health of racial and ethnic minorities is related to their disadvantaged socioeconomic position. Policy proposals should address the social welfare of minority populations.	Proposals include education (non-health), housing, residential integration, income support, employment policies, and income redistribution.	"Aids short-term supported housing and services demonstration – Amends the Stewart B. McKinney Homeless Assistance Act to authorize the Secretary to make grants for programs to prevent homelessness among persons with AIDS and to provide them with short-term supported housing and related services. Provides for minority outreach" (H.R. 3423, 1989).
Government capacity and accountability	Policies should establish new institutions, planning processes, or systems for gathering information on health disparities.	Proposals include the establishment of offices of minority health in federal and state bureaucracies, mandating strategic plans, and improving data collection on health disparities.	"Associate Director for minority concerns – Establishes…the position of Associate Director for minority concerns within the National Institute of Mental Health" (S. 1177, 1980).

Community participation	Policies should ensure that members of local and minority communities participate in the planning of minority health initiatives.	Proposals include attempts to ensure that members of local and minority communities participate in the planning of health care provision, public health interventions, and research on health disparities.	"Activities carried out by such a project shall include the following: (1) Planning, organizing, and conducting a symposium of all major elements of the community to identify the best ways to reach and influence African-American individuals in the community" (H.R. 1218, 2001).
Biomedical research (biomedical sub-package)	Same as biomedical	Proposals include conducting research on particular diseases and on biological differences among minority groups; including and protecting minorities in research trials; and recruiting and training minority biomedical researchers.	"Requires the Director to...conduct or support research to expand the understanding of the causes of, and to find a cure for, lupus, including research to determine the reasons underlying the elevated prevalence of the disease among African American and other women" (H.R. 1111, 1997).
Biomedical access (biomedical sub-package)	Same as biomedical	Proposals include increasing insurance coverage for minorities; setting up clinics in neighborhoods, schools and public housing; and ensuring that health care facilities are located in areas that serve minorities.	"Medically Underserved Access to Care Act of 1999...To require managed care organizations to contract with providers in medically underserved areas" (H.R. 1860, 1999).
Biomedical quality (biomedical sub-package)	Same as biomedical	Proposals include increasing the linguistic and cultural competence of health care providers and institutions, enforcing anti-discrimination laws, and recruiting and training minority health providers.	"Directs the Secretary to: (1) develop educational materials on providing health services in a culturally competent manner; (2) establish a Center for Linguistic and Cultural Competence in Health Care; and (3) carry out cultural competence demonstration projects at two hospitals" (H.R. 5595, 2000).

Table 2. (*Continued*)

Package	Position	Summary of Proposals	Sample Signature Elements
Clinical preventive services (public health sub-package)	Same as public health	Proposals include immunization and vaccination, and the screening, monitoring and early diagnosis of diseases.	"Amends the Public Health Service Act to authorize the Secretary of Health and Human Services to...assist States in preventing or reducing morbidity and premature mortality resulting from diabetes, with particular emphasis on Hispanics and other populations at risk" (H.R. 3259, 1987).
Health promotion (public health sub-package)	Same as public health	Proposals include reducing unhealthy or risky individual behaviors relating to drugs, alcohol, tobacco, risky sexual behaviors, diet, exercise, homicide, suicide, and accidents.	"Expands the purposes for which the Secretary may make grants to public and nonprofit private entities to include alcoholism treatment and prevention services, with emphasis on underserved racial and ethnic minorities..." (S. 3184, 1976).
Health protection (public health sub-package)	Same as public health	Proposals include interventions such as the legal regulation of guns, crime, drugs, alcohol, and tobacco, efforts to ensure auto and highway safety, food safety, sanitation, occupational health and safety, and environmental regulation and cleanup.	"Environmental Justice Act of 2002 – Requires Federal agencies to include achieving environmental justice in their missions through identifying and addressing any disproportionately high and adverse human health or environmental effects of their activities on minority and low-income communities" (H.R. 5637, 2002).

The biomedical model "typically refers to a unidirectional, biological cause-and-effect relationship between an agent and host. Its focus is individuals and its goal is the medical cure of disease."

Our Biomedical package includes three sub-packages: biomedical research, access and utilization of medical and mental health care (including dental care), and the quality and equality of medical and mental health care. Proposals within the *Biomedical Research* sub-package include conducting research on particular diseases, conducting research on biological differences between racial and ethnic groups, including and protecting minorities in research trials, and recruiting and training minority biomedical researchers. Proposals within the *Biomedical Access* sub-package include increasing insurance coverage for minorities; setting up clinics in neighborhoods, schools, and public housing; and ensuring that health care facilities are located in areas that serve minorities. The *Biomedical Quality* sub-package includes proposals on increasing the linguistic and cultural competence of health care providers and institutions, enforcing anti-discrimination laws, and recruiting and training minority health providers.

Public Health Package

The Public Health package also contains three sub-packages: clinical preventive services, health promotion, and health protection. The *Clinical Preventive Services* sub-package includes immunization and vaccination, and the screening, monitoring and early diagnosis of diseases. Proposals within the *Health Promotion* sub-package include reducing unhealthy or risky individual behaviors relating to drugs, alcohol, tobacco, sexual behaviors, diet, exercise, homicide, suicide, and accidents. The *Health Protection* sub-package includes proposals on the reduction of health risks through population-level rather than individual-level interventions. Such interventions include the legal regulation or taxation of guns, crime, drugs, alcohol, and tobacco, as well as efforts to ensure auto and highway safety, food safety, sanitation, and occupational health and safety. This category also includes environmental regulation and cleanup.

Non-Health Social Welfare Package

Relevant policies within the Non-Health Social Welfare package include education (non-health), housing, residential integration, income support, employment policies, and income redistribution. This package is no doubt under-represented because we only analyze bills that explicitly address health. To do otherwise would expand the scope of the project beyond our resources.

Government Capacity and Accountability Package

The Government Capacity and Accountability package includes establishing offices of minority health in federal and state bureaucracies, mandating strategic plans, and improving data collection on health disparities.

Community Participation Package

Proposals within the Community Participation package include attempts to promote the participation of members of local and minority communities in the planning of health care provision, in public health interventions, and in research on health disparities.

Below, we present data on the prevalence of these packages, paying particular attention to the interplay of biomedical and public health approaches in minority health policy. First, however, an overview of the history of minority health policy-making is in order. As our subsequent discussion of policy legacies shows, a complex interaction of historical forces has driven the trends in minority health policy over the past three decades. A better understanding of this history can help us to explain these trends.

AN OVERVIEW OF MINORITY HEALTH POLICY-MAKING

In this section, we detail major events in minority health policy-making, including executive actions, legislative enactments, and focusing events (see Table 3). In the section that follows this one, we focus not only on legislative *enactments*, but on all 147 bills introduced in Congress.

The Ford and Carter Administrations

In the 1970s, attention to minority health was minimal and most enactments were biomedical. The 94th Congress enacted an alcoholism treatment and

Table 3. Enactments of Bills Targeting Minority Health, 1975–2002.

Year	Congress	Biomedical	Public Health
1975–1976	94	S. 3184	S. 3184
1977–1978	95	S. 2466	
1979–1980	96	S. 525, S. 1177, S. 7203	S. 525
1981–1982	97	S. 1086	S. 1086
1983–1984	98	S. 2603	S. 2603
1985–1986	99		
1987–1988	100	H.J.RES. 119, H.R. 5210, S. 769, S. 2889	H.J.RES. 119
1989–1990	101	H.R. 5112, H.R. 5702, S. 2946	H.R. 5702
1991–1992	102	H.R. 2967, H.R. 3508, S. 1306, H.R. 5194	H.R. 2967, H.R. 5194
1993–1994	103	H.R. 3313, S. 1, S. 1284	
1995–1996	104	S. 641	S. 1316
1997–1998	105	H.R. 2202, S. 1722, S. 1754	
1999–2000	106	H.R. 782, S. 1880	H.R. 782
2001–2002	107	S. 1789	
Total		28	10

Note: Bills can contain both biomedical and public health proposals.

prevention bill that targeted minorities (S. 3184), and in the 95th Congress, a health care research and statistics bill called for regular assessment of the health problems of low-income and minority groups (S. 2466).

In 1979, the Surgeon General released the first *Healthy People* report, establishing five broad national health goals but none of these goals targeted racial and ethnic or income-based health disparities (U.S. Department of Health Education and Welfare, 1979). However, the following year, when it established 219 objectives for the attainment of these goals, the Public Health Service named five specific objectives for reducing racial and ethnic or income-based health disparities (in infant mortality, maternal mortality, low-weight births, prenatal care, and homicide).

Meanwhile, the 96th Congress enacted three minority health bills. It enacted a drug abuse, prevention, and treatment bill that targeted minorities and people with limited English-language skills, created the position of Associate Director for Underserved Populations in the National Institute on Drug Abuse (NIDA) and required state drug abuse plans to address the needs of minorities. It also established the position of Associate Director for Minority Concerns within the National Institute of Mental Health and required data collection on the supply of minority health personnel (S. 525, S. 1177 and S. 7203).

The Reagan Administration

In the early 1980s, attention to minority health remained low and enactments incorporated both public health and biomedical approaches. The 97th and 98th Congresses revised the Older Americans Act (OAA) of 1965 (which includes nutrition and long-term care services) to target minorities. The 97th Congress required services under the Act to be linguistically competent (S. 1086). The 98th Congress required the Office on Aging to consult with national minority organizations to develop training packages to help states reach elderly minority groups, called for the inclusion of minorities on advisory councils, and directed agencies to expand outreach to minorities (S. 2603).

A shift in minority health policy occurred in the mid-1980s, owing in large part to HHS Secretary Margaret M. Heckler. In 1984, Heckler released the department's annual report on the nation's health status and noted that minority groups suffered a "persistent and continuing disparity in the burden of death, illness, and disability." She disputed critics who argued that Reagan's budget cuts had contributed to a widening in these disparities. She then announced the creation of a task force on minority health to be directed by Thomas E. Malone, the African-American deputy director of the NIH (*New York Times*, January 18, 1984, p. A17; *Washington Post*, January 18, 1984, p. A2).

In October 1985, Malone's group released a seven-volume report that likely went beyond the Reagan Administration's wishes (U.S. Department of Health and Human Services, 1985). It estimated 60,000 "excess" deaths among African Americans each year. Eighty percent of these were the result of disparities in six major causes of death: cancers; cardiovascular disease; homicide, suicide and unintentional injuries; diabetes; infant mortality and cirrhosis. The report also showed differences in death rates between whites and Hispanics and Native Americans. Although the report mentioned poverty, lack of health insurance, and poor prenatal care as causes of health disparities, Heckler, under Administration orders, did not propose new funds or programs. She did allocate $3 million for a new Office of Minority Health (OMH) in the HHS that would target existing funds and monitor minority health.

In response to the report, black and minority health was a major subject at the 1986 annual convention of the Congressional Black Caucus. That same year, the Association of Minority Health Professions Schools (AMHPS), a group of eight historically black schools of medicine, pharmacy, and dentistry, teamed up with organizations of black medical professionals and the Children's Defense Fund to form the National Health Coalition for Minorities. The Coalition fought Reagan Administration budget cuts that threatened Medicaid and Medicare, research on minority health, and the training of minority health professionals. The most visible individual in this coalition was Dr. Louis W. Sullivan, President of the Morehouse School of Medicine (*Washington Post*, April 12, 1986, p. A7; *Washington Post*, October 14, 1986, p. Z17).

The Malone report resulted in a flood of legislation in the late 1980s. The 100th Congress enacted four minority health bills. It established a "National Minority Cancer Awareness Week". It mandated state grants for demonstration projects to provide drug treatment targeted to minorities. It gave grants to health professions schools for the education of minorities. And the omnibus public health service bill required the NIH to include minority groups in AIDS research, mandated research on the supply of minority health professionals, and required a study of the availability of language-appropriate health care for Hispanics (H.J.RES. 119, H.R. 5210, S. 769, and S. 2889).

In 1988, the state of Ohio established the first state office on minority health. Several other states soon followed. In all, 35 states have established minority health offices and seven others have designated minority health liaisons. Only seven states have done neither (Alaska, Colorado, Idaho, Kansas, North Dakota, South Dakota, and Washington) (Office of Minority Health Resource Center, 2002).

The Bush Administration

President Bush appointed Sullivan, life-long Democrat and friend, to head HHS. Sullivan pledged to improve the health of minorities, but in his first year he was widely perceived as an ineffective outsider with only weak ties to the White House. His stock rose, however, when he began a series of public attacks on the tobacco industry for marketing cigarettes to African Americans and working-class women.

The 101st Congress enacted three minority health bills. It expanded perinatal facilities in states where infant mortality rates for the poor and minorities were above the national average. It required the National Bone Marrow Donor Registry to increase the number of minorities in the donor pool. It also enacted the *Disadvantaged Minority Health Improvement Act of 1990*. The $112 million Act legislatively established the already existing Office of Minority Health within HHS; mandated the creation of an information clearinghouse on minority health; provided funding for primary care and counseling in public housing projects; established grants to increase the number of minority health professionals; directed the National Center for Health Statistics to collect data on minority health; and reauthorized community and migrant health centers (H.R. 5112, S. 2946, and H.R. 5702).

In 1991, the Public Health Service released the *Healthy People 2000* report. In contrast to the 1979 report, the reduction of health disparities was one of three major goals. The report devoted considerable attention to "special populations" – people with low income, racial and ethnic minorities, and people with disabilities. Of its 300 objectives, 50 targeted special populations. Typically, these objectives represented a narrowing of the gaps in health status between special populations and the general population, but they did not seek to eliminate those gaps (U.S. Department of Health and Human Services, 1991).

The 102nd Congress enacted four minority health bills. It authorized substance abuse treatment demonstration projects targeted to minorities. It required Older Americans Act state agencies to set specific goals for providing services and developing advocacy and outreach programs for low-income and minority individuals. It provided grants to health professions schools to increase the number of minority faculty and students. And it approved training Head Start personnel to provide services to children from non-English language backgrounds (S. 1306, H.R. 2967, H.R. 3508, and H.R. 5194).

The Clinton Administration

In 1992, the NIH Office of Research on Minority Health (ORMH) launched its Minority Health Initiative, funding biomedical and behavioral research at an initial budget of $45 million (Office of Research on Minority Health, 2002). In the same year, the Clinton Administration released its annual report on the nation's health. As usual, the report showed major racial and ethnic health disparities. HHS Secretary Donna Shalala argued that the disparities demonstrated the need for passage of the Administration's health reform plan (*Los Angeles Times*, September 16, 1993, p. A18).

The 103rd Congress required state developmental disabilities plans to include assurances of minority participation. It also required the Veterans' Administration to include women and minorities in clinical research. The NIH Revitalization Act formally established the Office of Research on Minority Health (ORMH) and required that all NIH-sponsored phase III clinical trials include enough women and minorities to perform valid subset analyses (S. 1284, H.R. 3313, S. 1).

The election of a Republican majority resulted in a decline in minority health proposals – especially in public health. The 104th Congress enacted two bills with minority health provisions. It required Ryan White planning councils to reflect the demographics of HIV. It also directed the EPA to identify groups at greater risk from contaminants in drinking water (S. 641, S. 1316).

In the late 1990s, minority health received new impetus from the White House. In May 1997, President Clinton apologized for the Tuskegee experiment, in which the syphilis of 400 African-American men went untreated so that PHS researchers could observe the trajectory of the disease. The next month, Clinton launched the President's Initiative on Race, leading to the publication of a chart book that included health indicators broken down by race and ethnicity. In 1998, Clinton made minority health disparities the subject of a Saturday radio broadcast and established the goal of eliminating them by 2010. In February of that year, he announced the HHS Initiative to Eliminate Racial and Ethnic Disparities in Health. The initiative included the Racial and Ethnic Approaches to Community Health program (REACH 2010), which was funded at $10 million in its first year and provided grants to 32 community coalitions to reduce health disparities in 18 states. The initiative also called for public–private public collaboration and established an HHS taskforce on disparities. Subsequently, HHS established goals to eliminate disparities in six areas by 2010: infant mortality, cancer, cardiovascular disease, diabetes, HIV/AIDS, and immunizations.

The 105th Congress required the bone marrow donor registry to give priority to minorities. It called on the NIH to research the causes of cardiovascular disease among women and, in particular, among African Americans and other minorities. It also reauthorized grants to health professions schools for minority recruitment, established an advisory committee for the Office of Minority Health in HHS, and funded data collection on minority health by the National Center for Health Statistics (H.R. 2202, S. 1722, and S. 1754).

In 1999, the Clinton Administration and the Congressional Black and Hispanic caucuses developed the Minority HIV/AIDS Initiative. The package of programs provided $156 million in grants administered by OMH, Centers for Disease Control and Prevention (CDC), NIH, the Substance Abuse and Mental Health Services Administration (SAMHSA), the Indian Health Services (IHS), and the Health Services and Resources Administration (HSRA) (COSMOS Corporation, 2000). That same year, the Institute

of Medicine (IOM) released a report finding that the NIH's efforts to research cancer among minorities were inadequate (U.S. Institute of Medicine, 1999). Senator Bill Bradley made racial and ethnic health disparities an
important issue in his presidential campaign.

The 106th Congress enacted two minority health bills. The first was an
amendment to the Older Americans Act that required the Administration
on Aging to take corrective action if new co-payments reduced participation
by minorities. The second was a $350 million bill that upgraded the Office of
Research on Minority Health in the NIH to center status. The bill also set
up "Centers of Excellence" for research on health disparities and the training of minority health professionals, established extramural loans for this
research, requested a report of NIH resources devoted to disparities research, required health care disparities research by Agency for Healthcare
Research and Quality, directed the Institute of Medicine to study HHS data
collection on race and ethnicity, and required HHS to undertake a public
awareness campaign (H.R. 782, S. 1880).

In his January 2000 State of the Union Address, President Clinton decried
racial and ethnic health disparities and touted the NIH center bill (*Washington
Post*, April 10, 2001, p. A17). In the same year, PHS released its *Healthy
People 2010* report. Eliminating health disparities was one the report's two
central goals. While the previous *Healthy People* report had contained separate targets for special populations and the general population, accepting
that a gap would persist, the latest report included the same targets for both.

The George W. Bush Administration

In March 2002, the IOM issued a report finding that racial and ethnic
minorities receive lower-quality health care regardless of income or insurance status. The report suggested that the HHS Office of Civil Rights receive
more money to adequately enforce anti-discrimination laws in health care
(U.S. Institute of Medicine, 2003). Meanwhile, the 107th Congress required
the inclusion of minorities in Food and Drug Administration (FDA) pediatric studies (S. 1789).

This historical overview reveals ebbs and flows in attention to minority
health, the number of legislative enactments, and the degree to which they
incorporated public health or biomedical proposals. Table 3 summarizes bill
enactments over the 28-year period. As the table shows, Congress enacted 28
bills containing biomedical proposals, but only 10 bills containing public
health proposals. Between 1993 and 2002, Congress enacted 10 bills

containing biomedical proposals, but only 2 bills containing a public health proposal.

In the following section, we move away from a focus on legislative enactments and executive branch activity to focus on the proposals (enacted or not) considered by Congress over the same period. These proposals reveal how Congress thought about minority health and how it tried to address it.

TRENDS IN MINORITY HEALTH PROPOSALS, 1975–2002

An analysis of minority health bills from 1975 to 2002 reveals considerable variation in their frequency and content over time. As Fig. 1 shows, there were approximately 5 bills on minority health per Congress until 1987–1988 when the number of bills doubled and eventually peaked at just over 20 bills in 1993–1994. In 1995–1996 and 1997–1998, the number of bills declined, but began to rise again in 1999–2000.

Turning to the content of the bills, approximately 43 percent focused primarily on minority health while the remaining 57 percent dealt mainly with the health of the general population or low-income people while targeting minorities in some way. If we sort the minority health bills into the five packages and six sub-packages discussed above, access and utilization of medical (and mental health) care was the most prevalent, followed by government capacity and accountability, health promotion, quality of medical care, and biomedical research (see Fig. 2). Only a small number of bills dealt with clinical preventive services, health protection, non-health social welfare policies or community participation. Because of the complexity of many of the bills, we included some in more than one package – a common approach in studies of this type (Burstein, Bricher, & Einwohner, 1995). Within these packages and sub-packages, the most common individual proposals were as follows: creating new government institutions (including advisory committees) (39 bills), recruiting and training minority health providers (31), targeting biomedical research toward diseases with large disparities (21), improving data collection on health disparities (21), improving cultural competence of health providers (including language competence) (20), drug abuse prevention and awareness (18), alcohol abuse prevention and awareness (13), recruitment and training of minority biomedical researchers (11), inclusion of minorities in biomedical research trials (9), and prevention of pregnancy and sexually transmitted diseases (9).

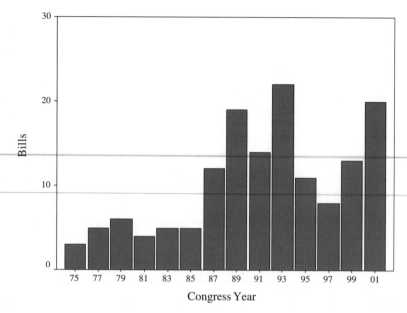

Fig. 1. Minority Health Bills, Two-Year Congressional Terms, 1975–2002.

If we divide the bills into the two packages of biomedicine and public health, we find that 84 percent of the bills contained biomedical proposals while only 46 percent contained public health proposals. Thirty-three percent of the bills contained both types of proposals. In addition to the prevalence of biomedical bills, an indicator of biomedical dominance is that 61 percent of biomedical proposals appeared in bills without public health proposals. By contrast, only 30 percent of public health proposals appeared in bills without biomedical proposals. In other words, public health proposals most often appeared in combination with biomedical proposals, but biomedical proposals most often appeared alone.

Examining the two packages over time, our analysis suggests five relatively distinct periods for minority health proposals (see Fig. 3). In the first (1975–1980 – the Ford and Carter administrations), there were few bills of either type, but bills containing biomedical proposals outnumbered those containing public health proposals. During the second period (1981–1986 – the first 6 years of the Reagan Administration), there were still few minority health bills, but there were roughly equal numbers of each type of proposal. An upsurge in minority health bills occurred in the third period (1987–1994).

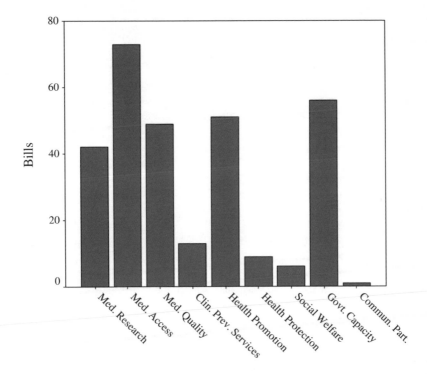

Fig. 2. Proposal Packages of Minority Health Bills, 1975—2002. (*Note:* Some bills are included in multiple packages.)

This was the period immediately following the release of the Malone report and included the Bush and early Clinton administrations. The number of both types of bills increased, but the number of biomedical bills increased much more than public health bills. In the fourth period (1995–1998) with a new Republican congressional majority, both types of bills declined, but public health bills declined more sharply. In the fifth period (1999–2002), the number of minority health bills rose again as the Clinton Administration committed to eliminating health disparities by 2010. Both types of bills increased, but biomedical bills continued to outpace public health ones. Surveying all five periods, biomedical bills outnumbered public health bills in every period, but public health bills were still fairly well represented, and there were about the same number of both types of bills during the second period and the early part of the third.

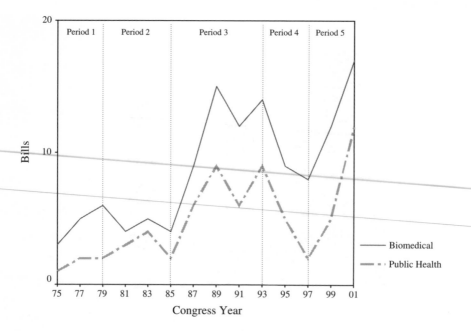

Fig. 3. Minority Health Bills Containing Biomedical or Public Health Proposals, Two-Year Congressional Terms, 1975—2002. (*Note:* Some bills are included in multiple packages.)

Dividing the biomedical package into the biomedical research sub-package and medical care (the biomedical access and biomedical quality sub-packages) offers a more nuanced view of the trends. Fig. 4 indicates that there were very few biomedical research bills until the 1987–1988 Congress when the number of these bills began to increase. After that time, biomedical research bills accounted for a large portion of the gap between biomedical and public health bills. These trends provoke three main questions. First, the biomedical package is dominant in most years. What accounts for this dominance? Second, although the biomedical package was dominant in most years, this was not uniformly the case. Notably, in the early 1980s, public health proposals were almost as numerous as their biomedical counterparts. What accounts for this period of relative parity? Third, when the minority health issue achieved national prominence in the late 1980s and early 1990s (Period 3 of our analysis), Congress responded with more biomedical proposals than public health ones, and an important component

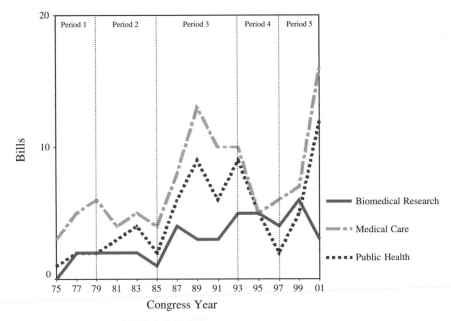

Fig. 4. Minority Health Bills Containing Biomedical Research, Medical Care, and Public Health Proposals, Two-Year Congressional Terms, 1975—2002. (*Note:* Some bills are included in multiple packages.)

of this increase was an increase in biomedical *research* proposals. Given the skepticism of many in the scientific community about the existence of innate, biological differences among racial or ethnic groups (Foster & Sharp, 2002), what explains the marked ascendancy of biomedical research initiatives for addressing racial/ethnic health disparities during this period?

THE "NEW PERSPECTIVE ON HEALTH" AND PUBLIC HEALTH PARITY

Within the last three decades of minority health policy, the early 1980s appear to be anomalous in that public health proposals in Congress nearly equaled those with a biomedical orientation. To understand this period in minority health history, we must return to the decade immediately preceding it. Beginning in the 1970s, numerous scholars argued that medical care was only a small determinant of population health in comparison with factors such as sanitation, nutrition, healthy behaviors, environmental and work-place conditions, and income inequality (Fuchs, 1975; Marmot, Shipley, & Rose, 1984; McKeown, 1976). The "new perspective on health", as it was then called, became influential in academia, medicine, public health, state bureaucracies, and Congress. It was enshrined in government reports in Canada, Britain, and the U.S. (e.g. the Healthy People Report) (Great Britain Department of Health and Social Security, 1980; LaLonde, 1974; U.S. Department of Health Education and Welfare, 1979).

The new perspective attracted the attention of progressives, who empha-sized the need for greater structural changes and saw in it opportunities to ameliorate social conditions that lead to bad health for the poor and mi-norities. At the same time, the new perspective attracted the attention of neo-conservatives, who emphasized personal responsibility for minority health outcomes and saw in it opportunities to cut health spending (Marmor, Barer, & Evans, 1994).

This conflict played itself out in the aftermath of the 1985 Malone report. The report had concluded that many health disparities were preventable and stressed efforts to educate minority groups on ways to reduce health risks. According to HHS Secretary Margaret Heckler, "much of the health gap suffered by minority Americans – perhaps even most of it – is related to knowledge and lifestyle. Smoking, alcohol, diet, and obesity are clearly linked to the higher cancer, cirrhosis, cardiovascular, infant mortality, and other disease rates affecting our minorities." A critic from the Children's Defense Fund complained that "the report is misleading in its emphasis on self-help because it suggests that self-help is going to significantly narrow the gap between blacks and whites." Others complained it was hypocritical for the Reagan Administration to release its report while attempting to cut spending on Medicaid, community health centers, family planning and public health programs (*Washington Post*, October 17, 1985, p. A1; *New York Times*, October 17, 1985, p. A16).

The conflict between progressive and conservative versions of the "new perspective" was also evident within minority communities themselves. Many liberals and African Americans criticized HHS Secretary Sullivan for his emphasis on personal responsibility for health. In March 1990, Sullivan told a mostly black audience that African Americans "cannot hope to solve the problems confronting our young black men until we put a halt to the finger-pointing and the scape-goating and understand that it is primarily up to us – individually, our families, our communities, our institutions, our traditional ethical standards, and cultural strengths – to save our young men. We must build our vision for a better future on the solid rock of personal and community responsibility" (*Boston Globe*, May 20, 1990, p. 22). Although the National Association for the Advancement of Colored People (NAACP) and the National Medical Association (NMA) credited Sullivan for raising the nation's consciousness about minority health disparities, they criticized his opposition to national health insurance and other progressive reforms (*Washington Post*, August 18, 1990, p. A4). Thus, the rise in public health approaches during the 1980s was likely the result of the development of "the new perspective on health" and its embrace by both progressives and conservatives during a period of conservative government.

SOCIAL MOVEMENTS AND BIOMEDICAL RESEARCH

While the events above help explain why public health proposals reached parity with biomedical proposals in the early 1980s, they cannot account for the expansion of biomedical research proposals in the late 1980s and early 1990s. This was a period of fairly stagnant NIH funding (though funding would eventually double between 1998 and 2003), so it is unlikely that the increase was the result of new levels of enthusiasm for biomedical research. Instead, we need to look at the experience of two contemporaneous social movements—the HIV/AIDS movement and the women's health movement. These movements increased both the visibility of biomedical research and demands for its accountability during the late 1980s (Epstein, 1996, 2004; Weisman, 1998). HIV/AIDS activists pushed for the inclusion of more women and minorities in clinical trials because such trials offered access to otherwise unobtainable experimental treatments. And women's health activists questioned whether the findings of clinical trials with only male participants could be extrapolated to women (Epstein, 2004). Both movements ended up producing minority health proposals. The women's health movement pushed several bills that sought the inclusion of women and minorities in NIH and FDA clinical trials. And other bills sought the inclusion of minorities in AIDS research. The minority health movement largely embraced and echoed these demands. Some within it, however, argued that requirements for the inclusion of minorities in clinical research actually fostered racism because they were predicated on the notion that race is a biological rather than a social category and that there are significant biological differences among races (Epstein, 2004).

Though the new perspective on health and contemporaneous social movements can help us to understand the period of parity between bio-medical and public health bills and the rise in biomedical research pro-posals at the end of the 1980s, they cannot explain why biomedical proposals have been dominant for most of the period under consideration and remain so into the 21st century. For this, the concept of policy legacies is required.

POLICY LEGACIES AND BIOMEDICAL DOMINANCE

Policy legacy arguments suggest that new proposals will build on previous policies – using them as positive or negative examples. They also suggest that existing policies may affect political actors' resources, incentives, cog-nitions, and access to information, as well as their normative beliefs about the legitimacy of certain practices, forms of organization, and organizations themselves (see Amenta, 1998; Bonastia, 2000; Esping-Andersen, 1990; Halfmann, 2003; Hall, 1986, 1989; Heclo, 1974; Pierson, 1992, 1994; Skocpol, 1992; Steinmo, Thelen, & Longstreth, 1992; Weir, 1992).

This theoretical orientation suggests that legacies of existing general health and minority health policies would have profound effects on the content of subsequent minority health proposals. Our data support this claim and suggest multiple mechanisms whereby policy legacies shaped the content of minority health proposals. We show that policy legacies have operated in four distinct ways. They have: (1) structured the minority health interest group sector (2) provided opportunities for the attachment of mi-nority health proposals to broader bills (3) provided opportunities for the incremental expansion of minority health policies, and (4) shaped the cog-nitions of policy-makers and interest groups.

Structuring the Minority Health Interest Group Sector

The United States spends more on health than any other country (14.6 percent of GDP in 2002) and approximately 45 percent of this is government spending. Spending on public health and prevention is minimal. Estimates range from 1 to 5 percent of all health spending (Brown, Corea, Luce, Elixhauser, & Sheingold, 1992; OECD, 2004; U.S. Public Health Service, 1993). In other words, the United States has a policy legacy of massive government investment in medical care and minimal investment in public health and prevention. This policy legacy has provided resources for the formation of medical interest groups and incentives for their participation in policy-making. As a result, the most numerous and most influential interest groups in minority health policy-making are offshoots of the medical care system (for a similar argument about general health policy, see Lavis & Sullivan, 2000). Of 36 national groups active on minority health, 44 percent are organizations of medical professionals. Another 8 percent are not made up of health care professionals but are solely devoted to medical care issues (*Gale Group Associations Unlimited*).

The group that has been the most successful in influencing Congress is AMHPS. A founder and former President of the organization, Louis Sullivan, served as the Secretary of HHS during the first Bush Administration, and a former AMHPS board member, David Satcher, served as the Surgeon General and the Assistant Secretary for Health during the Clinton Administration. Employing a full-time Washington lobbyist and working closely with Congressman Louis Stokes (D-OH), AMHPS has secured the enactment of more minority health legislation than any other single actor. The two most important enactments, the Disadvantaged Minority Health Act of 1990 and the creation of the NIH Center on Minority Health and Health Disparities, were both proposed by AMHPS and resulted in considerable resource flows to its institutional members. After AMHPS, the most influential group in minority health is the NMA, an organization of African American doctors. NMA officials are well represented in the Congressional Black Caucus (CBC) Health Brain Trust and, according to one congressional staff member, any major new piece of legislation on minority health must first be discussed with the NMA.

Several scholars have argued that the medical industry supports increased expenditure on medical care and opposes prevention and public health initiatives that might cut into that expenditure (Lavis & Sullivan, 2000; Marmor et al., 1994; McGinnis, Williams-Russo, & Knickman, 2002). In the case of minority health policy, the main effect of medical interest groups has not been to oppose legislation, but to propose it. When we asked members of Congress and their staffs why they had introduced particular proposals, they often answered that an interest group (usually a medical one) had come to them with the idea. Richard Hall (2000) argues that because of extreme demands on their time and attention, congresspersons rely heavily on interest groups for policy ideas and proposals. Interest groups bear most of the costs of bill introduction – providing an informational and labor subsidy to members of Congress. Often an interest group develops the proposal, drafts the bill, helps write the congressperson's speeches and press releases, and develops strategies for passing the bill. Our interviews uncovered a great deal of this type of behavior.

Providing Opportunities for Attaching Minority Health Proposals to Broader Bills

Approximately 57 percent of minority health proposals were attached to bills with a broader purpose than minority health. Our research indicates that proposal attachment occurred in three different ways. First, a legislator (or interest group) decided to add a provision targeting minorities to her own broader bill – either because the legislator had an interest in minority health, or because doing so provided an additional selling point or coalitional opportunity for the bill. Second, a legislator (or interest group) became aware of a broader bill and lobbied to have it target minorities. Third, a legislator (or interest group) sought to have her pre-existing minority health proposal attached to a broader bill.

An example of the first type of attachment is provided by the demands of the women's health movement for the inclusion of women in NIH and FDA clinical trials. The movement also demanded that minorities be included in such trials, apparently without being specifically requested to do so by minority health advocates. Thus, the women's health activism accounted for part of the increase in biomedical research proposals among minority health bills from 1989 to 1994 (103rd Congress, S. 1).

An example of the second type of attachment is provided by the Ryan White Care Act. In 1990, the Act provided primary care and supportive services to people with HIV/AIDS (P.L. 101–381). After the Act was implemented, minority interest groups complained that not enough Ryan White money was going to minorities. As a result, the 1996 reauthorization of the Act required that the health services planning councils that provide advice on Ryan White grant distribution be reflective of the demographics of the epidemic in their geographic area (104th Congress, S. 641). In another example, when the NIH budget doubled from 1998 to 2003, legislators concerned about minority health sought to ensure that a portion of the new money went to research on minority health. When we asked one legislative aide why his congressman had advocated for the expansion of the minority health office in NIH rather than in some other part of HHS, he replied, "Because that's where the money is."

An example of the third type of attachment is provided by Senator Matsunaga's (D-HI) bill to make the Assistant Secretary of the Veterans'

Administration (VA) responsible for monitoring and promoting minority access to VA services and benefits (101st Congress, S. 564). This bill was referred to the committee and later became part of a much broader veterans' health care bill that passed the Senate (S. 13).

These examples suggest that the pool of broader bills available for attachment helps determine what types of minority health proposals are put forward. This pool is heavily dependent upon existing policies since much of policy-making involves building on existing bills or reauthorizing them. In fact, in his study of the reauthorization process, Hall (2002) found that the vast majority of bills introduced in Congress are related to pending reauthorizations. Since there are more biomedical policies in need of reauthorization than there are public health ones, the pool of bills available for attachment has a strong biomedical skew.

Providing Opportunities for Incremental Expansion of Minority Health Policies

Not only were minority health proposals attached to bills that addressed broader health issues, but minority health proposals also built on existing minority health policies. Since most of these policies had a biomedical focus, new proposals did too. For example, in 1987, four historically black health professions schools received federal funding for the establishment of Centers of Excellence for the training of medical care providers (100th Congress, S. 769). A few years later, Hispanic and Native American groups successfully sought such funding as well (100th Congress, H.R. 5702). To cite another example, in 1992, Congress established the Office of Research on Minority Health in NIH (103rd Congress, S. 1). In 2000, minority health advocates successfully upgraded this office to the National Center on Minority Health and Health Disparities (106th Congress, S. 1880).

Shaping the Cognitions of Policy-Makers and Interest Groups

Policy legacies are also located in the minds of policy-makers and interest groups. As "bounded rationality" theorists note, policy-makers act under conditions of uncertainty and ambiguity and have limited time, resources, and information. As a result, they rarely canvass all possible options, but instead rely on short lists, heuristics, and rules-of-thumb. One insight of bounded rationality theory is that policy-makers often rely on old solutions to solve new problems (Cohen, March, & Olsen, 1972; Kingdon, 1984;

Lavis, 2002; Zahariadis, 1999). In this case, the old solution is medical care. Despite widespread acceptance within academia of the proposition that medical care is only a minor determinant of disparities in health status, members of Congress and their staffs and representatives of minority health interest groups rarely mention non-medical interventions as a method of reducing disparities.

When we asked congressional informants how they prioritized or chose among different means of addressing minority health – biomedical, public health, or non-health social welfare policies – the question typically drew stammers or blank stares. We think this occurred for two reasons. First, although our informants in federal bureaucracies and academia had clearly spent a great deal of time thinking about this question, congressional informants seemed to think more at the level of individual proposals than at the level of these broader, somewhat abstract, categories. Second, as a rule, members of Congress and their staffs do not *explicitly* budget their time and attention between issues. Instead, they react to each individual issue on its own merits as it comes along. Our interviews uncovered few attempts by legislators to develop strategic plans or priority lists for addressing minority health. Some of this did take place within the Congressional Black Caucus, but it is not clear that this led to much legislation. The absence of abstract discussion of policy options and the reactive allocation of time and attention to proposals suggest that policy-makers do not so much brainstorm a set of new solutions for a particular policy problem as evaluate proposed solutions (often with the help of interest groups) to determine if those proposals serve their policy and political goals. This practice serves to reinforce the use of old tools since these are the proposals that policy-makers are exposed to through incremental policy-making and the reauthorization of existing policies.

Furthermore, interest groups are adept at framing their preferred policy outcomes as solutions to the problems that legislators wish to solve. One interest group representative pointed out that AMHPS was particularly skilled at this:

> Is the establishment of a national center the appropriate response to health disparities, or is the establishment of a national center the appropriate response to an IOM study that comes out and says that the Cancer Institute is not spending enough money on minority cancer research? It was AMHPS's solution to that problem. The establishment of a national center was their solution to any number of things that came up that they could use to demonstrate the need for the [Center]...You asked a lot about pipeline [minority recruitment to the health professions] and why have these solutions been put in place in response to these problems and the answer is because those are the solutions that AMHPS has been pushing.

The informant made a similar comment about AMHPS's role in the Disadvantaged Minority Health Improvement Act of 1990:

> They've been talking about health status; they've been talking about disparities; they've been talking about improving access and all those kinds of things that you hear about at the Black Caucus. The trick that they've been able to perform is to say, okay, you've got these things out there, you've got these issues, you've got these challenges, here's a solution that's in the national interest.

CONCLUSION

In this study, we examined proposals for improving the health of racial and ethnic minorities that reached the congressional agenda from 1975 to 2002. We found that biomedical proposals dominated in most years and that a large part of the biomedical dominance after 1988 involved an increase in biomedical research proposals, spurred in part by the HIV/AIDS and women's health movements. There was a brief period of parity between biomedical and public health proposals during the early 1980s, which was related to the emergence of the "new perspective on health" and its embrace by both progressives and conservative budget cutters during the Reagan Administration.

We also argued that policy legacies have been and continue to be a key determinant of biomedical dominance in minority health policy-making. Policy legacies affected the interests, opportunities, and ideas of policy-makers and interest groups. They structured the minority health interest group sector, provided opportunities for attaching minority health proposals to broader bills, provided opportunities for the incremental expansion of minority health policies, and shaped the cognitions of policy-makers and interest groups. All of these mechanisms served to fuel the momentum of the biomedical package during the late 1980s and early 1990s. These mechanisms should prove useful in the study of other policy domains as well.

The policy legacy mechanisms discussed here present pitfalls for minority health policy-making. Because of them, rational actors may not always produce rational outcomes for those whom their policies are meant to assist. Racial and ethnic health disparities persist and most observers agree that biomedical solutions alone will not eliminate them. Our study suggests that, in order for health disparities to be reduced or eliminated, policy legacies that inhibit innovation and reinforce biomedical dominance will need to be overcome.

Future research should compare the congressional arena with others, such as federal and state bureaucracies, state legislatures, the courts, philanthropy, academia, and the media, in order to determine if biomedical dominance is equally pronounced in those arenas and if policy legacies play a similar role. Future research should also add a cross-national component – examining discourse and policy-making on health disparities in other nations in order to determine the degree of biomedical dominance in minority health policy-making in other contexts and the forces that produce it.

NOTES

1. For the purpose of this paper, we use the language of Congress without interrogation. Thus, we use terms such as "minority", "race", "ethnicity", and "Hispanic" without examining their problematic social construction. (For such an examination, see Cornell & Hartman, 1998; Omi & Winant, 1994; Ramaga, 1992; Wilkinson, 2000.)

ACKNOWLEDGMENTS

We thank Rashi Fein, Rick Hall, Jim House, Paula Lantz, Catherine Lee, Andrew Levine, Mark Mizruchi, David Mechanic, and Mark Peterson for their useful comments. We thank Deepali Pallegar, Brian Swierczek, Gail Pieknik, Theresa Ramirez, Paula Song, Bridget Metzler, Tracy Finlayson, and Alyssa Pozniak for research assistance. We acknowledge funding from the Robert Wood Johnson Foundation, the Horowitz Foundation for Social Policy, the UC-Davis Institute for Governmental Affairs, and the UC-Davis Committee on Research.

REFERENCES

Amenta, E. (1998). *Bold relief: Institutional politics and the origins of modern American social policy*. Princeton: Princeton University Press.
Bonastia, C. (2000). Why did affirmative action in housing fail during the Nixon era? Exploring the institutional homes of social policies. *Social Problems, 47*(4), 523–542.
Brown, R., Corea, J., Luce, B., Elixhauser, A., & Sheingold, S. (1992). Effectiveness in disease and injury prevention: Estimated national spending on prevention, 1988. *Morbidity and Mortality Weekly Report, 24*(July), 529–531.
Burstein, P., Bricher, R. M., & Einwohner, R. L. (1995). Policy alternatives and political change: Work, family, and gender on the congressional agenda, 1945–1990. *American Sociological Review, 60*(1), 67–83.

Cohen, M., March, J., & Olsen, J. (1972). A garbage can model of organizational choice. *Administrative Science Quarterly, 17*(March), 1–25.

Congressional Research Service. (1975). *Digest of public general bills and resolutions.* Washington, DC: Library of Congress.

Cornell, S., & Hartman, D. (1998). *Ethnicity and race: Making identities in a changing world.* Thousand Oaks, CA: Pine Forge Press.

COSMOS Corporation. (2000). *Assessment of State minority health infrastructure and capacity to address issues of health disparity.* Washington, DC: Office of Minority Health, Office of Public Health and Science, U.S. Department of Health and Human Services.

Epstein, S. (1996). *Impure science: AIDS, activism, and the politics of knowledge.* Berkeley: University of California Press.

Epstein, S. (2004). Bodily differences and collective identities: The politics of gender and race in biomedical research in the United States. *Body and Society, 10*(2), 183–203.

Esping-Andersen, G. (1990). *Three worlds of welfare capitalism.* Princeton, NJ: Princeton University Press.

Foster, M. W., & Sharp, R. R. (2002). Race, ethnicity, and genomics: Social classifications as proxies of biological heterogeneity. *Genome Research, 12*(6), 844–850.

Fuchs, V. R. (1975). *Who shall live? Health, economics, and social choice.* New York: Basic Books.

Gamson, W. A., & Modigliani, A. (1987). The changing culture of affirmative action. *Research in Political Sociology, 3*, 137–177.

Gamson, W. A., & Modigliani, A. (1989). Media discourse and public opinion on nuclear power: A constructionist approach. *American Journal of Sociology, 95*(1), 1–37.

Great Britain Department of Health and Social Security. (1980). *Inequalities in health: Report of a working group chaired by Sir Douglas Black.* London: Department of Health and Social Security.

Halfmann, D. (2003). Historical priorities and the responses of doctors' associations to abortion reform proposals in Britain and the United States, 1960–1973. *Social Problems, 50*, 567–591.

Hall, P. (1989). *The political power of economic ideas: Keynesianism across countries.* Princeton: Princeton University Press.

Hall, P. A. (1986). *Governing the economy: The politics of State intervention in Britain and France.* Oxford: Oxford University Press.

Hall, R. L. (2000). Lobbying as legislative subsidy. Paper presented at the Annual meeting of the American Political Science Association, Washington, DC.

Hall, T. (2002). *When things really happen: The role of reauthorizations in the process of policy change.* Ph.D. thesis, University of Georgia, Athens.

Heclo, H. (1974). *Modern social politics in Britain and Sweden.* New Haven, CN: Yale University Press.

Kingdon, J. (1984). *Agendas, alternatives and public policies.* Boston: Little, Brown.

LaLonde, M. (1974). *A new perspective on the health of Canadians.* Ottawa: Minister of Supply and Services.

Lavis, J., & Sullivan, T. (2000). The State as a setting. In: B. Poland, L. Green & I. Rootman (Eds), *Settings for health promotion: Linking theory and practice.* Newbury Park, CA: Sage.

Lavis, J. N. (2002). Ideas at the margin or marginalized ideas? Nonmedical determinants of health in Canada. *Health Affairs, 21*(2), 107.

Marmor, T. R., Barer, M. L., & Evans, R. G. (1994). The determinants of a populations health: What can be done to improve a democratic Nation's health status. In: R. G. Evans, M. L. Barer & T. R. Marmor (Eds), *Why are some people healthy and others not?: The determinants of health of populations* (pp. 217–230). New York: A. de Gruyter.

Marmot, M. G., Shipley, M. J., & Rose, G. (1984). Inequalities in death – specific explanations of a general pattern? *Lancet, 1*, 1003–1006.

McGinnis, J. M., Williams-Russo, P., & Knickman, J. R. (2002). The case for more active policy attention to health promotion. *Health Affairs, 21*(2), 78.

McKeown, T. (1976). *The modern rise of population.* New York: Academic Press.

OECD. (2004). *OECD Health data.* Paris: OECD.

Office of Minority Health Resource Center. (2002). *State minority health liaisons: Office of Minority Health Research Center.* U.S. Department of Health and Human Services.

Office of Research on Minority Health. (2002). *ORMH history.* U.S. Department of Health and Human Services, National Institutes of Health, Office of Research on Minority Health Website.

Omi, M., & Winant, H. (1994). *Racial formation in the United States: From the 1960s to the 1990s.* New York: Routledge.

Pierson, P. (1992). 'Policy feedbacks' and political change: Contrasting Reagan's and Thatcher's pension – reform initiatives. *Studies in American Political Development, 6*, 359–390.

Pierson, P. (1994). *Dismantling the welfare State? Reagan, Thatcher and the politics of retrenchment.* New York: Cambridge University Press.

Ramaga, P. V. (1992). Relativity of the minority concept. *Human Rights Quarterly, 14*(1), 104–119.

Skocpol, T. (1992). *Protecting soldiers and mothers.* Cambridge, MA: Harvard University Press.

Steinmo, S., Thelen, K., & Longstreth, F. (1992). *Structuring politics: Historical institutionalism in comparative analysis.* Cambridge: Cambridge University Press.

U.S. Department of Health and Human Services. (1985). *Report of the Secretary's task force on Black and minority health.* Washington, DC: U.S. Government Printing Office.

U.S. Department of Health and Human Services. (1991). *Healthy people 2000: National health promotion and disease prevention objectives, full report with commentary.* Washington, DC: U.S. Government Printing Office.

U.S. Department of Health Education and Welfare. (1979). *Healthy people: The Surgeon General's report on health promotion and disease prevention.* Washington: U.S. Government Printing Office.

U.S. Institute of Medicine. (1999). *The unequal burden of cancer: An assessment of NIH research and programs for ethnic minorities and the medically underserved.* Washington, DC: National Academies Press.

U.S. Institute of Medicine. (2003). *Unequal treatment: Confronting racial and ethnic disparities in health care.* Washington, DC: National Academies Press.

U.S. Public Health Service. (1993). Health care reform: A paper on population-based core functions. *Journal of Public Health Policy, 19*(4), 394–419.

Weir, M. (1992). *Politics and jobs: The boundaries of employment policy in the United States.* Princeton, NJ: Princeton University Press.

Weisman, C. S. (1998). *Women's health care: Activist traditions and institutional change.* Baltimore: Johns Hopkins University Press.

Wilkinson, D. (2000). Rethinking the concept of "minority": A task for social scientists and practitioners. *Journal of Sociology and Social Welfare, 27*(1), 115–132.

Zahariadis, N. (1999). Ambiguity, time and multiple streams. In: P. A. Sabatier (Ed.), *Theories of the policy process*. Boulder, CO: Westview Press.

METHODOLOGICAL APPENDIX

We attempted to identify all relevant congressional bills from 1975 to 2002 that addressed the health of racial and ethnic minorities (contact authors for search criteria). We uncovered 400 bills. We then excluded bills that dealt solely with Native Americans since this group is small and more importantly has a unique political situation related to tribal governments, treaties, and the Indian Health Service. We also excluded appropriations and budget reconciliation bills, and bills that, although indexed as relating to minorities and health, did not actually address minority health. We included bills if they referred to minorities, particular racial or ethnic groups, diversity, un-der-represented groups, or border areas. We did not include bills that re-ferred to the medically underserved, since these included low-income whites and residents of rural areas. After excluding these various bills, we were left with 219. We double-checked our dataset against the "minorities" index of the *Digest of Public General Bills and Resolutions* – up until 1990 when the *Digest* ends (Congressional Research Service, 1975). This index did not in-clude any bills that our dataset did not and missed many bills that our dataset did include. It was quite common for multiple bills in the same Congress to contain identical or highly similar proposals for addressing minority health. Legislators often introduce the same bill in both houses so that it may proceed concurrently in each and initial bills are often folded into later ones. We excluded 72 duplicate bills in order to avoid over-counting the proposals that they contained. This left us with 147 bills. Many bills contained more than one proposal, and many proposals could be cat-egorized with multiple codes. As a result, some bills received as many as nine topic codes – though 70 percent received three codes or fewer. In most instances, bill summaries were sufficient for our coding purposes but, when necessary, we consulted the full text of the bill.

LITERACY: INFLUENCE ON ACCESS AND USE OF THE HEALTH CARE SYSTEM

Karen Seccombe, Richard S. Lockwood and Stephen Reder

ABSTRACT

The striking number of persons with low levels of literacy in the United States is a major public-health concern. This study examines the relationship between literacy levels and both (1) access to health care and (2) use of specific health care services among adults. The data are collected from in-person interviews with a representative sample of adults aged 18–44 in Portland, Oregon, who are proficient English speakers, and have not completed high school nor have a GED. Adults with lower levels of literacy are less likely to have a usual provider, to have health insurance, and they have trouble understanding written medical directions, more difficulty getting needed care, and poorer health. They also use physician services, overnight hospital stays, and emergency rooms more frequently, controlling for education, access, health, and sociodemographic characteristics. Literacy is conceptually distinct from education and independently affects the way in which adults seek health care.

Health Care Services, Racial and Ethnic Minorities and Underserved Populations: Patient and Provider Perspectives
Research in the Sociology of Health Care, Volume 23, 277–295
ISSN: 0275-4959/doi:10.1016/S0275-4959(05)23013-2

The high number of Americans with limited literacy is a serious social problem and public policy concern. The ability to read and write is fundamental to navigate innumerable tasks of daily living. Beyond mere inconvenience, low literacy has harmful consequences for health and well-being. Persons with low literacy have significantly poorer health than do those with higher levels of literacy, independent of the effects of education, income, and other relevant socioeconomic conditions.

While research has established the link between literacy and health, significantly less is known about the manner in which access to health care may be limited among persons with low reading skills, and the ways in utilization patterns may differ. Our fundamental goal is to expand our understanding of the role that literacy plays in obtaining the health care that is necessary to promote good health, safety, and well-being.

INTRODUCTION

The Department of Education (DOE) reveals that approximately 40 million adult Americans have limited or extremely limited reading and quantitative skills. Another 50 million Americans have marginal skills, with difficulty using basic reading, writing, and computational skills for everyday activities (Kirsch, Jungeblut, Jenkins, & Kolstad, 1993; National Center for Educational Statistics, 1999; Reder, 1998). For example, adults scoring in the lowest category of the 5-level typology created by the DOE (Level 1) can usually sign their name and identify brief pieces of information in a clearly written newspaper article. However, they cannot locate an intersection on a street map, write a letter explaining an error on a bill, identify and enter background information on a social security card application, calculate total costs of purchase from an order form, or use a calculator to determine a 10 percent discount. They have only rudimentary reading and writing skills. About 4 percent of the adult population, or about 8 million people, cannot perform even the simplest literacy tasks.

Literacy allows a person to locate information, understand instructions, solve problems, interpret data, and integrate multiple pieces of information. Lower literacy generally means limited employment opportunities, greater risk of poverty, and an overall lower quality of life. For example, nearly half of the adults scoring in the DOE's Level 1 category lived in poverty, compared with only 4–8 percent of those adults scoring in Levels 4 and 5. Three in four recipients of the welfare program Temporary Assistance to Needy Families (TANF) performed in the two lowest literacy levels, as did seven in ten men and women in our nation's jails and prisons (National Center for Educational Statistics, 1999; Educational Testing Service, 1995; U.S. Department of Education, 1994).

LITERACY AND HEALTH

One serious, but poorly understood implication of widespread low literacy is its effect upon health. Meanwhile, the relationship between *education* and health has been firmly established, elaborated upon in such reports as *Healthy People 2010* by the U.S. Department of Health and Human Services. Persons with lower levels of education have poorer levels of self-reported health and functioning, and higher rates of infectious disease, chronic diseases, and have shorter life expectancy (see Ross & Wu, 1995 for a review of the literature). Explanations for the relationship include such factors as (1) *the nature of work and economic conditions*, including employment and work conditions, income, or fulfillment from work; (2) *social–psychological resources*, such as a sense of control and social support resources; and (3) *the degree of health lifestyle*, including smoking, exercise, drinking, or obtaining regular check-ups (Ross & Wu, 1995). Ross and Wu test these relationships using data from two nationally representative samples; the first sample was collected in 1990 and contains 2,031 respondents aged 18–90, and the second sample contains 3,025 respondents aged 20–64 who were interviewed in 1979 and then again in 1980 (2,436 respondents). Ross and Wu found that high educational attainment improves health directing, and it improves health indirectly through work and economic condition, social–psychological resources, and health lifestyle.

Noticeably absent from the sociological literature is an interest in the role that *literacy* plays in understanding the relationship between education and health. Nonetheless, a growing number of researchers and practitioners in other disciplines are beginning to tease out literacy from education, and suggest that education level by itself is an imprecise proxy for literacy (Rudd & Moeykens, 1999; Rudd & Colton, 1998; Weiss & Coyne, 1997).

It appears that people with low levels of literacy also have significantly poorer health than those with stronger reading and writing skills (Baker, Parker, Williams, Clark, & Nurss, 1997; Davis et al., 1996; National Work Group on Literacy and Health, 1998; Rudd & Moeykens, 1999; TenHave et al., 1997; Weiss, Hart, McGee, & D'Estelle, 1992), persisting after controlling for confounding sociodemographic characteristics, including education. TenHave et al. (1997) examined the relationship between literacy levels and a reported history of heart attack and hospitalization for a heart condition and diabetes, and found that individuals with low levels of literacy were significantly more likely to report having all of these conditions after controlling for educational attainment. Weiss et al. (1992) analyzed the physical and psychosocial health of a random sample of subjects enrolled in a publicly funded literacy-training program in Arizona. They found that subjects with extremely low reading levels had significantly poorer physical and psychosocial health than did subjects with higher levels.

Why do people with limited reading and computational skills have poorer health beyond the effects of education? It is generally believed that literacy influences the ability to understand and use key medical information, whether it involves navigating the health care system, comprehending illness-related information, following instructions, taking medicines as prescribed, learning about illness prevention and health promotion, or filling out insurance forms (Baker et al., 1996; Roter, Rudd, & Comings, 1998; Williams et al., 1995). Beaver and Luker (1997) examined the readability of 50 information booklets available to women with breast cancer and found that they are not suitable for the majority of women because they presume too high a reading level. Davis, Crouch, Wills, Miller, and Abdehou (1990) reviewed the match between the reading skills of 151 ambulatory care patients and the educational materials in five different ambulatory care settings. The average reading comprehension of the patients was 6th grade, while the education materials required between an 11th and a 14th grade reading level.

Likewise, because consent procedures generally contain complex legal and medical jargon, low literacy may preclude an individual from participating in certain procedures or medical research (Agre, McKee, Gargon, & Kurtz, 1997; Baker & Taub, 1983; Davis, Holcome, Berkel, Pramanik, & Divers, 1998). Reviews of consent forms indicate that their reading level ratings ranged from 8th grade to college graduate levels, beyond the comprehension of most adults.

Literacy may also affect the ability to understand information and follow directions. Davis et al. (1996) examined the relationship between literacy and the knowledge of and attitudes toward screening mammography among a sample of 445 low-income women aged 40 and over. Women with lower literacy skills were significantly less knowledgeable about screening mammography, which may contribute to the underutilization of this diagnostic test. Bennett et al. (1998) examined the relationship between literacy and stage of presentation among 212 low-income men with prostate cancer. They report that men with literacy levels below the 6th grade were more likely to present with advanced-stage prostate cancer. While race was also a significant predictor of stage of presentation, the effects of race disappeared when controlling for literacy, geographic region, and age. Emergency department discharge instructions have also been assessed for their readability levels. Instruction materials range from a 6th grade reading level to a level above grade 13, which could affect their ability to follow instructions correctly (Jolly, Scotte, & Sanford, 1995; Powers, 1988).

These studies suggest that literacy levels may affect the way that a person uses the health care system. Persons with low reading skills may postpone or forgo needed care because they have failed to access crucial information. Yet, surprisingly, few studies have tested this relationship systematically and within a variety of health care contexts. In fact, a study by Weiss et al. (1994) based on a sample of 401 randomly selected Medicaid patients, found that annual health care costs did *not* differ significantly by literacy skills – the mean health care costs were $4,574 per person. Thus, if people with lower reading skills navigate the system differently than those with stronger reading skills, it is not clear how this difference is manifested, under what conditions it occurs, and what the consequences of this difference are.

A few studies provide some preliminary insights into the ways in which literacy may influence the use of health services. Baker, Parker, and Clark (1998) examined the relationship between literacy, health status, and hospital admissions. Using 1,000 English-speaking patients seeking non-urgent care at an urban public hospital, they found that persons with inadequate functional literacy (measured as "adequate," "marginal," and "inadequate") were more than twice as likely to have been hospitalized as those persons whose literacy skills were evaluated as adequate (51.7 percent vs. 21.3 percent, respectively), after controlling for age, gender, race, health status, income, and insurance. Another study by Baker et al. (1997), based on subjects from two urban public hospitals, examined the relationship between literacy, self-reported health, and number of hospital and physician visits, and whether the patient had a usual source of care. They found that literacy was not related to having a regular source of care or number of physician visits, but patients with inadequate literacy at one of the hospitals were more likely than other patients to report a hospitalization in the previous year.

Purpose of this Research

These findings are suggestive, but the samples consist entirely of people already known to use the health care system. Our goal is to examine the effect of literacy upon individual ability to access the health care system, and individual use of several specific health services. We hypothesize (1) that individuals with lower levels of literacy have less access and greater impediments using the health care system; (2) persons with lower literacy skills use particular health services differently; they are relatively less likely to have a usual source of health care; to use the emergency room more frequently; to more frequently use serious and costly services such as overnight hospitalization; and are more likely to forgo care altogether; and (3) we anticipate that these relationships will persist even after controlling for the effects of education level.

METHODS

Sample

Data are collected from in-person interviews with adults participating in the ongoing Longitudinal Study of Adult Learning (LSAL) funded by the U.S. Department of Education for the National Center for the Study of Adult Learning and Literacy (NCSALL). The target population is residents of the Portland, Oregon metropolitan area who at Wave 1 of the survey are aged 18–44, proficient (not necessarily native) speakers of English, do not have a high school diploma or equivalent, and are not currently in high school. Participants will be interviewed five times over a period of 7 years. The data used here are from Waves 1 and 2 of the survey.

The LSAL panel consists of a representative sample of 934 respondents. Respondents were sampled through two frames. The first frame consisted of the general target population; individuals were randomly selected, screened for eligibility, and recruited for the study through random-digit-dialing and computer-assisted telephone interviewing (CATI) methods. The second frame used to oversample participants in adult education programs consisted of members of the target population who recently enrolled in adult basic or adult secondary education courses at one of the three community colleges offering such classes in the metropolitan area. Potential respondents in both the student and the general frames were contacted, screened, and recruited for participation through the same CATI method, and are in all respects treated identically throughout the longitudinal study. Approximately, equal number of respondents was sampled in each frame and sampling weights were constructed for respondents in each frame.

Eight hundred forty-one respondents completed Waves 1 and 2. The analytic sub-sample used in this study includes 768 respondents with complete data on all five dependent variables. Sample weights were proportionally adjusted for this sub-sample. The weighted proportions of respondents from each sampling frame changed very little from the original sample.

Study participants were interviewed in their homes. The sessions last about 2 h, and consist of approximately 60-min interviews followed by paper-and-pencil assessment of functional literacy proficiency (i.e., Tests of Adult Literacy Skills (TALS)) and other cognitive assessments. The interview explores a wide variety of individuals' education and employment activities, histories, goals, and barriers, including issues surrounding health and health care. The health modules asked respondents about their health status; access and barriers to getting care; and use of health services.

Measures

The LSAL includes the following variables relevant to our analysis. Our dependent variable, use of health services, is measured by asking respondents how many times in the last year they have used five different types of health services: (1) doctor's office or outpatient clinic; (2) overnight hospital stay; (3) prescription medicines; (4) telephone contact with a nurse or doctor; and (5) emergency room visits. Responses were coded as continuous variables.

Literacy is measured using the TALS. This standardized scale is commonly used in literacy studies, included by the DOE for the 1992 National Adult Literacy Survey. It consists of 3 separate tests: prose, document, and quantitative literacy. The document portion of TALS was used because it effectively combines elements of all three tests. Documents consist of structured prose and quantitative information, in complex arrays of rows and columns, such as tables, data forms, lists, charts, and maps. Literacy with documents means that people can read and locate information, integrate information from various parts of a document, and write new information as requested in appropriate places in a document.

The scale ranges from 0 to 500. In multivariate analyses, literacy is coded as a continuous variable. For other analyses, we use the ordinal transformation employed by the DOE that bins the data into five levels, using cut points along the continuous scale. In this research, the upper two levels have been combined because of their small sample sizes. Level 1 ranges from 0 to 225; Level 2 from 226 to 275; Level 3 from 276 to 325; and Levels 4 and 5 range from 326 to 500.

Access to health care is measured by the following items: (1) Is there a specific person or place that you usually go to when you are sick and need

advice about your health? (1 = yes, 0 = no); (2) Do you currently have
health insurance? (1 = yes, 0 = no); (3) Over the past year, did you or anyone in your household delay seeking medical care because of worry about
the cost? (1 = yes, 0 = no); (4) When the doctors or staff give you written
material about your general health or about a health problem, would you
say that it is easy, somewhat difficult, or difficult to read and understand the
material? (easy = 1, somewhat difficult = 2, difficult = 3); (5) Over the past
year was there any time when you or someone in your household needed
medical or dental care but did not get it? (1 = yes, 0 = no).

Health status is measured by the following item: "Overall, how would you
rate your health – (1) excellent, (2) very good, (3) good, (4) fair, or (5) poor?"

Several demographic variables are used as controls because these may
affect the ability to access the health care system. Controlling for education
level completed (continuous, ranging from 1–12) allows us to isolate the
unique effects of literacy beyond education. Household Income ((1) less
than $5,000; (2) $5,000 but less than $20,000; (3) $20,0000 but less than
$30,000; (4) $30,000 but less than $40,000; (5) $40,000 and over), Age (continuous), and Gender (1 = male, 0 = female) are highly correlated with the
use of health care services. Living arrangement (1 = alone, 0 = living with
others), and owning or having access to a working motor vehicle (1 = yes,
0 = no) represent possible structural constraints to seeking care.

RESULTS

The characteristics of the sample are presented in Table 1. We see that 11.8
percent of respondents fall into the lowest literacy level (Level 1), and 31.4
percent score in Level 2. Adults in these two categories have difficulty in
using basic reading and computational skills for common everyday activities. Because of the small number of individuals falling into levels 4 and 5
(19.5 percent), these two levels have been combined in analyses. Almost 30
percent of the sample have completed only 9th grade or less (recall that the
sample consists of persons with less than a high school diploma or GED).

Many respondents appear to have some difficulty accessing health care.
Nearly one in five respondents (19.8 percent) do not have a usual source of
care. Nearly one-third did not have health insurance at the time of the
interview (31.6 percent). Likewise, nearly one-third reportedly have experienced a delay in getting needed care because of cost (30.5 percent). One in
five respondents report having at least some difficulty understanding written

Table 1. Sample Characteristics.

	%	N
TALS level		
Level 1; 0–225	11.8	91
Level 2; 226–275	31.4	241
Level 3; 276–325	37.3	286
Level 4 and 5; 326–500	19.5	150
Grade complete		
8th grade or less	12.6	96
9th grade	16.1	123
10th grade	27.1	208
11th grade	42.9	330
Unknown	1.4	11
Usual provider		
No	19.8	153
Yes	80.2	615
Missing	0	0
Insurance		
No	31.6	153
Yes	68.4	615
Missing	0	0
Delay		
No	69.5	534
Yes	30.5	234
Missing	0	0
Written		
Easy	79.7	612
Somewhat difficult	14.8	114
Difficult	5.5	42
Missing	0	0
Get care		
No	68.7	528
Yes	31.3	241
Missing	0	0
Health status		
Excellent	17.4	134
Very good	31.2	240
Good	26.4	203
Fair	14.4	110
Poor	2.3	18
Missing	8.3	64

Table 1. (*Continued*)

	%	N
Age		
18–20	27.1	208
21–29	32.7	251
30–39	29.0	222
40–44	11.2	86
Missing	0.3	3
Family income		
<$5,000	5.1	39
$5,000–19,999	30.4	234
$20,000–29,999	17.8	137
$30,000–39,999	15.7	120
>$39,999	27.3	210
Missing	3.6	28
Gender		
Female	51.5	396
Male	48.1	370
Missing	0.3	3
Living arrangement		
Alone	9.8	75
With others	90.2	693
Missing	0	0
Motor vehicle		
No	28.2	217
Yes	71.5	549
Missing	0.03	3

materials from providers (20.3 percent), and nearly one-third claim to have gone without medical or dental care when they needed it (31.3 percent).

The health of respondents tends to be poorer than national averages. Nearly one in five report that their health is only fair or poor (16.7 percent). Less than one in five report excellent health (17.4 percent).

The ages of our respondents range from 18 to 44, and most are under age 30 (59.8 percent). Over half have household incomes under $30,000 per year (53.3 percent). Males and females are nearly equally represented in the sample (48.1 percent and 51.5 percent, respectively; data is missing for three respondents). Only one in 10 respondents live alone (9.8 percent) and over one-quarter do not own or have access to a reliable motor vehicle (28.2 percent).

Table 2 reports the degree of access to health care across TALS level. These data reveal that, generally, adults with lower literacy are less likely to have a usual provider ($p = 0.001$), are less likely to have health insurance ($p = 0.004$), are more likely to have some degree of difficulty understanding written instructions from a doctor or other medical staff ($p < 0.001$), and they are more likely to have gone without needed care ($p = 0.002$). There is little difference across TALS score in whether respondents have delayed seeking care because of cost. Finally, Table 2 examines differences in the use of health status across TALS level. Consistent with previous research, the data reveal a positive relationship between health and literacy ($p < 0.001$).

Table 3 reports the mean (and median) use of five different health services, across TALS level. The data suggest that adults with lower levels of literacy use many health care services more frequently. For example, examining the data for doctor visits reveals that persons who score in the TALS level 1 averaged 14.2 visits during the previous year, whereas persons who score in levels 4 and 5 averaged 6.5 visits ($p < 0.001$). We see this pattern as well with overnight hospital stays (0.3 vs. 0) ($p = 0.006$), the use of prescription medicines (3.6 vs. 2.8) ($p = 0.021$), telephone contact with doctors or nurses (13.2 vs. 3.6) ($p < 0.001$), and emergency room visits (3.7 vs. 0.6) ($p < 0.001$). Multivariate regression isolates the independent effects of literacy on each of these specific health services.

Tables 4–8 report the standardized coefficients of literacy, education, access variables, health status, and demographic characteristics as they are regressed on each of the five utilization variables: The number of (1) physician visits; (2) overnight hospital stays; (3) prescription medicines; (4) telephone contacts; and (5) emergency room visits over the past year.

The data suggest that literacy is associated with three of the five health care services examined here, independent of education, access, health status, and demographic characteristics. First, with respect to physician visits, adults with lower levels of literacy have a greater number of visits when controlling for confounding effects of grade completed, access variables, health status, and demographics. Delaying care in the past due to cost, having a lower income, being a female, and owning a vehicle or having access to one are also associated with a greater use of physician services.

Literacy is also negatively associated with the number of overnight hospital stays in a multivariate context. Persons with lower levels of literacy report more overnight hospital stays than do persons with higher levels. Higher levels of education are also associated with hospital stays. With respect to access, having health insurance is the only access variable associated with a greater number of overnight hospital stays. The model also

Table 2. TALS Level by Access to Health Care (*n*, %).

	TALS 1	TALS 2	TALS 3	TALS 4/5
Usual provider				$\chi^2 = 15.59$
				df $= 3$
				$p = 0.001$
Yes	70 (76.9)	208 (86.3)	211 (73.8)	127 (84.7)
No	21 (23.1)	33 (13.7)	75 (26.2)	23 (15.3)
Total	91 (100)	241 (100)	286 (100)	150 (100)
Health insurance				$\chi^2 = 13.13$
				df $= 3$
				$p = 0.004$
Yes	46 (63.9)	129 (80.6)	131 (67.2)	77 (79.4)
No	26 (36.1)	31 (19.4)	64 (32.8)	20 (20.6)
Total	72 (100)	160 (100)	195 (100)	97 (100)
Delay from cost				$\chi^2 = 0.926$
				df $= 3$
				$p = 0.819$
Yes	27 (29.7)	78 (32.4)	82 (28.7)	47 (31.3)
No	64 (70.3)	163 (67.6)	204 (71.3)	103 (68.7)
Total	91 (100)	241 (100)	286 (100)	150 (100)
Understand written material				$\chi^2 = 56.6$
				df $= 6$
				$p < 0.001$
Easy	60 (65.9)	193 (79.8)	217 (75.6)	142 (95.3)
Somewhat difficult	17 (18.7)	46 (19)	47 (16.4)	4 (2.7)
Difficult	14 (15.4)	3 (1.2)	23 (8)	3 (2)
Total	91 (100)	242 (100)	287 (100)	149 (100)
Difficulty getting care				$\chi^2 = 15.01$
				df $= 3$
				$p = 0.002$
Yes	32 (35.6)	89 (36.8)	91 (31.8)	28 (18.8)
No	58 (64.4)	153 (63.2)	195 (68.2)	121 (81.2)
Total	90 (100)	242 (100)	286 (100)	149 (100)
Health status				$\chi^2 = 59.18$
				df $= 12$
				$p < 0.001$
Excellent	17 (21.3)	55 (25.6)	45 (17.2)	16 (10.8)
Very good	14 (17.5)	59 (27.4)	96 (36.8)	72 (48.9)
Good	21 (26.3)	66 (30.7)	86 (33)	29 (19.6)
Fair	22 (27.5)	30 (14)	33 (12.6)	25 (26.9)
Poor	6 (7.5)	5 (2.3)	1 (0.4)	6 (4.1)
Total	80 (100)	215 (100)	261 (100)	148 (100)

Table 3. Mean (median) Use of Health Services[a] by TALS Level.

	TALS 1	TALS 2	TALS 3	TALS 4/5	Total	
Doctor/Clinic visit	14.2 (3)	12.6 (4)	6.8 (4)	6.5 (2.8)	9.4 (4)	$F = 8.23$ df $= 3$ $p < 0.001$
Overnight hospital stay	0.3 (0)	0.5 (0)	0.2 (0)	0.0 (0)	0.3 (0)	$F = 4.14$ df $= 3$ $p = 0.006$
Prescription medicines	3.6 (2)	4.4 (3)	3.1 (1)	2.8 (1)	3.5 (2)	$F = 3.25$ df $= 3$ $p = 0.021$
Telephone contact	13.2 (3)	7.2 (3)	5.8 (2)	3.6 (1)	6.7 (2)	$F = 9.49$ df $= 3$ $p < 0.001$
Emergency room visits	3.7 (1)	1.8 (1)	1.4 (1)	0.6 (0)	1.6 (1)	$F = 12.59$ df $= 3$ $p < 0.001$

[a]Self-reported frequency of use.

Table 4. Standardized Coefficients of Effects of Literacy, Education, Access, Health Status, and Demographics on Physician Visits.

	Model 1	Model 2	Model 3	Model 4
TALS	−0.160*	−0.160*	−0.155*	−0.139*
Grade completed	−0.150*	−0.133*	−0.092*	−0.057
Access				
Provider		0.123*	0.096*	0.057
Insurance		0.080*	0.061	0.059
Delay		0.105*	0.120*	0.104*
Written		−0.009	−0.003	0.023
Get care		−0.042	−0.032	−0.052
Health status			0.098*	0.076
Demographics				
Age				0.058
Family income				−0.114*
Gender				−0.153*
Living arrangement				−0.059
Motor vehicle				0.090*
Adjusted R^2	0.051	0.078	0.074	0.110
N	764	764	703	703

*$p < 0.05$.

Table 5. Standardized Coefficients of Effects of Literacy, Education, Access, Health Status, and Demographics on Overnight Hospital Stays.

	Model 1	Model 2	Model 3	Model 4
TALS	−0.142*	−0.140*	−0.156*	−0.146*
Grade completed	0.094*	0.078*	0.070	0.091*
Access				
Provider		0.030	0.039	0.073
Insurance		0.080*	0.086*	0.108*
Delay		−0.029	−0.023	−0.019
Written		−0.030	−0.046	−0.046
Get care		−0.024	−0.023	−0.024
Health status			−0.050	−0.043
Demographics				
Age				−0.106*
Family income				−0.097*
Gender				0.015
Living arrangement				0.161*
Motor vehicle				0.004
Adjusted R^2	0.023	0.030	0.035	0.078
N	764	764	703	703

*$p < 0.05$.

Table 6. Standardized Coefficients of Effects of Literacy, Education, Access, Health Status, and Demographics on Prescription Medications.

	Model 1	Model 2	Model 3	Model 4
TALS	−0.033	−0.033	−0.040	−0.031
Grade completed	−0.151*	−0.108*	−0.095*	−0.050
Access				
Provider		0.117*	0.078*	0.069
Insurance		0.069	0.060	0.078*
Delay		0.192*	0.220*	0.207*
Written		0.014	0.020	0.030
Get care		−0.024	−0.031	−0.055
Health status			0.021	0.022
Demographics				
Age				−0.083*
Family income				−0.144*
Gender				−0.123*
Living arrangement				0.015
Motor vehicle				0.080*
Adjusted R^2	0.022	0.065	0.065	0.104
N	764	764	703	703

*$p < 0.05$.

Table 7. Standardized Coefficients of Effects of Literacy, Education, Access, Health Status, and Demographics on Telephone Contact.

	Model 1	Model 2	Model 3	Model 4
TALS	−0.138*	−0.131*	−0.084*	−0.067
Grade completed	−0.027	−0.011	0.021	0.056
Access				
Provider		−0.025	0.028	0.003
Insurance		0.181*	0.120*	0.120*
Delay		0.005	−0.034	−0.053
Written		−0.068	−0.048	−0.033
Get care		0.116*	0.100*	0.087*
Health status			0.149*	0.135*
Demographics				
Age				−0.013
Family income				−0.064
Gender				−0.167*
Living arrangement				0.043
Motor vehicle				0.018
Adjusted R^2	0.018	0.054	0.050	0.075
N	764	764	703	703

*$p < 0.05$.

Table 8. Standardized Coefficients of Effects of Literacy, Education, Access, Health Status, and Demographics on Emergency Room Visits.

	Model 1	Model 2	Model 3	Model 4
TALS	−0.163*	−0.155*	−0.114*	−0.101*
Grade completed	−0.191	−0.183*	−0.104*	−0.088*
Access				
Provider		−0.057	−0.005	−0.007
Insurance		0.132*	0.080*	0.083*
Delay		−0.006	−0.028	−0.031
Written		−0.034	0.041	0.053
Get care		0.084*	0.114*	0.110*
Health status			0.073	0.061
Demographics				
Age				0.011
Family income				−0.069
Gender				−0.045
Living arrangement				0.046
Motor vehicle				0.015
Adjusted R^2	0.068	0.082	0.052	0.055
N	764	764	703	703

*$p < 0.05$.

reveals that those adults who are younger, have lower incomes, and who live alone also report a greater number of overnight hospital stays.

Literacy is not significantly associated with the use of prescription medicines, when controlling for the effects of other variables. The data suggest that having health insurance, reporting a delay in seeking care because of cost, having a lower income, being a female, and having access to a reliable vehicle are associated with more frequent use of prescription medicines.

Literacy is also not associated with the frequency of telephone contact with a doctor or nurse in a multivariate context. With respect to access variables, having insurance and reportedly not getting needed care in the past because of cost are associated with more frequent telephone contact. Those persons in poorer health, and females make greater telephone contact.

Adults with lower levels of literacy have a greater number of emergency room visits, net the effect of background factors. Adults with less education, those who have health insurance, those who have gone without needed care in the past are more likely to use emergency rooms. Self-reported health status is not significant in a multivariate context.

CONCLUSION

This study examines the effect of literacy upon individual ability to access the health care system, and their use of several specific health services. Due to the close match of the demographics and sampling proportions between the original sample and the sub-sample analyzed here, these results are generalizable to the target population of individuals in the Portland, Oregon metropolitan area. Several notable findings have emerged from these analyses.

First, in support of the first hypothesis, adults with the lowest levels of literacy do face a number of obstacles in accessing health care. For example, they are five times as likely as those scoring in the highest level to say that they have difficulty understanding the written materials that the doctor or staff may give them. This has a number of important implications in securing health care – difficulty in reading appointment slips, understanding medical regimes, grasping the information in medical booklets, understanding informed consent, and securing follow-up care. It may also cause adults to forgo needed care. Persons scoring in the lowest literacy level report nearly twice as often that they have been unable to get the health care that they need.

Second, in support of the second hypothesis, literacy levels do affect many ways in which adults utilize the health care system. Lower literacy is associated with a greater number of doctor or clinic visits, more frequent overnight stays in a hospital, and an increase in emergency room visits over a 1-year period when the effects of education, access, health status, and demographic characteristics are controlled.

Third, these data suggest that the influence of literacy extends beyond that of education level. Although education is used frequently as a proxy for the concept of socioeconomic status, we should not ignore the unique position that literacy plays in securing good health, and access to health care. Literacy and education have unique independent affects on access to health care and use of the health care system. We suggest that attention be refocused toward the influence of varying literacy levels. With approximately 40 million adults in the United States suffering from extremely limited reading skills, and another 50 million with only marginal skills, the health care professionals cannot assume that those they are intended to serve understand their written materials. Difficulty in comprehending traditionally written medical materials is a significant problem that contributes to barriers in accessing care and using the health care system differently. Assuming high levels of patient literacy is likely to cause undue personal hardship, not to mention tremendous financial costs to the health care industry itself.

We see self-determination as a fundamental right of patients, given that we as a society place a high value on equity in health care (Richardson, 1999). Yet, millions of Americans are being denied these fundamental rights by their inability to read these materials. Just as interpreter services, and coordination with traditional or alternative healers are becoming increasingly viewed as important mechanisms to ameliorate disparate health outcomes among groups of people (Brach & Fraser, 2000), so too should we become attuned to alternative ways of presenting written health information. Literacy does indeed affect access to and use of a variety of health care services.

ACKNOWLEDGMENTS

These data are from the Longitudinal Study of Adult Learning (LSAL), a project of the National Center for the Study of Adult Learning and Literacy (NCSALL). NCSALL, a partnership between Harvard University, Portland State University, Rutgers University, the University of Tennessee, and World Education, is funded by the, Educational Research and Centers Program, U.S., Department of Education, Award Number R309B60002.

Stephen Reder is the Principal Investigator for the LSAL. The authors assume all responsibility for the findings reported here. We thank Clare Strawn, Jordan Durbin, Renato Carletti, M. Cecil Smith, Robin Timmermans, and many others for their countless hours devoted to data collection, management, and analysis.

REFERENCES

Agre, P., McKee, K., Gargon, N., & Kurtz, C. (1997). Patient satisfaction with an informed consent process. *Cancer Practice, 5*, 162–167.

Baker, D. W., Parker, R. M., & Clark, W. S. (1998). Health literacy and the risk of hospital admission. *Journal of General Internal Medicine, 13*, 791–798.

Baker, D. W., Parker, R. M., Williams, M. V., Clark, W. S., & Nurss, J. (1997). The relationship of patient reading ability to self-reported health and use of health services. *American Journal of Public Health, 87*, 1027–1030.

Baker, D. W., Parker, R. M., Williams, M. V., Ptikin, K., Parikh, N. S., Coates, W., & Mwalimu, I. (1996). The health experience of patients with low literacy. *Archives of Family Medicine, 5*, 329–334.

Baker, M. T., & Taub, H. A. (1983). Readability of informed consent forms for research in a veterans administration medical center. *JAMA, 250*, 2646–2648.

Beaver, K., & Luker, K. (1997). Readability of patient information booklets for women with breast cancer. *Patient Education & Counseling, 31*, 95–102.

Bennett, C. L., Ferreira, M. R., Davis, T. C., Kaplan, J., Weinberger, M., Kuzel, T., Seday, M. A., & Sartor, O. (1998). Relation between literacy, race, and stage of presentation among low-income patients with prostate cancer. *Journal of Clinical Oncology, 16*, 3101–3104.

Brach, C., & Fraser, I. (2000). Can cultural competency reduce racial and ethnic disparities? A review and conceptual model. *Medical Care Research and Review, 57*, 181–217.

Davis, T. C., Arnold, C., Berkel, H. J., Nandy, I., Jackson, R. H., & Glass, J. (1996). Knowledge and attitude on screening mammography among low-literate, low-income women. *Cancer, 78*, 1912–1920.

Davis, T. C., Crouch, M. A., Wills, G., Miller, S., & Abdehou, D. M. (1990). The gap between patient reading comprehension and the readability of patient education materials. *Journal of Family Practice, 35*, 533–538.

Davis, T. C., Holcome, R. F., Berkel, H. J., Pramanik, S., & Divers, S. G. (1998). Informed consent for clinical trials: A comparative study of standard versus simplified forms. *Journal of The National Cancer Institute, 90*, 669–674.

Educational Testing Service. (1995). *Literacy and dependency: The literacy skills of welfare recipients in the United States.* Washington, DC: U.S. Department of Education.

Jolly, B. T., Scotte, J. L., & Sanford, S. M. (1995). Simplification of emergency department discharge instructions improves patient comprehension. *Annals of Emergency Medicine, 26*, 443–446.

Kirsch, I.S., Jungeblut, A., Jenkins, L., & Kolstad, A. (1993). *Adult literacy in America.* Educational Testing Service. Washington, DC: U.S. Department of Education.

National Center for Educational Statistics. 1992. (1999). *National Adult Literacy Survey: Overview.* Available online: http://nces.ed.gov/naal/naal92/overview.html Accessed 2/9/2000.

National Work Group on Literacy and Health. (1998). Communicating with patients who have limited literacy skills: Report of the national work group on literacy and health. *Journal of Family Practice, 46*, 168–176.

Powers, R. D. (1988). Emergency department patient literacy and the readability of patient-directed materials. *Annals of Emergency Medicine, 17*, 124–126.

Reder, S. (1998). *The state of literacy in America: Estimates at the local, state, and national levels*. Washington, DC: National Institute for Literacy.

Richardson, L. D. (1999). Patients' rights and professional responsibilities: The moral case for cultural competence. *Mt Sinai Journal of Medicine, 66*, 267–270.

Ross, C. E., & Wu, C. (1995). The links between education and health. *American Sociological Review, 60*, 719–745.

Roter, D. L., Rudd, R. E., & Comings, J. P. (1998). Patient literacy: A barrier to quality care. *Journal of General Internal Medicine, 13*, 850–851.

Rudd, R.E., Colton, T. (1998). *An overview of medical and public health literature addressing literacy issues: An annotated bibliography*. NCSALL Reports No. 7, August.

Rudd, R. E., & Moeykens, B. A. (1999). *Findings from a national survey of adult educators: Health and Literacy*. NCSALL Reports. Cambridge, MA: NCSALL.

TenHave, T. R., Van Horn, B., Kumanyika, S., Askov, E., Matthews, Y., & Adams-Campbell, L. L. (1997). Literary assessment in a cardiovascular nutrition education setting. *Patient Education & Counseling, 31*, 139–150.

U.S. Department of Education. (1994). *Literacy behind prison walls*. National Center for Education Statistics, October, Washington, DC: U.S. Dpartment of Education.

Weiss, B. D., Blanchard, J. S., McGee, D. L., Hart, G., Warren, B., Burgoon, M., & Smith, K. J. (1994). Illiteracy among medicaid recipients and its relationship to health care costs. *Journal of health Care for the Poor and Underserved, 5*, 99–111.

Weiss, B. D., & Coyne, C. (1997). Communicating with patients who cannot read. *The New England Journal of Medicine, 337*, 272–274.

Weiss, B. D., Hart, G., McGee, D. L., & D'Estelle, S. (1992). Health status of illiterate adults: Relation between literacy and health status among persons with low literacy skills. *Journal of the American Board of Family Practice, 5*, 257–264.

Williams, M. V., Parker, R. M., Baker, D. W., Parikh, K., Coates, W. C., & Nurss, J. R. (1995). Inadequate functional literacy among patients at two public hospitals. *JAMA, 2714*, 1677–1682.

SET UP A CONTINUATION ORDER TODAY!

Did you know that you can set up a continuation order on all Elsevier-JAI series and have each new volume sent directly to you upon publication? For details on how to set up a **continuation order**, contact your nearest regional sales office listed below.

To view related series in Sociology, please visit:

www.elsevier.com/sociology

The Americas
Customer Service Department
11830 Westline Industrial Drive
St. Louis, MO 63146
USA
US customers:
Tel: +1 800 545 2522 (Toll-free number)
Fax: +1 800 535 9935
For Customers outside US:
Tel: +1 800 460 3110 (Toll-free number).
Fax: +1 314 453 7095
usbkinfo@elsevier.com

Europe, Middle East & Africa
Customer Service Department
Linacre House
Jordan Hill
Oxford OX2 8DP
UK
Tel: +44 (0) 1865 474140
Fax: +44 (0) 1865 474141
eurobkinfo@elsevier.com

Japan
Customer Service Department
2F Higashi Azabu, 1 Chome Bldg
1-9-15 Higashi Azabu, Minato-ku
Tokyo 106-0044
Japan
Tel: +81 3 3589 6370
Fax: +81 3 3589 6371
books@elsevierjapan.com

APAC
Customer Service Department
3 Killiney Road #08-01
Winsland House I
Singapore 239519
Tel: +65 6349 0222
Fax: +65 6733 1510
asiainfo@elsevier.com

Australia & New Zealand
Customer Service Department
30-52 Smidmore Street
Marrickville, New South Wales 2204
Australia
Tel: +61 (02) 9517 8999
Fax: +61 (02) 9517 2249
service@elsevier.com.au

30% Discount for Authors on All Books!

A 30% discount is available to Elsevier book and journal contributors on all books *(except multi-volume reference works)*.

To claim your discount, full payment is required with your order, which must be sent directly to the publisher at the nearest regional sales office above.